Integrated Anesthesia and Nutrition Approaches to Enhanced Recovery after Surgery

Prasanta Kumar Bhattacharyya
Nidhi Kumari • Ravi Yadav
Debasrita Banerjee
Editors

Integrated Anesthesia and Nutrition Approaches to Enhanced Recovery after Surgery

Clinical Perspectives and Patient Care

Springer

Editors
Prasanta Kumar Bhattacharyya
Department of Plastic Surgery
K.P.C. Medical College & Hospital
Kolkata, West Bengal, India

Nidhi Kumari
Department of Anesthesiology
NC Medical College
Panipat, Haryana, India

Ravi Yadav
Department of Anesthesia & Operation Theater Technology
Medhavi Skills University
School of Health Sciences & Technology
Singtam, Sikkim, India

Debasrita Banerjee
Department of Nutrition and Dietetics
Medhavi Skills University
Singtam, Sikkim, India

ISBN 978-981-92-3293-2 ISBN 978-981-92-3294-9 (eBook)
https://doi.org/10.1007/978-981-92-3294-9

This Springer imprint is published by the registered company Springer Nature Singapore Pte Ltd.
The registered company address is: 152 Beach Road, #21-01/04 Gateway East, Singapore 189721, Singapore

Preface

Major surgery remains one of the most powerful physiological stressors encountered in clinical practice. Surgical patients today are older, frailer, and more comorbid than in previous decades, and a growing body of evidence shows that unmitigated surgical stress contributes to complications, prolonged recovery, impaired quality of life, and even adverse oncologic outcomes. Enhanced Recovery After Surgery (ERAS) pathways have emerged as one of the most important perioperative innovations of the last two decades, demonstrating that coordinated, multimodal care can attenuate the stress response, reduce complications, shorten length of stay, and optimize resource utilization across diverse surgical specialties.

Despite this progress, the scientific and clinical literatures on anesthesia and perioperative nutrition have largely evolved in parallel streams. Anesthetic techniques are often discussed separately from nutritional optimization, and ERAS guidelines are frequently implemented in silos, with anesthesiologists, surgeons, nutritionists, and allied health professionals working with overlapping but insufficiently integrated protocols. Yet the physiology of surgical stress does not respect disciplinary boundaries: nociception, neuroendocrine activation, inflammation, endothelial dysfunction, and hypermetabolism are tightly interlinked with substrate availability, body composition, immunonutrition, and glycemic control. Without a shared conceptual framework, opportunities to synergize anesthetic strategies and nutritional interventions are easily missed.

This volume, *Integrated Anesthesia and Nutrition Approaches to Enhanced Recovery After Surgery: Clinical Perspectives and Patient Care*, was developed to address this critical gap. It brings together expertise from anesthesia, surgery, clinical nutrition and dietetics, intensive care, and allied health sciences to present ERAS not merely as a checklist of perioperative elements, but as a deliberately designed physiological intervention that acts simultaneously on inflammatory, neuroendocrine, metabolic, and functional axes. The book emphasizes how evidence-based anesthetic techniques—such as regional anesthesia, multimodal and opioid-sparing analgesia, hemodynamic optimization, and lung-protective ventilation—interact with carbohydrate loading, early high-protein feeding, immunonutrition, and metabolic modulation to "flatten and shrink" the surgical stress curve.

The early chapters (Chaps. 1, 2, and 3) provide the conceptual foundation by outlining the historical evolution from Selye's general adaptation syndrome to contemporary ERAS frameworks and detailing the molecular, cellular, and systems physiology of surgical stress and recovery. Particular attention is given to damage-associated molecular patterns, thromboinflammation, neuroendocrine stress axes, insulin resistance, sarcopenia, and organ-specific manifestations, thereby equipping readers with a mechanistic understanding of why integrated perioperative care matters. Subsequent chapters (Chaps. 4, 5, 6, 7, 8, and 9) focus on perioperative nutritional assessment, prehabilitation, fasting and carbohydrate-loading protocols, management of insulin resistance, and nutrition in high-risk and malnourished surgical populations, with practical algorithms and protocols grounded in recent guidelines and high-quality evidence.

The middle section of the book (Chaps. 10, 11, and 12) applies these principles to specialty-specific ERAS pathways in colorectal, cardiac, and orthopedic surgery, demonstrating how anesthesia and nutrition can be co-designed along procedure-specific trajectories. These chapters emphasize real-world implementation, including considerations for resource-limited settings, and highlight how adherence to integrated pathways can translate into measurable improvements in complications, length of stay, functional recovery, and costs. Cross-cutting chapters on multimodal analgesia, postoperative pain, early mobilization, and team-based implementation (Chaps. 13 and 14) reinforce the central role of pain control, functional restoration, and interprofessional collaboration in optimizing long-term outcomes.

The final chapters (Chaps. 15 and 16) look toward the future of "precision ERAS," discussing emerging biomarkers, sarcopenia and frailty assessment tools, digital health and remote monitoring, and AI-enabled decision support, alongside case-based vignettes that illustrate typical challenges and solutions in integrated ERAS programs. Across all chapters, we have sought to maintain a consistent structure—abstract, learning objectives, core content, tables and algorithms, key points, case vignettes, and review questions—to support both busy clinicians and postgraduate learners.

This book is primarily intended for anesthesiologists, surgeons, clinical nutritionists and dietitians, intensivists, perioperative nurses, and allied health professionals involved in the care of surgical patients. It is also designed to serve as a graduate-level reference for trainees in anesthesiology, general and specialty surgery, clinical nutrition and dietetics, critical care, and operation theatre technology, particularly in competency-based curricula that emphasize ERAS, regional anesthesia, multimodal analgesia, glycemic control, and perioperative nutrition. We hope that readers will find in these pages not only an up-to-date synthesis of evidence but also pragmatic tools—protocols, checklists, quality indicators, and case examples—that can be readily adapted to their institutional context.

The development of this volume has been a truly interdisciplinary effort involving contributors from diverse institutions and practice environments. We are deeply grateful to all authors who have shared their expertise and to the mentors, colleagues, and institutional leaders who have supported ERAS implementation in their own settings. It is our sincere hope that this book will assist clinicians and teams in delivering safer, more efficient, and more patient-centered surgical care, and that it will contribute in a small way to the ongoing evolution of integrated perioperative medicine.

On behalf of all the Editors

Singtam, Sikkim, India Ravi Yadav

Acknowledgments

The preparation of *Integrated Anesthesia and Nutrition Approaches to Enhanced Recovery After Surgery: Clinical Perspectives and Patient Care* has been a collective effort, and the editors wish to express their profound gratitude to the many individuals and institutions who have contributed to its development.

We are deeply indebted to all chapter authors and contributors, who generously shared their time, expertise, and clinical experience while balancing the demands of patient care, teaching, and research. Their scholarly work, critical appraisal of the literature, and willingness to refine chapters through multiple rounds of revision have been central to the scientific quality and practical relevance of this volume. We are equally grateful to the peer reviewers and senior colleagues who provided constructive feedback on individual chapters and on the overall structure of the book.

We acknowledge the support of *Medhavi Skills University, School of Health Sciences & Technology, Singtam, Sikkim, India*, whose academic environment and encouragement for interdisciplinary collaboration between anesthesia technology and nutrition have provided fertile ground for the conception of this project. We also extend our thanks to *K.P.C. Medical College & Hospital, Kolkata*, and *NC Medical College, Panipat*, for fostering strong perioperative and surgical services that exemplify the kind of integrated care this book seeks to promote.

The editors would like to thank their students, trainees, and clinical teams in the operating theatre, intensive care units, and wards, whose daily questions and clinical challenges have informed the choice of topics, case vignettes, and algorithms included in these chapters. Their commitment to applying ERAS principles under real-world constraints has been a constant source of motivation. We are also grateful to the nurses, dietitians, physiotherapists, and allied health professionals whose work at the bedside demonstrates that enhanced recovery is truly a multidisciplinary endeavor.

We appreciate the guidance and professionalism of the publishing team, whose editorial support and patience throughout the proposal, review, and production stages have been invaluable. Finally, we thank our families for their understanding and encouragement during the many evenings and weekends devoted to writing, editing, and revising this book. Without their unwavering support, this project would not have been possible.

On behalf of the Editors

Contents

About the Editors

Prasanta Kumar Bhattacharyya is Professor and Head of Plastic Surgery at K.P.C. Medical College & Hospital, Kolkata, India, with over three decades of post-MS general surgical practice and more than two decades of experience in plastic surgery. He holds multiple advanced qualifications, including D.Ortho, MS (General Surgery), M.Ch (Plastic Surgery), M.Ch (Orthopaedics), an M.Phil in Regenerative Medicine and Translational Sciences, and a Ph.D. on diabetic lower limb ulcers from the West Bengal University of Health Sciences. He has authored more than 30 peer-reviewed publications on diabetic complications, burns, reconstructive techniques, and gastrointestinal surgery and has delivered invited lectures at state, national, and international meetings. He has held leadership roles in several professional bodies, including President of the Association of Plastic Surgeons of West Bengal, President of the Burns Association of West Bengal, and senior positions in the Indian Medical Association. His long-standing engagement with multidisciplinary surgical care and organizational leadership provides a broad clinical and systems-level perspective to this integrated ERAS text. He also serves as the Honorary Secretary of the Journal of the Indian Medical Association (JIMA), one of India's most widely circulated medical journals, currently indexed in Scopus, Embase, and Index Copernicus and published by Jaypee Brothers Medical Publishers.

Nidhi Kumari is Associate Professor of Anesthesiology at NC Medical College & Hospital, Israna, Panipat, India. She completed her MD in Anesthesiology and Critical Care from Government Medical College, Patiala, and earned her MBBS degree from Government Medical College, Azmritsar. With a distinguished blend of clinical expertise, academic excellence, and research experience, she has established herself in the field of anesthesiology and perioperative critical care. She has more than three years of senior residency experience at Dr. Ram Manohar Lohia Hospital, New Delhi, where she managed a diverse range of surgical and critically ill patients in high-acuity settings. She also served as an Assistant Professor at NC Medical College & Hospital, Israna, Panipat, actively contributing to medical education, clinical training, and patient-centered perioperative care. Her clinical interests encompass general and regional anesthesia, advanced airway management, opioid-free and opioid-sparing anesthetic techniques, perioperative optimization of high-risk hypertensive and cardiac patients, and critical care medicine. She has a special interest in evidence-based anesthetic practices and Enhanced Recovery After Surgery (ERAS) protocols aimed at improving surgical outcomes and patient recovery. She has authored and co-authored several publications in reputed peer-reviewed indexed journals, including the *African Journal of Paediatric Surgery, Global Journal for Research Analysis, Research and Opinion in Anesthesia and Intensive Care, Indian Journal of Anesthesia and Analgesia, Asian Journal of Medical Sciences*, and *Adesh University Journal of Medical Sciences and Research*. Her research work primarily focuses on perioperative outcomes, hemodynamic responses, and innovations in anesthetic and critical care management. Her extensive frontline experience, academic contributions, and commitment to advancing perioperative medicine significantly strengthen the anesthetic and ERAS perspectives presented in this volume.

Ravi Yadav is an Assistant Professor & Head of Department in the Department of Anesthesia & Operation Theatre Technology at Medhavi Skills University, Singtam, Sikkim, India. He holds a B.Sc. in Operation Theatre Technology and an M.Sc. in Anesthesia Technology and is registered under the National Commission for Allied and Healthcare Professions (NCAHP) and the National Health Authority, Government of India. With a strong blend of clinical expertise, academic leadership, and research excellence, he has gained extensive experience across reputed healthcare and academic institutions in India. His clinical training and professional experience include Max Smart Super Specialty Hospital, New Delhi; NC Medical College Hospital, affiliated with PGIMS Rohtak; and the National Institute of Medical Sciences, Jaipur. In addition to his clinical contributions, he has served in key academic leadership positions, including Head of Department, where he has played an instrumental role in curriculum development, student mentorship, and advancement of allied healthcare education.

He has authored and co-authored more than 25 peer-reviewed indexed research publications in reputed international and national journals, including the *Indian Journal of Critical Care Medicine, Perioperative Care and Operating Room Management, Journal of Emergency Practice and Trauma, Acta Anaesthesiologica Belgica, Discover Public Health, Middle East Fertility Society Journal*, and *Discover Neuroscience*. His scholarly contributions primarily focus on perioperative care, neuroanesthesia, patient safety, difficult airway management, Enhanced Recovery After Surgery (ERAS) protocols, and the integration of emerging technologies in anesthesia and operation theatre practice. He also holds two patents in healthcare technology, reflecting his commitment to innovation and advancement in perioperative and allied healthcare sciences. He currently serves as the Joint Secretary of the Indian Society of Technologists (Anesthesia and Operation Theatre Technology) and is the editor of Advances in Surgical Science: Techniques, Innovations, and Clinical Applications. His multidisciplinary expertise, research contributions, and dedication to academic and clinical excellence continue to contribute significantly to the advancement of anesthesia technology, perioperative sciences, and patient-centered surgical care.

Debasrita Banerjee is an Assistant Professor in the Department of Nutrition and Dietetics at Medhavi Skills University, Singtam, Sikkim, and a freelance clinical dietitian. He earned his B.Sc. and M.Sc. in Dietetics and Applied Nutrition from Amity University, Haryana, where he received an Academic Silver Medal at the undergraduate level and a Gold Medal at the postgraduate level. He is pursuing a Ph.D. in Dietetics and Applied Nutrition and has qualified the UGC-NET (Home Science) for lectureship. He has held prior academic positions in West Bengal and Andhra Pradesh and has also worked as a Quality Analyst (Nutrition & Nursing), reflecting his interest in educational quality assurance. His research and publications span therapeutic nutrition, metabolic disorders, obesity, functional food products, and systematic reviews in clinical nutrition, with book chapters on probiotics in cancer chemoprevention and antioxidants in diabetes. His expertise in evidence-based perioperative nutrition and product development underpins the nutritional components of this ERAS-focused volume.

Introduction to Enhanced Recovery After Surgery (ERAS)

1

Jatin Kataria and Ravi Yadav

Abstract

Enhanced recovery after surgery (ERAS) has revolutionized the perioperative pathway by changing the conventional, piecemeal approaches to a more integrated, evidence-based, and multimodal approach. The major goal of ERAS is to minimize the stress of surgery, ensure physiological stability, and promote a quick recovery. First described in colorectal surgery in the 1990s by Henrik Kehlet's "fast-track" concept, ERAS has now transformed into evidence-based guidelines for specific procedures by the ERAS Study Group and ERAS Society. These guidelines have been applied in a variety of surgeries, including hepatobiliary, urological, gynecological, obstetric, orthopedic, thoracic, and organ transplantation procedures. There has been robust evidence supporting the efficacy of ERAS, with recent meta-analyses confirming reduced length of stay and significantly reduced complication rates without increasing readmission or mortality rates.

In this chapter, the main concepts, physiological rationale, and historical development of ERAS, in addition to a critical evaluation of evidence and guidelines, are discussed. Emphasis is given to the interdisciplinarity of ERAS, especially in relation to anesthesiologists and clinical nutrition experts. Anesthesiologists are highlighted in relation to multimodal, opioid-minimizing analgesic strategies, optimization of fluids, and hemodynamic stability, whereas dietitians are central in relation to nutritional screening, nutritional support, carbohydrate loading, and early postoperative nutrition. Finally, implementation

J. Kataria
School of Allied Health Sciences, Department of Anesthesia & Operation Theater Technology, Noida International University, Greater Noida, Uttar Pradesh, India

R. Yadav (✉)
Department of Anesthesia & Operation Theater Technology, Medhavi Skills University, School of Health Sciences & Technology, Singtam, Sikkim, India

P. K. Bhattacharyya et al. (eds.), *Integrated Anesthesia and Nutrition Approaches to Enhanced Recovery after Surgery*,
https://doi.org/10.1007/978-981-92-3294-9_1

strategies and future perspectives, including personalized ERAS, digital health technologies, and ERAS in complex conditions such as organ transplantation and cirrhosis, are presented, serving as a base for further discussion on anesthesia and nutrition in ERAS.

Keywords

Perioperative care · Multimodal approach · Fast-track surgery · Postoperative recovery

1.1 Introduction and Conceptual Framework

The traditional perioperative care process has been associated with the following: prolonged fasting before and after surgery, liberal fluid administration, nasogastric decompression, delayed ambulation, and cautious reintroduction of oral fluids. It is vital to note that such approaches have been based on traditional rather than evidence-based medicine (Parks et al. 2018; Melnyk et al. 2011). It is imperative to note that such approaches may impair the neuroendocrine response of the body to stress and may result in insulin resistance, increased metabolic rate, and respiratory dysfunction, among other complications (Sharma et al. 2022).

On the contrary, Enhanced Recovery After Surgery (ERAS), which is a multimodal, evidence-based perioperative care process, is described as the combination of preoperative optimization, intraoperative care, and postoperative rehabilitation strategies designed to reduce the impact of surgical stress, hasten the restoration of normal physiological function, and thereby enhance the speed of recovery (Table 1.1) (Fearon et al. 2005; Ljungqvist et al. 2017). ERAS is not a single intervention but rather a combination of multiple components, each making a small

Table 1.1 Representative ERAS elements across the perioperative continuum

Perioperative phase	Domain	Key elements	Rationale/evidence summary
Preoperative	Patient education and expectation management	Procedure-specific counseling; mobilization and feeding milestones; analgesia plan; discharge criteria	Reduces anxiety, improves adherence, and facilitates earlier mobilization and discharge in colorectal and gynecologic ERAS programs
Preoperative	Risk stratification and prehabilitation	Frailty and cardiopulmonary assessment; smoking/alcohol cessation; exercise training; nutrition supplementation	Improves functional capacity and may reduce complications and length of stay in high-risk patients

(Continued)

Table 1.1 (Continued)

Perioperative phase	Domain	Key elements	Rationale/evidence summary
Preoperative	Nutrition and metabolic optimization	Validated nutrition screening (e.g., NRS-2002); enteral supplementation 7–14 days when feasible; abbreviated fasting with carbohydrate drinks	Mitigates catabolism and insulin resistance and is associated with fewer infections and shorter hospitalization in GI oncology
Intraoperative	Surgical approach	Laparoscopic/robotic techniques where safe; minimal tissue trauma; avoidance of routine drains and nasogastric tubes	Reduces pain, ileus, and length of stay when embedded in high-compliance ERAS pathways
Intraoperative	Anesthetic management and analgesia	Short-acting anesthetics; neuraxial or regional blocks; acetaminophen and NSAIDs; limited systemic opioids; PONV prophylaxis	Decreases opioid consumption, nausea, ileus, and promotes early mobilization across GI, gynecologic, and orthopedic surgery
Intraoperative	Fluid and temperature management	Goal-directed fluid therapy; avoidance of both liberal and overly restrictive regimens; active warming measures	Maintains organ perfusion while limiting interstitial edema, reduces complications, and supports early recovery
Postoperative	Early mobilization	Out-of-bed mobilization on day of surgery or postoperative day 1; progressive ambulation targets	Associated with lower pulmonary and thromboembolic complications and shorter length of stay
Postoperative	Early oral intake and nutrition support	Clear liquids on day of surgery; rapid advancement to full diet; high-protein supplements; early enteral feeding when needed	Early feeding within 24 h is safe after GI surgery and reduces infectious complications and length of stay
Postoperative	Catheter, drain, and tube management	Avoidance of routine nasogastric tubes; selective drains with early removal; early urinary catheter removal	Reduces pneumonia, urinary tract infection, and facilitates mobilization and feeding
Postoperative	Standardized discharge and follow-up	Function-based criteria (pain control on oral agents, mobilization, diet tolerance) and structured post-discharge contact	Enables safe early discharge without higher readmission rates and improves patient experience

Abbreviations: *ERAS* enhanced recovery after surgery, *NRS-2002* nutrition risk screening 2002, *GI* gastrointestinal, *NSAIDs* nonsteroidal anti-inflammatory drugs, *PONV* postoperative nausea and vomiting

contribution to the final outcome, which, when combined in a synergistic fashion, provides a larger effect than the sum of the individual parts (Altman et al. 2019; Golder and Papalois 2021; Sauro et al. 2024).

1.2 Pathophysiology of Surgical Stress and Rationale for ERAS

1.2.1 Neuroendocrine and Metabolic Response

Major surgeries induce afferent neural and humoral signals from the injured tissues, culminating in the activation of the hypothalamic-pituitary-adrenal axis and the sympathetic nervous system. This culminates in the production of stress-related hormones such as cortisol, catecholamines, glucagon, and proinflammatory cytokines (Desborough 2000; Kehlet and Wilmore 2002). This has the overall effect of inducing hyperglycemia, negative nitrogen balance, and the loss of skeletal and visceral proteins. In addition, the process of endothelial dysfunction and changes in the immune response makes the patients more susceptible to infections and fluid shifts that induce tissue edema (Thorell et al. 1999; Varadhan et al. 2010).

The degree and duration of insulin resistance are closely related to the degree of surgical trauma. These are critical factors that influence postoperative outcomes such as infection rates, impaired wound healing, and increased hospital stay in colorectal, orthopedic, and hepatobiliary surgical procedures (Thorell et al. 1999; Joliat et al. 2023; Tong et al. 2022). From a theoretical perspective, the implementation of ERAS guidelines is aimed at correcting this abnormal metabolic response to surgical stress using a variety of interventions such as pain control, regional anesthesia, minimal preoperative fasting with carbohydrate loading, fluid management, normothermia, and early enteral nutrition. Figure 1.1 shows the conceptual intensity of the surgical stress response along the timeline of the perioperative period, comparing standard care with the ERAS pathway.

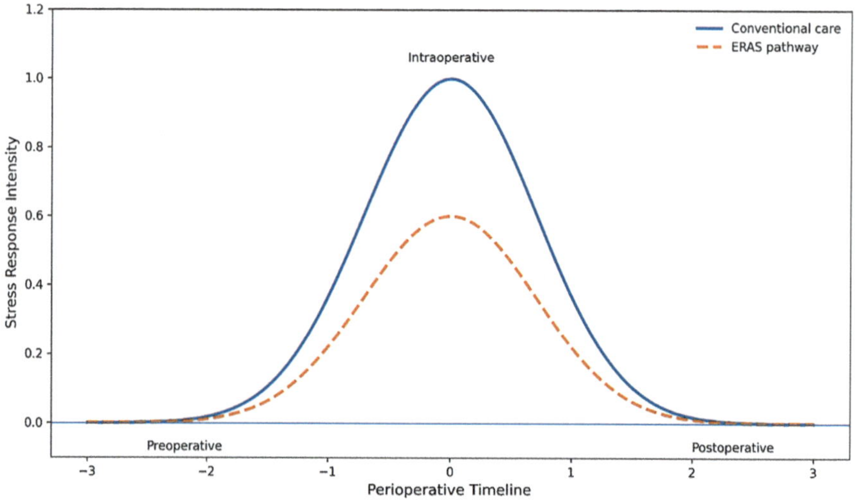

Fig. 1.1 Surgical stress response. (Original figure created by the authors using MS Excel 2021)

1.2.2 Organ-Specific Considerations

The respiratory function is frequently impaired in the perioperative period because of various factors such as anesthesia, recumbent position, pain-induced splinting, and opioid-induced hypoventilation. These factors predispose patients to various complications such as atelectasis and pneumonia. Therefore, various elements of ERAS, such as early mobilization of patients, implementation of mechanical ventilation, avoidance of nasogastric tubes, and opioid-free multimodal analgesia, are crucial in maintaining respiratory function and reducing postoperative respiratory complications in abdominal and thoracic surgeries (Feldheiser et al. 2016; Fiore Jr et al. 2016).

In the same way, gastrointestinal dysfunction following a surgical process is associated with the sympathetic stress response, inflammation, bowel manipulation, and the action of opioids. This may manifest as postoperative ileus. ERAS has been shown to mitigate gastrointestinal dysfunction through various strategies such as the use of minimally invasive procedures, early oral feeding, early removal of nasogastric tubes and drains, reduced opioid use, and the use of chewing gum. All these strategies can assist in the early recovery of gastrointestinal functions and the reduction of the incidence of postoperative ileus (Melnyk et al. 2011; Parks et al. 2018).

Hemodynamically, excessive crystalloid resuscitation can lead to interstitial edema, tissue compartment syndromes, and compromise of anastomoses, whereas hypovolemia can lead to compromised organ perfusion. Goal-directed fluid therapy (GDFT) with dynamic preload indices and cardiac output monitoring to aim for euvolemia has been associated with reduced complications and shorter lengths of stay in high-risk patients undergoing major abdominal surgery, especially with ERAS implementation (Minto et al. 2015; Joliat et al. 2023; Varadhan et al. 2010).

1.3 Historical Evolution of ERAS

1.3.1 From "Fast-Track" Surgery to ERAS

The modern concept of ERAS has its origins in Henrik Kehlet's research in the late 1990s, which demonstrated that "fast-track" pathways involving epidural analgesia, early mobilization, and early feeding could be used to safely reduce length of stay to 2 days after an open sigmoidectomy, a significant departure from conventional practice (Kehlet 1997; Kehlet and Mogensen 1999). Further randomized trials in colorectal surgery have demonstrated that such pathways reduce complications and shorten stay by 2–5 days compared to conventional care (Varadhan et al. 2010; Zhuang et al. 2013).

Such research has helped to shift focus from individual interventions (e.g., epidurals, laparoscopic procedures) to the concept of integrated perioperative care bundles as being central to improving outcomes. These studies also highlighted the substantial "gap" between evidence and practice in European centers, where perioperative care was highly variable and often not evidence-based (Wind et al. 2006; Golder and Papalois 2021).

1.3.2 ERAS Study Group and ERAS Society

In 2001, Ken Fearon and Olle Ljungqvist established the ERAS Study Group with the aim of performing systematic reviews of perioperative care in patients undergoing colorectal resection and in 2005 developed the first guidelines for patients undergoing colonic resection (Fearon et al. 2005). This is the first set of guidelines that incorporates the three phases of perioperative care and emphasizes the importance of a multi-modal and multi-disciplinary approach in the care of patients undergoing resection of the colon.

In 2010, the ERAS Study Group transformed into the ERAS Society, a non-profit organization with the aim of producing guidelines for various procedures, encouraging the implementation of the guidelines, and assisting with the auditing process through the ERAS Interactive Audit System (EIAS) (Brindle et al. 2020; Ljungqvist et al. 2017). To date, the ERAS Society has developed guidelines for various procedures such as colorectal resection, liver resection, pancreaticoduodenectomy, gastrectomy, radical cystectomy, gynecologic oncology, cesarean delivery, esophagectomy, and many more (Gustafsson et al. 2019; Cerantola et al. 2013; Lassen et al. 2012).

In the quest to standardize the methodology used in guidelines, Brindle et al. (2020) advocated for the development of ERAS-specific standards that include the development of guidelines by multidisciplinary guideline development groups, systematic review of the literature, assessment of evidence using the GRADE (Grading of Recommendations, Assessment, Development, and Evaluations) system, and the development of guidelines that are regularly updated as new evidence emerges.

1.3.3 Expansion Across Specialties and Settings

From its origins in elective colorectal surgery, ERAS has now expanded to include hepatobiliary and pancreatic surgery, urology, gynecology and obstetrics, thoracic surgery, bariatric and upper gastrointestinal oncology, breast cancer and head and neck cancer surgery, and, more recently, solid organ transplantation (Altman et al. 2019; Golder and Papalois 2021; Parks et al. 2018). Evidence from several reviews supports the fact that when ERAS is implemented and audited appropriately, it reduces length of stay and complications without compromising safety in all these specialties (Hughes et al. 2014; Ahmed et al. 2018; Bisch et al. 2021).

ERAS has now been applied to emergency laparotomy, cesarean delivery, and neonatal and pediatric surgery, necessitating further changes but retaining the core principles of stress reduction, mobilization, and nutrition (Altman et al. 2019; Joliat et al. 2023).

1.4 Evidence Base and Clinical Impact

1.4.1 Global Meta-Analytic Evidence

The most comprehensive recent evidence is derived from the 2024 meta-analysis conducted by Sauro et al., which was published in JAMA Network Open. This study consisted of 74 randomized clinical trials involving 9076 adult patients across nine ERAS-guided surgical procedures (Table 1.2) (Sauro et al. 2024). When comparing conventional care with ERAS, a reduction of 1.88 days in hospital length of stay and 2.83 days in postoperative length of stay was observed. Additionally, complications were reduced by 29%. This is equivalent to a 0.71 relative risk. No increase in readmission rates and mortality within 30 days postoperatively was noted.

It is also notable that the benefit of using ERAS is dependent on the type of surgical procedure and the implementation of the ERAS. More benefit is obtained when there is a greater implementation of the ERAS elements. This is demonstrated by a greater reduction in hospital length of stay when more elements of ERAS are used (Sauro et al. 2024).

Table 1.2 Selected meta-analyses and guideline-based estimates of ERAS impact on clinical outcomes

Surgical domain/ procedure	Key source (year)	Study type/ size	Main outcome effects under ERAS	Notes
Multispecialty (9 procedures)	Sauro et al., JAMA Netw Open (2024)	Meta-analysis of 74 RCTs (9076 adults)	≈2-day reduction in total/postoperative length of stay; ≈30% relative reduction in overall complications; no increase in readmission or mortality	Effect sizes larger in pathways with more ERAS elements and higher protocol compliance
Elective open colorectal surgery	Varadhan et al., Clin Nutr (2010); Zhuang et al., Dis Colon Rectum (2013)	Meta-analyses of randomized trials	2–3-day shorter length of stay and lower overall complication rates with ERAS vs conventional care	Benefits consistent across centers when multimodal bundles are implemented as standardized pathways
Upper gastrointestinal surgery	Huang et al., BMC Surg (2020)	Meta-analysis of upper GI procedures	Reduced length of stay and costs without higher anastomotic leak or mortality	Supports application of ERAS principles beyond colorectal surgery

(Continued)

Table 1.2 (Continued)

Surgical domain/ procedure	Key source (year)	Study type/ size	Main outcome effects under ERAS	Notes
Liver resection	Hughes et al., HPB (2014); Joliat et al., World J Surg (2023)	Systematic review and ERAS guideline synthesis	Lower complication rates, shorter hospitalization, and favorable cost-effectiveness in hepatectomy	Strong recommendations for early feeding, selective drain use, and hemodynamic optimization in liver surgery ERAS pathways
Gynecologic oncology and cesarean delivery	Altman et al., CMAJ (2019); Bisch et al., Gynecol Oncol (2021)	Systematic reviews and health-economic analyses	Shorter length of stay, fewer complications, and marked reductions in opioid use	High patient satisfaction and favorable return on investment when implemented at the system level

Similar results have been observed in previous meta-analyses concerning colorectal surgery. Varadhan et al. (2010) and Zhuang et al. (2013) observed a reduction in postoperative stay by 2–3 days and significant reductions in overall complications with ERAS compared to conventional care. Another meta-analysis concerning upper gastrointestinal surgery in 2020 observed a reduction in postoperative stay and costs with ERAS, with no increase in leak or mortality. ERAS Society guidelines are strongly in favor of the implementation of ERAS, with the only questions remaining concerning how to improve compliance with ERAS and which components are the key in different situations.

1.4.2 Specialty-Specific Outcomes

1.4.2.1 Colorectal Surgery

The updated ERAS Society guidelines for colorectal surgery, based on evidence from randomized trials and large cohorts, suggest that there are approximately 20–25 elements in the care pathway. High-compliance ERAS programs, where more than 80% of elements are delivered, demonstrate a consistent reduction in complication rates by 30–50% and a reduction in hospital stay by 2–4 days, with minimal readmissions (Nelson et al. 2016; Thanh et al. 2020).

1.4.2.2 Liver Surgery

The 2022 ERAS liver surgery guideline update by Joliat et al. (2023) is a synthesis of 240 studies that generated 25 recommendations, 16 of which were given a strong recommendation grade (e.g., early oral intake, no routine nasogastric tubes or drains in uncomplicated hepatectomy, low central venous pressure with Goal-Directed Fluid Therapy) (Joliat et al. 2023). Results of meta-analyses have demonstrated that

ERAS in hepatectomy decreases complications, hospital stay, and costs. These are more pronounced when minimal invasive techniques are used together with high rates of ERAS compliance (Hughes et al. 2014; Joliat et al. 2023).

1.4.2.3 Urologic Oncology

In radical cystectomy, a procedure with a traditional complication rate of 60–70%, and a prolonged hospital stay, ERAS protocols with reduced bowel preparation, standardized feeding regimens, and multimodal analgesia have reduced the length of stay and the incidence of ileus without increasing the incidence of leaks or mortality (Melnyk et al. 2011; Cerantola et al. 2013). A meta-analysis in 2023 has confirmed the benefits of reduced complications, transfusions, and re-admissions with the use of ERAS in cystectomy patients (Zhou et al. 2023.

1.4.2.4 Gynecology and Obstetrics

In gynecologic oncology, Altman et al. (2019) and Nelson et al. (2019) have demonstrated that ERAS protocols reduce hospital stay, decrease complications, and significantly reduce opioid use while maintaining or improving patient-reported outcomes. Systematic reviews in cesarean delivery have demonstrated that ERAS (ERAC) pathways, including long-acting opioids with non-opioid adjuncts, early feeding, and mobilization, reduce hospital stay and improve maternal satisfaction without adverse effects on maternal and neonatal outcomes (Bisch et al. 2021; Sauro et al. 2024).

1.4.2.5 Transplantation

The implementation of ERAS in solid organ transplantation (SOT) has been poor so far. However, emerging evidence in liver and kidney transplant procedures is promising. Golder and Papalois (2021) have documented pilot studies on liver transplant procedures using ERAS protocols that demonstrated a reduction in length of stay by approximately 47%, with low rates of re-intubation and readmission. Renal transplant studies have demonstrated a reduction in length of stay, opioid usage, and delayed graft function with ERAS-style pathways.

1.4.3 Health-System and Economic Impact

Because ERAS decreases both complications and hospital stay—a major cost driver—its cost-effectiveness is consistently demonstrated despite initial costs of staff training and audit. In Canadian colorectal and gynecologic ERAS programs, every dollar spent generated a return of 3–4 dollars via resource savings (Thanh et al. 2020; Altman et al. 2019). A cost analysis in the Canadian Medical Association Journal (CMAJ) calculated that every patient benefited by approximately $2200–$2500 due to ERAS implementation in major abdominal surgery (Altman et al. 2019). These cost savings have also been demonstrated in pancreaticoduodenectomy and hepatobiliary surgery (Joliat et al. 2015; Hughes et al. 2014).

In resource-poor hospitals, ERAS can help relieve bed pressures without requiring large capital expenditure, although staffing for early mobilization and audit can be difficult (Parks et al. 2018; Sauro et al. 2024).

1.4.4 ERAS in Emerging and Highly Specialized Fields

1.4.4.1 Spine Surgery

Surgical treatment for the spine. The ERAS protocol used for spinal surgeries seeks to mitigate postoperative pain, long-term opioid consumption, and fear of movement in cognitive behavior therapy that delays recovery (Wainwright et al. 2020). Major practices entail thorough psychological counseling before surgery to minimize anxiety related to pain, minimally invasive procedures, opioid-free anesthesia with multiple approaches, and fast postoperative mobilization within 6 h (Debono et al. 2021). These programs have consistently shown shortened hospital stays and less postoperative pain while not causing more surgical complications, readmissions, or cost escalation (Magableh et al. 2024).

1.4.4.2 Head and Neck Surgery

The implementation of an ERAS protocol in oncological head and neck surgery presents special challenges due to the potential complications related to airways, difficulty in swallowing, and complicated surgeries like free tissue transfer (Dort et al. 2017). The key points include preoperative optimization of nutrition and avoiding tracheostomy wherever possible, as well as goal-directed fluid administration to avoid edema and underperfusion of the flap (Coyle et al. 2016). The postoperative period requires prompt introduction of enteral nutrition using nasogastric feeding or PEG, along with specialized pain management protocols designed specifically to counteract metabolic stress caused by large surgical resections (Nieminen et al. 2024).

1.4.4.3 Orthopedic Surgery

Orthopedic ERAS pathways have mainly been used in elective joint replacement surgeries in the hips and knees, placing great importance on preoperative optimization and education of the patients to ensure that their expectations after the surgery are managed (Soffin and YaDeau 2016). The intraoperative phase involves the application of neuraxial and regional nerve block anesthesia rather than general anesthesia, along with goal-directed fluid therapy, to minimize surgical stress (Wainwright et al. 2020). Rapid mobilization is therefore possible, leading to low thromboembolic events and early discharge from the hospital (Salamanna et al. 2022).

1.4.4.4 Breast Surgery

In relation to oncological and reconstructive breast surgeries, ERAS guidelines have been proven to effectively transition a number of large-scale operations from an inpatient admission to an outpatient or same-day discharge approach (Temple-Oberle et al. 2017). Such programs focus on regional anesthetic approaches (paravertebral, pectoral nerve blocks), PONV prevention, and opioid-sparing multimodal pain relief (Rojas et al. 2018). Literature studies show that such guidelines can reduce hospitalization periods and narcotics utilization without increasing the number of complications or admissions (Mui et al. 2024).

1.4.4.5 Thoracic Surgery

The application of the ERAS concept in thoracic surgery is closely associated with the development of VATS, since the aim of both practices is to avoid causing additional harm to patients during surgery (Batchelor et al. 2019). The key aspects of intraoperative care include the use of lung-protecting ventilation with low tidal volume and regional anesthesia in order to avoid the respiratory depression caused by opioids (Semenkovich et al. 2018). Early removal of chest drains together with intensive physiotherapy contributes to rapid mobilization and reduces risks for pulmonary complications (Dinic et al. 2018).

1.4.4.6 Cardiac Surgery

The implementation of ERAS programs for cardiac surgery involves integrating state-of-the-art physiological management principles designed to address the huge inflammatory response created by the use of cardiopulmonary bypasses and sternotomies (Engelman et al. 2019). Key components consist of aggressive blood conservation techniques, such as cell-salvage and viscoelastic testing aimed at reducing transfusion needs, strict glucose control, and fast-track anesthesia practices involving early extubation (Williams et al. 2019). Contemporary research confirms the significant reduction of ICU days, ventilation requirements, and hospital costs as well as enhanced results among high-risk individuals undergoing ERAS for cardiac surgery (Gunaydin et al. 2024).

1.5 Core Principles and Components of ERAS

1.5.1 Preoperative Phase

1.5.1.1 Patient Education and Expectation Management

High-quality ERAS care provides counseling that helps the patients understand the surgical process, pain levels, mobilization and feeding milestones, and discharge criteria, hence reducing their level of anxiety and ensuring that their expectations are met in the process of early recovery (Altman et al. 2019). Education concerning stoma care, catheters, and drains is also effective in reducing barriers to discharge and is particularly beneficial in colorectal and urologic oncology (Altman et al. 2019; Parks et al. 2018).

1.5.1.2 Risk Stratification, Smoking, and Alcohol Cessation

According to the ERAS guidelines, the assessment of comorbidities, functional status, frailty, and psychosocial status should be performed, with special attention paid to modifiable risks such as smoking, hazardous drinking, anemia, and poorly controlled diabetes (Altman et al. 2019; Joliat et al. 2023). Smoking and hazardous drinking increase pulmonary and infectious complications, and quitting at least 4 weeks before the operation significantly reduces the risks of pulmonary and infectious complications and is now a strong recommendation in the ERAS guidelines for liver surgery (Joliat et al. 2023).

1.5.1.3 Prehabilitation

Multimodal prehabilitation has shown positive outcomes in terms of improvements in cardiopulmonary fitness and quality of life and a reduction in complications and lengths of stay, particularly in frail and high-risk patients (Dagorno et al. 2022; Joliat et al. 2023). Although evidence is still emerging in trials of prehabilitation in liver and colorectal surgery, the ERAS Society Liver Guidelines recommend prehabilitation in high-risk patients if time allows (Joliat et al. 2023).

1.5.1.4 Nutrition Risk Screening and Optimization

These conditions independently predict infections, anastomotic dehiscence, prolonged Length of stay (LOS), and mortality in patients undergoing gastrointestinal (GI) oncology, vascular, and liver surgery (Weimann et al. 2021; Joliat et al. 2023). ERAS protocols thus, recommend the implementation of validated nutritional screening tools like NRS-2002, Malnutrition Universal Screening Tool (MUST), prognostic nutritional index, and preoperative enteral nutrition for 7–14 days in high-risk patients whenever possible (Weimann et al. 2021; Melnyk et al. 2011).

1.5.1.5 Fasting and Carbohydrate Loading

Modern guidelines have moved away from traditional "Nil per oral after midnight" to more evidence-based guidelines, allowing for fasting of solids for 6 h and clear liquids for 2 h before anesthesia is given (Practice Guidelines for Preoperative Fasting 2017; Joliat et al. 2023). This is a more scientific understanding of how physiology works in the perioperative period, minimizing the adverse effects of fasting on metabolism.

Evidence exists for the administration of preoperative carbohydrate-rich clear fluids, given in a dose of 800 mL on the evening before surgery and a further dose of 400 mL 2–3 h before induction of anesthesia. This has been shown to be beneficial in minimizing insulin resistance, preserving lean body mass, and improving patient comfort by reducing thirst and hunger without increasing gastric residual volumes or aspiration risk (Smith et al. 2014; Tong et al. 2022).

A recent Bayesian network meta-analysis by Tong et al. concluded that ingestion of low-dose oral carbohydrates (10–50 g) significantly reduced insulin resistance compared to fasting and placebo, although a favorable ranking profile was obtained; conversely, hard clinical endpoints of complications and length of stay showed heterogeneous effects (Tong et al. 2022). In summary, carbohydrate loading is weakly to moderately recommended by ERAS guidelines for metabolic optimization in major abdominal surgeries, although it is still relatively contraindicated in type 1 diabetes and gastroparesis (Joliat et al. 2023; Melloul et al. 2016).

1.5.2 Intraoperative Phase

1.5.2.1 Minimally Invasive Surgery

These techniques have been associated with less tissue trauma, inflammation, pain, and ileus, as well as earlier mobilization and discharge, especially in colorectal and hepatobiliary surgery, as demonstrated in the study by Gustafsson et al. (2019) and Hughes et al. (2014). However, the benefits are dependent on the expertise available in the institutions, with ERAS guidelines emphasizing that minimally invasive techniques should not be adopted as dogma.

1.5.2.2 Anesthetic Management and Multimodal Analgesia

Anesthesiologists have a critical role to play in translating the principles of ERAS into practice. ERAS-consistent anesthesia techniques include the use of short-acting agents, depth of anesthesia monitoring, multimodal opioid-sparing analgesia techniques such as neuraxial blocks, TAP blocks, local infiltration techniques, acetaminophen, NSAIDs, gabapentinoids selectively, and aggressive Postoperative Nausea and Vomiting (PONV) prophylaxis. Current evidence from systematic reviews shows that multimodal regimens reduce opioid requirements, pain scores, nausea, ileus, and length of stay for a variety of procedures including colorectal, gynecologic, and orthopedic procedures (Teeuwen et al. 2010; Bisch et al. 2021).

1.5.2.3 Fluid Management and Hemodynamic Optimization

The ERAS guidelines strongly advise against liberal fluid strategies as well as overly restrictive approaches that may compromise renal perfusion (Myles et al. 2018; Minto et al. 2015). In the study conducted by the Restrictive versus Liberal Fluid Therapy in Major Abdominal Surgery (RELIEF) trial, there is a significant association between acute kidney injury and overly restrictive fluid strategies (Myles et al. 2018). In the management of patients undergoing liver surgeries, low central venous pressure in parenchymal transection and the use of goal-directed fluid therapy in the postoperative period are strongly recommended in minimizing blood loss while maintaining organ perfusion (Joliat et al. 2023).

1.5.2.4 Temperature Management and Thromboprophylaxis

Inadvertent hypothermia can worsen coagulopathy, wound infection, and cardiovascular complications. Forced-air blankets and warmed fluids are an essential part of ERAS (Joliat et al. 2023; Madrid et al. 2016). Venous thromboembolism prophylaxis using pharmacologic and mechanical methods is strongly recommended for major abdominal, pelvic, and orthopedic surgery. Extended prophylaxis is recommended for cancer surgery at 28 days (Joliat et al. 2023; Sauro et al. 2024).

1.5.3 Postoperative Phase

1.5.3.1 Early Mobilization

Early and progressive mobilization is also an important part of ERAS and is associated with fewer pulmonary, thromboembolic, and functional complications, as well as shorter hospital stays (Altman et al. 2019; Golder and Papalois 2021). Mobilization is also associated with improved respiratory mechanics, circulation, and rapid restoration of preoperative functional status.

Large observational studies have demonstrated that lack of mobilization on the first postoperative day is associated with increased complications and longer hospital stay (Grass et al. 2018; Fiore Jr et al. 2016). Optimal mobilization is a complex process that requires pain control, removal of intravenous lines and catheters when appropriate, and early input from physiotherapists to facilitate patient mobilization.

1.5.3.2 Early Oral Intake and Nutrition

Early introduction of oral fluids on the day of surgery, followed by a quick transition to a regular diet, is a major component of the ERAS protocol in colorectal, hepatobiliary, gynecological, and urological surgeries (Altman et al. 2019; Joliat et al. 2023). Several systematic review studies have proven that the introduction of oral feeding in the first 24 h after gastrointestinal surgery is safe and does not increase the risk of anastomotic leakage (Lewis et al. 2009; Andersen et al. 2006). Early oral feeding also reduces the occurrence of infections and the length of stay in the hospital (Andersen et al. 2006).

Dietitians have a vital role to perform in the ERAS protocol by assessing the needs of the patients for proteins and energy, the administration of oral supplements, and the initiation of enteral feeding in patients in whom oral feeding alone may not be sufficient, especially in high-risk patients (Parks et al. 2018).

1.5.3.3 Catheter, Drain, and Tube Management

Routine nasogastric decompression and prophylactic use of surgical drains have not been found to confer any advantages in colorectal, hepatobiliary, and urological surgeries. On the contrary, they have been associated with an increased risk of pneumonia, discomfort for the patient, and delayed oral feeding (Melnyk et al. 2011; Petrowsky et al. 2004). Therefore, it has been advocated in the ERAS guidelines to avoid nasogastric tube placement and drain placement, apart from specific situations where they are clinically indicated. The focus is on early removal of such tubes (Joliat et al. 2023; Gustafsson et al. 2019).

Similarly, early removal of urinary catheters is advocated, as it has been associated with decreased rates of urinary tract infection. Again, this is dependent on good nursing care and clear protocols, especially in patients who have undergone neuraxial analgesia (Altman et al. 2019).

1.5.3.4 Standardized Discharge Criteria and Follow-up

ERAS programs highlight the importance of the use of functional discharge criteria rather than time-based criteria. In this context, the criteria for discharge are effective pain control using oral analgesics, sufficient oral intake, the ability to mobilize independently, and the absence of unresolved complications requiring inpatient care. The patient-centered approach facilitates timely discharge without compromising the quality of care (Altman et al. 2019; Parks et al. 2018; Sauro et al. 2024).

The importance of post-discharge follow-up as part of ERAS programs cannot be emphasized enough. ERAS programs usually recommend the use of phone calls, telemedicine services, or early outpatient visits as part of the post-discharge follow-up process. The approach helps in the early identification of complications, ensures the patient follows the required post-operative care plan, and provides reassurance to the patient during the post-operative period at home (Altman et al. 2019; Parks et al. 2018; Sauro et al. 2024).

1.5.4 Perioperative Patient Positioning Within ERAS Pathways

Although positioning during surgery is based on the principle of providing optimal visualization of the anatomical structure, excessively difficult positioning may cause substantial physiological disturbances, including hemodynamic disturbance, respiratory difficulty, and potential for developing pressure ulcers or nerve damage. The ERAS pathways use specific measures that counteract stress reactions caused by these various postures:

1.5.4.1 Trendelenburg and Lithotomy Position

Frequently utilized during colorectal, gynecological, and urological procedures that involve surgery in the pelvis region, especially with robotic and laparoscopic techniques, the Trendelenburg position with pneumoperitoneum has significant effects on cardiorespiratory physiology. In addition to raising central venous, intracranial, and intraocular pressures, it significantly decreases the compliance of lungs (Kalmar et al. 2010). In ERAS protocols, anesthesiologists respond to these issues through goal-directed fluid therapy (GDFT) aimed at avoiding fluid overload that would result in serious facial, laryngeal, and airway edema. Also, specific ventilatory strategies, including low volumes with PEEP are consistently applied, and DVT prevention is vigorously pursued (Ljungqvist et al. 2017).

1.5.4.2 Prone Position

Used frequently in spinal surgeries, the prone position comes with its own set of issues, such as reduced venous return owing to the compression of the inferior vena cava and POVL resulting from compromised ocular perfusion (Depasse et al. 2015). ERAS protocols for spinal surgeries require the use of special operating tables

(Jackson table), along with specific padding, to ensure that the abdomen remains free-hanging. In turn, this helps prevent the distension of the epidural venous plexus, greatly minimizing intraoperative blood loss (Wainwright et al. 2020). Other important ERAS protocols include maintaining a neutral head position and limiting the infusion of crystalloids to avoid POVL and facial edema.

1.5.4.3 Lateral Decubitus Position

Widely used for operations on the thorax and kidneys, the position of lateral decubitus creates V/Q mismatching due to the gravitational effect, where there is adequate perfusion of the dependent part of the lungs while its ventilation is inadequate (Batchelor et al. 2019). ERAS thoracic surgery guidelines stress that the management of one-lung ventilation in this position should be done very carefully. It implies limiting the fraction of inspiratory oxygen concentration to avoid absorption atelectasis, using PEEP in the dependent part of the lungs, and aggressive pain management through regional blocks (Gonfiotti et al. 2018).

1.5.4.4 Sitting or "Beach Chair" Position

Commonly applied in shoulder surgery as well as certain types of neurosurgical operations, the beach chair position is associated with a very high probability of occurrence of cerebral hypoperfusion and severe bradycardia/hypotension (so-called Bezold-Jarisch reflex) caused by a pool of venous blood in the legs (Soffin and YaDeau 2016). The ERAS protocol for such operations requires that the continuous monitoring of blood pressure be performed using an invasive method, with brain-level measurement taken at the height of the external auditory meatus.

1.6 Multidisciplinary Organization, Compliance, and Implementation Science

ERAS is, by its very nature, a multidisciplinary approach where surgeons, anesthesiologists, nurses, dietitians, physiotherapists, pharmacists, and administrators work together to develop and implement standardized care pathways and audit tools (Altman et al. 2019; Parks et al. 2018). Dose-response relationships have been demonstrated in colorectal and liver surgery, where higher adherence to ERAS components results in reduced postoperative complications, shorter lengths of stay, and reduced readmission rates (Fig. 1.2) (Pędziwiatr et al. 2015; Nelson et al. 2016; Joliat et al. 2023).

Nevertheless, a study by Sauro et al. (2024) revealed that only about 20% of randomized trials documented their level of compliance, and many of them used fewer than 70% of the well-established components of ERAS. This indicates that the real-world efficacy of ERAS might be lower than documented. Implementation tools, such as Reporting on ERAS Compliance, Outcomes, and variation in Elements Research (RECOvER) checklist, "Reporting on ERAS Compliance, Outcomes, and Elements Research," and ERAS Interactive Audit System (EIAS), facilitate standardization of reporting and can be used for quality improvement (Elias et al., 2019).

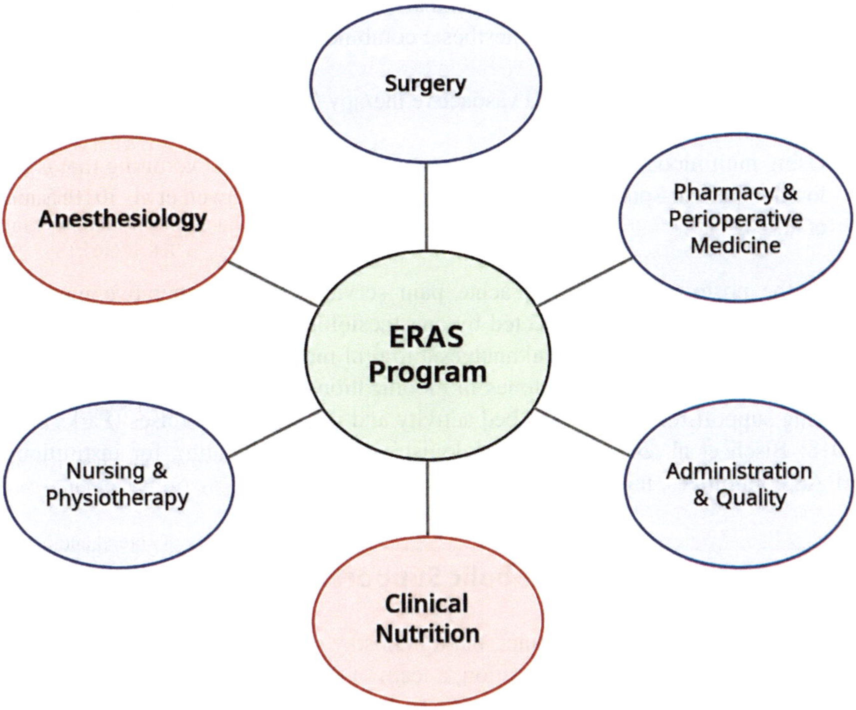

Fig. 1.2 Multidisciplinary ERAS framework. (Original figure created by the authors using MS PowerPoint 2021)

Some of the challenges in implementing ERAS include resistance to change of traditional practices, such as fasting, liberalizing fluids, and nasogastric tubes. There may be insufficient staff for early mobilization and nutrition support, and inadequate information technology infrastructure for real-time audit. Successful ERAS implementation has been associated with strong local champions, ERAS steering committees, and iterative education and feedback-driven refinement of ERAS protocols.

1.7 Central Role of Anesthesiology in ERAS

Anesthesiologists are at the center of preoperative evaluation, intraoperative care, and early postoperative management and are therefore critical to the process of ERAS implementation (Feldheiser et al. 2016; Golder and Papalois 2021). In this respect, preoperative anesthesia clinics are involved in the stratification of risks (sleep apnea, frailty, and cardiopulmonary reserve), optimization of comorbid conditions, patient counseling regarding fasting and analgesic requirements, and prehabilitation of smoking and alcohol cessation (Altman et al. 2019; Joliat et al. 2023).

Intraoperatively, anesthesiologists operationalize key ERAS goals by:

- Using short-acting anesthetic agents that can allow for early mobilization.
- Using neuraxial or regional anesthesia combined with non-opioid analgesics to reduce opioid requirements.
- Using goal-directed fluid and vasoactive therapy to optimize perfusion and minimize fluid overload.
- Using multimodal prophylaxis for postoperative nausea and vomiting that is tailored to patient-specific risks (Feldheiser et al. 2016; Teeuwen et al. 2010; Sauro et al. 2024).

In the postoperative period, acute pain services and perioperative medicine teams, often directed or codirected by anesthesiologists, manage the transition of care from epidural and regional analgesia to oral multimodal analgesia and adjust analgesia in response to milestones in mobilization, as well as physiotherapy and nursing support for early out-of-bed activity and respiratory exercises (Parks et al. 2018; Bisch et al. 2021). Anesthesiologists are now advocating for institutional ERAS committees, indicating the level of their engagement.

1.8 Nutrition and Metabolic Support Within ERAS

Nutrition is not seen as an adjunct, but a mainstay of ERAS. Beyond preoperative nutritional screening and optimization, a team of dietitians, surgeons, and anesthesiologists works together to ensure that:

- Fasting times before surgery are minimized.
- Preoperative carbohydrate loading is employed when necessary.
- Enteral nutrition is given preference over parenteral nutrition.
- The nutritional content is adjusted in accordance with catabolic stress, disease states, such as cirrhosis, and cancer cachexia.

Systematic reviews have shown that perioperative enteral nutrition and immunonutrition can decrease the risk of infections and the length of stay in GI cancer surgery, particularly in malnourished patients (Waitzberg et al. 2006). Nevertheless, routine immunonutrition is not recommended in the ERAS liver protocol because of heterogeneity and the absence of clear evidence of mortality reduction, with the emphasis being placed on further focused randomized trials (Joliat et al. 2023).

The changing carbohydrate loading literature represents an example of the ongoing evaluation of ERAS components. Small trials supported the benefits in the early stages, but the recent large network meta-analysis by Tong et al. (2022) refined our understanding, confirming improvements in metabolism (insulin resistance) but failing to show any effect on patient-reported outcomes or serious complications, again emphasizing the methodology limitations in the available evidence. Recommendations have therefore changed from unconditional to more qualified recommendations, especially in the context of liver disease and diabetes.

1.9 ERAS Across Populations, Settings, and the Care Continuum

1.9.1 Geriatric and Frail Patients

This is particularly true for older adults and frail patients who are at a particularly high risk of functional decline, delirium, and institutionalization following major surgeries (Hung et al. 2023; Joliat et al. 2023). ERAS care for this population has focused on the importance of comprehensive geriatric assessment, prevention of delirium (e.g., avoidance of benzodiazepines and promotion of sleep), prehabilitation, and early mobilization and enteral nutrition, all of which have been associated with improved functional outcomes and reduced complications (Lee et al. 2020; Feldheiser et al. 2016).

1.9.2 Low- and Middle-Income Countries

There are also challenges in the implementation of ERAS in low- and middle-income countries, including limited anesthesia and monitoring capabilities, limited access to regional anesthesia techniques, and limited physiotherapy and dietetics workforce availability (Parks et al. 2018). However, simplified ERAS pathways that include education, evidence-based fasting and fluid management, mobilization, and rational catheter and drain management have also resulted in significant reductions in length of stay without increasing the complication rate (Sauro et al. 2024; Altman et al. 2019). These studies indicate that the ERAS philosophy of evidence-based, patient-centered, and multi-disciplinary perioperative care with continuous audit may be applicable even in the absence of technology such as the Goal-Directed Fluid Therapy (GDFT) monitors.

1.9.3 Post-Discharge and Long-Term Outcomes

Although initial research in ERAS has centered on in-hospital outcomes, there is now greater emphasis on 30 and 90-day morbidities, quality of life, cognition, and oncologic outcomes. Improvement in early complications and maintenance of functional reserve may improve long-term survival, especially in cancer operations, although evidence is limited and biased (Sauro et al. 2024; Ljungqvist et al. 2017). The key point is that ERAS is not just about early discharge; it is actually earlier discharge as a result of safe and physiological recovery, not as a result of premature discharge.

1.10 Future Directions: Precision ERAS, Digital Health, and Research Agenda

Several converging trends are shaping the next generation of ERAS:

Precision and risk-stratified ERAS. Machine learning models utilizing data from EIAS and other data sets could potentially be used to predict individual risks for complications and length of stay, thus allowing for tailored prehabilitation strategies, analgesics, and nutrition (Sauro et al. 2024; Golder and Papalois 2021). For example, patients with high pain trajectory predictions could be given more aggressive regional anesthetic and non-opioid adjunct strategies, while those at highest risk for infection could be given more aggressive nutrition and glycemic strategies.

Digital patient engagement and remote monitoring. Smartphone apps and wearable technology are being integrated into ERAS pathways for providing educational content, monitoring step count and sleep, and promoting breathing exercises, as well as detecting abnormal recovery trends for early intervention (Parks et al. 2018; Altman et al. 2019). Initial results demonstrate improved compliance with mobilization and nutrition recommendations, as well as high levels of patient satisfaction.

Expansion to transplantation, cirrhosis, and complex oncologic resections. Ongoing research in liver and kidney transplant surgery is focused on developing ERAS protocols that are compatible with complex immunosuppression, organ allocation, and critical care dependency. ERAS guidelines for cirrhotic patients, high-risk pelvic exenteration, and multivisceral resection are research priorities.

Element-level optimization and de-implementation. The meta-analysis by Sauro et al. (2024) emphasized the fact that most studies combine various elements, making it hard to identify which elements are considered essential in various settings. Future studies using randomized and adaptive platform trials should aim to vary specific ERAS elements, such as carbohydrate loading, epidural vs. TAP blocks, and drain use, in order to identify the high-value elements and de-implement low-yield elements.

1.11 Conclusion

"Enhanced Recovery After Surgery" has revolutionized perioperative care from an art form based on tradition to a science based on physiology, randomized trial evidence, and continuous audit. Strong meta-analyses and excellent guidelines confirm that well-executed ERAS protocols can decrease complications, shorten lengths of stay, and lower healthcare costs in a broad range of surgeries without compromising safety. Anesthesiologists and nutrition experts are the conductors of this perioperative care process, designing strategies that minimize metabolic stress and maximize recovery and well-being.

As "Enhanced Recovery After Surgery" continues to develop and improve in terms of personalization, digitization, and globalization, it offers a potent platform for the integration of anesthesia and nutrition care into a holistic perioperative process with the potential for enhancing not only the short-term care of the surgical patient but also long-term health and value in the global community.

References

Ahmed OS, Rogers AC, Bolger JC, Mastrosimone A, Robb WB. Meta-analysis of enhanced recovery protocols in bariatric surgery. J Gastrointest Surg. 2018;22(6):964–72. https://doi.org/10.1007/s11605-018-3709-x.

Altman AD, Helpman L, McGee J, Samouëlian V, Auclair MH, Brar H, Nelson GS, Society of Gynecologic Oncology of Canada's Communities of Practice in ERAS and Venous Thromboembolism. Enhanced recovery after surgery: implementing a new standard of surgical care. CMAJ. 2019;191(17):E469–75. https://doi.org/10.1503/cmaj.180635.

Andersen HK, Lewis SJ, Thomas S. Early enteral nutrition within 24h of colorectal surgery versus later commencement of feeding for postoperative complications. Cochrane Database Syst Rev. 2006;4:CD004080. https://doi.org/10.1002/14651858.CD004080.pub2.

Practice guidelines for preoperative fasting and the use of pharmacologic agents to reduce the risk of pulmonary aspiration: application to healthy patients undergoing elective procedures: an updated report by the American Society of anesthesiologists task force on preoperative fasting and the use of pharmacologic agents to reduce the risk of pulmonary aspiration. Anesthesiology. 2017, 126(3), pp. 376–93. https://doi.org/10.1097/ALN.0000000000001452

Batchelor TJP, Rasburn NJ, Abdelnour-Berchtold E, Brunelli A, Cerfolio RJ, Gonzalez M, Ljungqvist O, Petersen RH, Popescu WM, Slinger PD. Guidelines for enhanced recovery after lung surgery: recommendations of the Enhanced Recovery After Surgery (ERAS®) Society and the European Society of Thoracic Surgeons (ESTS). Eur J Cardiothorac Surg. 2019;55(1):91–115. https://doi.org/10.1093/ejcts/ezy301.

Bisch SP, Jago CA, Kalogera E, Ganshorn H, Meyer LA, Ramirez PT, Dowdy SC, Nelson G. Outcomes of enhanced recovery after surgery (ERAS) in gynecologic oncology – a systematic review and meta-analysis. Gynecol Oncol. 2021;161(1):46–55. https://doi.org/10.1016/j.ygyno.2020.12.035.

Brindle M, Nelson G, Lobo DN, Ljungqvist O, Gustafsson UO. Recommendations from the ERAS® Society for standards for the development of enhanced recovery after surgery guidelines. BJS Open. 2020;4(1):157–63. https://doi.org/10.1002/bjs5.50238.

Cerantola Y, Valerio M, Persson B, Jichlinski P, Ljungqvist O, Hubner M, Kassouf W, Muller S, Baldini G, Carli F, Naesheimh T, Ytrebo L, Revhaug A, Lassen K, Knutsen T, Aarsether E, Wiklund P, Patel HR. Guidelines for perioperative care after radical cystectomy for bladder cancer: Enhanced Recovery After Surgery (ERAS(®)) Society Recommendations. Clin Nutr. 2013;32(6):879–87. https://doi.org/10.1016/j.clnu.2013.09.014.

Coyle MJ, Main B, Hughes C, Craven R, Alexander R, Porter G, Thomas S. Enhanced recovery after surgery (ERAS) for head and neck oncology patients. Clin Otolaryngol. 2016;41(2):118–26. https://doi.org/10.1111/coa.12482.

Dagorno C, Sommacale D, Laurent A, Attias A, Mongardon N, Levesque E, Langeron O, Rhaiem R, Leroy V, Amaddeo G, Brustia R. Prehabilitation in hepato-pancreato-biliary surgery: a systematic review and meta-analysis. A necessary step forward evidence-based sample size calculation for future trials. J Visc Surg. 2022;159(5):362–72. https://doi.org/10.1016/j.jviscsurg.2021.07.003.

Debono B, Wainwright TW, Wang MY, Sigmundsson FG, Yang MMH, Smid-Nanninga H, Bonnal A, Le Huec J-C, Fawcett WJ, Ljungqvist O, Lonjon G, de Boer HD. Consensus statement for perioperative care in lumbar spinal fusion: Enhanced Recovery After Surgery (ERAS®) Society recommendations. Spine J. 2021;21(5):729–52. https://doi.org/10.1016/j.spinee.2021.01.001.

Depasse JM, Palumbo M, Haque M, Eberson CP, Daniels AH, Palumbo MA. Complications associated with prone positioning in elective spinal surgery. World J Orthop. 2015;6(3):351–9. https://doi.org/10.5312/wjo.v6.i3.351.

Desborough JP. The stress response to trauma and surgery. Br J Anaesth. 2000;85(1):109–17. https://doi.org/10.1093/bja/85.1.109.

Dinic VD, Stojanovic MD, Markovic D, Cvetanovic V, Vukovic AZ, Jankovic RJ. Enhanced recovery in thoracic surgery: a review. Front Med. 2018;5:14. https://doi.org/10.3389/fmed.2018.00014.

Dort JC, Farwell DG, Findlay M, Huber GF, Kerr P, Shea-Budgell MA, Simon C, Uppington J, Zygun D, Ljungqvist O, Harris J. Optimal perioperative care in major head and neck cancer surgery with free flap reconstruction: a consensus review and recommendations from the Enhanced Recovery After Surgery Society. JAMA otolaryngology—head & neck surgery. 2017;143(3):292–303. https://doi.org/10.1001/jamaoto.2016.2981.

Elias KM, Stone AB, McGinigle K, Tankou JI, Scott MJ, Fawcett WJ, Demartines N, Lobo DN, Ljungqvist O, Urman RD, ERAS® Society and ERAS® USA. The reporting on ERAS compliance, outcomes, and elements research (RECOvER) checklist: a joint statement by the ERAS® and ERAS® USA Societies. World J Surg. 2019;43(1):1–8. https://doi.org/10.1007/s00268-018-4753-0.

Engelman DT, Ben Ali W, Williams JB, Perrault LP, Reddy VS, Arora RC, Roselli EE, Khoynezhad A, Gerdisch M, Levy JH, Lobdell K, Fletcher N, Kirsch M, Nelson G, Engelman RM, Gregory AJ, Boyle EM. Guidelines for perioperative care in cardiac surgery: Enhanced Recovery After Surgery Society Recommendations. JAMA Surg. 2019;154(8):755–66. https://doi.org/10.1001/jamasurg.2019.1153.

Fearon KC, Ljungqvist O, Von Meyenfeldt M, Revhaug A, Dejong CH, Lassen K, Nygren J, Hausel J, Soop M, Andersen J, Kehlet H. Enhanced recovery after surgery: a consensus review of clinical care for patients undergoing colonic resection. Clin Nutr. 2005;24(3):466–77. https://doi.org/10.1016/j.clnu.2005.02.002.

Feldheiser A, Aziz O, Baldini G, Cox BP, Fearon KC, Feldman LS, Gan TJ, Kennedy RH, Ljungqvist O, Lobo DN, Miller T, Radtke FF, Ruiz Garces T, Schricker T, Scott MJ, Thacker JK, Ytrebø LM, Carli F. Enhanced Recovery After Surgery (ERAS) for gastrointestinal surgery, part 2: consensus statement for anaesthesia practice. Acta Anaesthesiol Scand. 2016;60(3):289–334. https://doi.org/10.1111/aas.12651.

Fiore JF Jr, Bejjani J, Conrad K, Niculiseanu P, Landry T, Lee L, Ferri LE, Feldman LS. Systematic review of the influence of enhanced recovery pathways in elective lung resection. J Thorac Cardiovasc Surg. 2016;151(3):708–715.e6. https://doi.org/10.1016/j.jtcvs.2015.09.112.

Golder HJ, Papalois V. Enhanced recovery after surgery: history, key advancements and developments in transplant surgery. J Clin Med. 2021;10(8):1634. https://doi.org/10.3390/jcm10081634.

Gonfiotti A, Viggiano D, Bongiolatti S, Bertolaccini L, Solli P, Bertani A, Voltolini L, Crisci R, Droghetti A. Enhanced Recovery After Surgery (ERAS®) in thoracic surgical oncology. Future Oncol. 2018;14(6s):33–40. https://doi.org/10.2217/fon-2017-0471.

Grass F, Pache B, Martin D, Addor V, Hahnloser D, Demartines N, Hübner M. Feasibility of early postoperative mobilisation after colorectal surgery: a retrospective cohort study. Int J Surg. 2018;56:161–6. https://doi.org/10.1016/j.ijsu.2018.06.024.

Gunaydin S, Simsek E, Engelman D. Enhanced recovery after cardiac surgery and developments in perioperative care: a comprehensive review. Turk Gogus Kalp Damar Cerrahisi Derg. 2024;33(1):121–31. https://doi.org/10.5606/tgkdc.dergisi.2024.26770.

Gustafsson UO, Scott MJ, Hubner M, Nygren J, Demartines N, Francis N, Rockall TA, Young-Fadok TM, Hill AG, Soop M, de Boer HD, Urman RD, Chang GJ, Fichera A, Kessler H, Grass F, Whang EE, Fawcett WJ, Carli F, Lobo DN, et al. Guidelines for perioperative care in elective colorectal surgery: Enhanced Recovery After Surgery (ERAS®) Society Recommendations: 2018. World J Surg. 2019;43(3):659–95. https://doi.org/10.1007/s00268-018-4844-y.

Huang ZD, Gu HY, Zhu J, Luo J, Shen XF, Deng QF, Zhang C, Li YB. The application of enhanced recovery after surgery for upper gastrointestinal surgery: meta-analysis. BMC Surg. 2020;20(1):3. https://doi.org/10.1186/s12893-019-0669-3.

Hughes MJ, McNally S, Wigmore SJ. Enhanced recovery following liver surgery: a systematic review and meta-analysis. HPB (Oxford). 2014;16(8):699–706. https://doi.org/10.1111/hpb.12245.

Hung DSW, Chu CWH, Kwok KH. The enhanced recovery after surgery program in elderly patients over 75 years of age undergoing elective colorectal cancer surgery. Surg Pract. 2023;27(4):226–31. https://doi.org/10.1111/1744-1633.12661.

Joliat GR, Labgaa I, Petermann D, Hübner M, Griesser AC, Demartines N, Schäfer M. Cost-benefit analysis of an enhanced recovery protocol for pancreaticoduodenectomy. Br J Surg. 2015;102(13):1676–83. https://doi.org/10.1002/bjs.9957.

Joliat GR, Kobayashi K, Hasegawa K, Thomson JE, Padbury R, Scott M, Brustia R, Scatton O, Tran Cao HS, Vauthey JN, Dincler S, Clavien PA, Wigmore SJ, Demartines N, Melloul E. Guidelines for perioperative care for liver surgery: Enhanced Recovery After Surgery (ERAS) Society Recommendations 2022. World J Surg. 2023;47(1):11–34. https://doi.org/10.1007/s00268-022-06732-5.

Kalmar AF, Foubert L, Hendrickx JF, Mottrie A, Absalom A, Mortier EP, Struys MM. Influence of steep trendelenburg position and CO(2) pneumoperitoneum on cardiovascular, cerebrovascular, and respiratory homeostasis during robotic prostatectomy. Br J Anaesth. 2010;104(4):433–9. https://doi.org/10.1093/bja/aeq018.

Kehlet H. Multimodal approach to control postoperative pathophysiology and rehabilitation. Br J Anaesth. 1997;78(5):606–17. https://doi.org/10.1093/bja/78.5.606.

Kehlet H, Mogensen T. Hospital stay of 2 days after open sigmoidectomy with a multimodal rehabilitation programme. Br J Surg. 1999;86(2):227–30. https://doi.org/10.1046/j.1365-2168.1999.01023.x.

Kehlet H, Wilmore DW. Multimodal strategies to improve surgical outcome. Am J Surg. 2002;183(6):630–41. https://doi.org/10.1016/s0002-9610(02)00866-8.

Lassen K, Coolsen MM, Slim K, Carli F, de Aguilar-Nascimento JE, Schäfer M, Parks RW, Fearon KC, Lobo DN, Demartines N, Braga M, Ljungqvist O, Dejong CH, ERAS® Society, European Society for Clinical Nutrition and Metabolism, & International Association for Surgical Metabolism and Nutrition. Guidelines for perioperative care for pancreaticoduodenectomy: Enhanced Recovery After Surgery (ERAS®) Society recommendations. Clinical Nutri. 2012;31(6):817–30. https://doi.org/10.1016/j.clnu.2012.08.011.

Lee KC, Streid J, Sturgeon D, Lipsitz S, Weissman JS, Rosenthal RA, Kim DH, Mitchell SL, Cooper Z. The impact of frailty on long-term patient-oriented outcomes after emergency general surgery: a retrospective cohort study. J Am Geriatr Soc. 2020;68(5):1037–43. https://doi.org/10.1111/jgs.16334.

Lewis SJ, Andersen HK, Thomas S. Early enteral nutrition within 24 h of intestinal surgery versus later commencement of feeding: a systematic review and meta-analysis. J Gastrointest Surg. 2009;13(3):569–75. https://doi.org/10.1007/s11605-008-0592-x.

Ljungqvist O, Scott M, Fearon KC. Enhanced recovery after surgery: a review. JAMA Surg. 2017;152(3):292–8. https://doi.org/10.1001/jamasurg.2016.4952.

Madrid E, Urrútia G, Roqué i Figuls M, Pardo-Hernandez H, Campos JM, Paniagua P, Maestre L, Alonso-Coello P. Active body surface warming systems for preventing complications caused by inadvertent perioperative hypothermia in adults. Cochrane Database Syst Rev. 2016;4(4):CD009016. https://doi.org/10.1002/14651858.CD009016.pub2.

Magableh HM, Ibrahim S, Pennington Z, Nathani KR, Johnson SE, Katsos K, Freedman BA, Bydon M. Transforming outcomes of spine surgery: exploring the power of enhanced recovery after surgery protocol: a systematic review and meta-analyses of 15,198 patients. Neurosurgery. 2024;95(1):3–25. https://doi.org/10.1227/neu.0000000000002865.

Melloul E, Hübner M, Scott M, Snowden C, Prentis J, Dejong CH, Garden OJ, Farges O, Kokudo N, Vauthey JN, Clavien PA, Demartines N. Guidelines for perioperative care for liver surgery: Enhanced Recovery After Surgery (ERAS) Society Recommendations. World J Surg. 2016;40(10):2425–40. https://doi.org/10.1007/s00268-016-3700-1.

Melnyk M, Casey RG, Black P, Koupparis AJ. Enhanced recovery after surgery (ERAS) protocols: time to change practice? Can Urol Assoc J. 2011;5(5):342–8. https://doi.org/10.5489/cuaj.11002.

Minto G, Scott MJ, Miller TE. Monitoring needs and goal-directed fluid therapy within an enhanced recovery program. Anesthesiol Clin. 2015;33(1):35–49. https://doi.org/10.1016/j.anclin.2014.11.003.

Mui J, Cheng E, Salindera S. Enhanced recovery after surgery for oncological breast surgery reduces length of stay in a resource limited setting. ANZ J Surg. 2024;94(6):1096–101. https://doi.org/10.1111/ans.18901.

Myles PS, Bellomo R, Corcoran T, Forbes A, Peyton P, Story D, Christophi C, Leslie K, McGuinness S, Parke R, Serpell J, Chan MTV, Painter T, McCluskey S, Minto G, Wallace S, Australian and New Zealand College of Anaesthetists Clinical Trials Network and the Australian and New Zealand Intensive Care Society Clinical Trials Group. Restrictive versus liberal fluid therapy for major abdominal surgery. N Engl J Med. 2018;378(24):2263–74. https://doi.org/10.1056/NEJMoa1801601.

Nelson G, Kiyang LN, Crumley ET, Chuck A, Nguyen T, Faris P, Wasylak T, Basualdo-Hammond C, McKay S, Ljungqvist O, Gramlich LM. Implementation of Enhanced Recovery After Surgery (ERAS) across a provincial healthcare system: the ERAS Alberta colorectal surgery experience. World J Surg. 2016;40(5):1092–103. https://doi.org/10.1007/s00268-016-3472-7.

Nelson G, Bakkum-Gamez J, Kalogera E, Glaser G, Altman A, Meyer LA, Taylor JS, Iniesta M, Lasala J, Mena G, Scott M, Gillis C, Elias K, Wijk L, Huang J, Nygren J, Ljungqvist O, Ramirez PT, Dowdy SC. Guidelines for perioperative care in gynecologic/oncology: Enhanced Recovery After Surgery (ERAS) Society recommendations-2019 update. Int J Gynecol Cancer. 2019;29(4):651–68. https://doi.org/10.1136/ijgc-2019-000356.

Nieminen T, Tapiovaara L, Bäck L, Lindford A, Lassus P, Lehtonen L, Mäkitie A, Keski-Säntti H. Correction: Enhanced recovery after surgery (ERAS) protocol improves patient outcomes in free flap surgery for head and neck cancer. Eur Arch Otorhinolaryngol. 2024;281(6):3313–4. https://doi.org/10.1007/s00405-024-08520-4.

Parks L, Routt M, De Villiers A. Enhanced recovery after surgery. J Adv Pract Oncol. 2018;9(5):511–9. Enhanced Recovery After Surgery – PubMed.

Pędziwiatr M, Kisialeuski M, Wierdak M, Stanek M, Natkaniec M, Matłok M, Major P, Małczak P, Budzyński A. Early implementation of enhanced recovery after surgery (ERAS®) protocol – compliance improves outcomes: a prospective cohort study. Int J Surg. 2015;21:75–81. https://doi.org/10.1016/j.ijsu.2015.06.087.

Petrowsky H, Demartines N, Rousson V, Clavien PA. Evidence-based value of prophylactic drainage in gastrointestinal surgery: a systematic review and meta-analyses. Ann Surg. 2004;240(6):1074–85. https://doi.org/10.1097/01.sla.0000146149.17411.c5.

Rojas KE, Manasseh DM, Flom PL, Agbroko S, Bilbro N, Andaz C, Borgen PI. A pilot study of a breast surgery Enhanced Recovery After Surgery (ERAS) protocol to eliminate narcotic prescription at discharge. Breast Cancer Res Treat. 2018;171(3):621–6. https://doi.org/10.1007/s10549-018-4859-y.

Salamanna F, Contartese D, Brogini S, Visani A, Martikos K, Griffoni C, Ricci A, Gasbarrini A, Fini M. Key components, current practice and clinical outcomes of ERAS programs in patients undergoing orthopedic surgery: a systematic review. J Clin Med. 2022;11(14):4222. https://doi.org/10.3390/jcm11144222.

Sauro KM, Smith C, Ibadin S, Thomas A, Ganshorn H, Bakunda L, Bajgain B, Bisch SP, Nelson G. Enhanced recovery after surgery guidelines and hospital length of stay, readmission, complications, and mortality: a meta-analysis of randomized clinical trials. JAMA Netw Open. 2024;7(6):e2417310. https://doi.org/10.1001/jamanetworkopen.2024.17310.

Semenkovich TR, Hudson JL, Subramanian M, Kozower BD. Enhanced Recovery After Surgery (ERAS) in thoracic surgery. Semin Thorac Cardiovasc Surg. 2018;30(3):342–9. https://doi.org/10.1053/j.semtcvs.2018.06.001.

Sharma K, Akre S, Chakole S, Wanjari MB. Stress-induced diabetes: a review. Cureus. 2022;14(9):e29142. https://doi.org/10.7759/cureus.29142.

Smith MD, McCall J, Plank L, Herbison GP, Soop M, Nygren J. Preoperative carbohydrate treatment for enhancing recovery after elective surgery. Cochrane Database Syst Rev. 2014;2014(8):CD009161. https://doi.org/10.1002/14651858.CD009161.pub2.

Soffin EM, YaDeau JT. Enhanced recovery after surgery for primary hip and knee arthroplasty: a review of the evidence. Br J Anaesth. 2016;117(suppl 3):iii62–72. https://doi.org/10.1093/bja/aew362.

Teeuwen PH, Bleichrodt RP, Strik C, Groenewoud JJ, Brinkert W, van Laarhoven CJ, van Goor H, Bremers AJ. Enhanced Recovery After Surgery (ERAS) versus conventional postoperative care in colorectal surgery. J Gastrointest Surg. 2010;14(1):88–95. https://doi.org/10.1007/s11605-009-1037-x.

Temple-Oberle C, Shea-Budgell MA, Tan M, Semple JL, Schrag C, Barreto M, Blondeel P, Hamming J, Dayan J, Ljungqvist O, ERAS Society. Consensus review of optimal perioperative care in breast reconstruction: Enhanced Recovery after Surgery (ERAS) Society Recommendations. Plast Reconstr Surg. 2017;139(5):1056e–71e. https://doi.org/10.1097/PRS.0000000000003242.

Thanh N, Nelson A, Wang X, et al. Return on investment of the Enhanced Recovery After Surgery (ERAS) multiguideline, multisite implementation in Alberta, Canada. Can J Surg. 2020;63(6):E542–50. https://doi.org/10.1503/cjs.006720.

Thorell A, Nygren J, Ljungqvist O. Insulin resistance: a marker of surgical stress. Curr Opin Clin Nutr Metab Care. 1999;2(1):69–78. https://doi.org/10.1097/00075197-199901000-00012.

Tong E, Chen Y, Ren Y, Zhou Y, Di C, Zhou Y, Shao S, Qiu S, Hong Y, Yang L, Tan X. Effects of preoperative carbohydrate loading on recovery after elective surgery: a systematic review and Bayesian network meta-analysis of randomized controlled trials. Front Nutr. 2022;9:951676. https://doi.org/10.3389/fnut.2022.951676.

Varadhan KK, Neal KR, Dejong CH, Fearon KC, Ljungqvist O, Lobo DN. The enhanced recovery after surgery (ERAS) pathway for patients undergoing major elective open colorectal surgery: a meta-analysis of randomized controlled trials. Clinical Nutri. 2010;29(4):434–40. https://doi.org/10.1016/j.clnu.2010.01.004.

Wainwright TW, et al. Consensus statement for perioperative care in total hip replacement and total knee replacement surgery: Enhanced Recovery After Surgery (ERAS®) Society recommendations. Acta Orthop. 2020;91(3):363. https://doi.org/10.1080/17453674.2020.1724674.

Waitzberg DL, Saito H, Plank LD, Jamieson GG, Jagannath P, Hwang TL, Mijares JM, Bihari D. Postsurgical infections are reduced with specialized nutrition support. World J Surg. 2006;30(8):1592 604. https://doi.org/10.1007/s00268-005-0657-x.

Weimann A, Braga M, Carli F, Higashiguchi T, Hübner M, Klek S, Laviano A, Ljungqvist O, Lobo DN, Martindale RG, Waitzberg D, Bischoff SC, Singer P. ESPEN practical guideline: clinical nutrition in surgery. Clinical Nutri. 2021;40(7):4745–61. https://doi.org/10.1016/j.clnu.2021.03.031.

Williams JB, McConnell G, Allender JE, Woltz P, Kane K, Smith PK, Engelman DT, Bradford WD. One-year results from the first US-based enhanced recovery after cardiac surgery (ERAS cardiac) program. J Thorac Cardiovasc Surg. 2019;157(5):1881–8. https://doi.org/10.1016/j.jtcvs.2018.10.164.

Wind J, Polle SW, Fung Kon Jin PH, Dejong CH, von Meyenfeldt MF, Ubbink DT, Gouma DJ, Bemelman WA, Laparoscopy and/or Fast Track Multimodal Management Versus Standard Care (LAFA) Study Group, & Enhanced Recovery after Surgery (ERAS) Group. Systematic review of enhanced recovery programmes in colonic surgery. Br J Surg. 2006;93(7):800–9. https://doi.org/10.1002/bjs.5384.

Zhou Y, Li R, Liu Z, Qi W, Lv G, Zhong M, Liu X, Zhu M, Jiang Z, Chen S, Shi B, Zhu Y. The effect of the enhanced recovery after surgery program on radical cystectomy: a meta-analysis and systematic review. Front Surg. 2023;10:1101098. https://doi.org/10.3389/fsurg.2023.1101098.

Zhuang CL, Ye XZ, Zhang XD, Chen BC, Yu Z. Enhanced recovery after surgery programs versus traditional care for colorectal surgery: a meta-analysis of randomized controlled trials. Dis Colon Rectum. 2013;56(5):667–78. https://doi.org/10.1097/DCR.0b013e3182812842.

Physiological Basis of Surgical Stress and Recovery

2

Ravi Yadav and Debasrita Banerjee

Abstract

Background: Major surgery induces a coordinated stress response involving neuroendocrine, inflammatory, immune, metabolic, endothelial, and mitochondrial pathways that evolved to support short-term survival. In contemporary surgical populations characterized by aging, frailty, multimorbidity, and malnutrition, this response may become maladaptive, contributing to hyperglycemia, catabolism, immune dysfunction, organ injury, delirium, persistent postsurgical pain, and impaired long-term recovery. Excessive stress has also been linked to adverse oncologic outcomes, including increased risk of cancer recurrence.

Objectives: This chapter examines the molecular, cellular, and systems-level physiology of the surgical stress response, including emerging concepts such as thromboinflammation and mitochondrial damage-associated molecular patterns (mtDAMPs). It explores how Enhanced Recovery After Surgery (ERAS®) pathways use integrated anesthetic and nutritional strategies to attenuate stress and improve recovery, while addressing vulnerable populations, including frail, sarcopenic, emergency, and oncologic surgery patients. Future directions toward biomarker-driven precision ERAS are also discussed.

Methods: A narrative review was conducted using ERAS® Society guidelines, speciality consensus statements, systematic reviews, meta-analyses, randomized trials, and high-quality observational studies published over the last two decades through 2026. Evidence was drawn primarily from PubMed, major perioperative

R. Yadav
Department of Anesthesia & Operation Theater Technology, Medhavi Skills University, School of Health Sciences & Technology, Singtam, Sikkim, India

D. Banerjee (✉)
Department of Nutrition and Dietetics, Medhavi Skills University, Singtam, Sikkim, India

P. K. Bhattacharyya et al. (eds.), *Integrated Anesthesia and Nutrition Approaches to Enhanced Recovery after Surgery*,
https://doi.org/10.1007/978-981-92-3294-9_2

journals, and ERAS® resources, with emphasis on perioperative anesthesia, nutrition, immunology, metabolism, and implementation science.

Results: Surgical trauma triggers release of DAMPs and mtDAMPs, activating inflammatory cascades alongside sympathoadrenal and HPA-axis responses that promote insulin resistance, hypermetabolism, muscle proteolysis, and immune reprogramming. Endothelial dysfunction and thromboinflammation further contribute to organ injury. Biomarkers such as IL-6, CRP, cortisol, and glucose trajectories reflect stress intensity and predict complications. ERAS interventions—including multimodal anesthesia, carbohydrate loading, early high-protein feeding, immunonutrition, mobilization, and prehabilitation—attenuate stress responses, preserve immune and mitochondrial function, and reduce complications and length of stay.

Conclusions: The surgical stress response is a modifiable multi-axis phenomenon. Physiologically informed ERAS pathways integrating anesthesia, nutrition, mobilization, and frailty-focused strategies improve recovery and outcomes, while future precision ERAS models may enable more individualized perioperative care.

Keywords

Surgical stress response · Neuroendocrine response · Perioperative nutrition · Immunonutrition · Thromboinflammation · Mitochondrial dysfunction

2.1 Introduction

Surgery causes a systemic stress response involving almost all organs, as the body seeks to re-establish equilibrium after injury, blood loss, and risk of infection (Cusack and Buggy 2020). But in modern surgery, this response may become pathological because it occurs in patients who are older, frailer, and sicker than in the past, with common pre-existing cardiovascular, metabolic, and nutritional deficiencies (Golder and Papalois 2021; Guo et al. 2023). A dysregulated stress response to surgery drives hyperglycemia, muscle catabolism, immune dysfunction, organ failure, delirium, chronic pain, and cancer recurrence, which all prolong recovery and compromise long-term quality of life (Ljungqvist 2010; Jawa et al. 2011; Fuller et al. 2023).

Historical perioperative practices, including prolonged fasting and generous fluid resuscitation, deep general anesthesia with large doses of opioids, routine drainage and tube insertion, and delayed ambulation and feeding, tended to exaggerate rather than suppress stress responses, delaying ileus, promoting muscle catabolism, and increasing cardiovascular, respiratory, and infection complications (Kehlet and Wilmore 2008; Thiele et al. 2015). ERAS continues to develop perioperative care as a specific physiological intervention: a structured pathway of multidisciplinary, evidence-based care designed to limit stress and increase resilience by providing a coordinated package of anesthesia, surgery, nutrition, and rehabilitation (Nelson et al. 2023).

This understanding of the physiology of surgery at the molecular, cellular, and systems levels allows clinicians to apply ERAS strategies (particularly integrated anesthesia and nutrition) in a rational manner, to reduce the adverse responses, and to promote recovery, as opposed to merely treating complications after they occur (Kehlet 1997; Mithany et al. 2023; Jain et al. 2023).

2.2 Historical Evolution: From Selye's Stress to ERAS

The general adaptation syndrome described by Hans Selye was the first attempt to explain the stress response to noxious stimuli, with an emphasis on the HPA axis and sympathoadrenal system (Cusack and Buggy 2020). In surgical patients, observational studies from the mid-twentieth century reported massive increases in perioperative catecholamines and cortisol, as well as a large negative nitrogen balance following surgery, which suggested that the "stress of surgery" was a key driver of postoperative recovery (Ljungqvist 2010; Jawa et al. 2011).

Kehlet and others played a pivotal role in demonstrating that this response can be modified: the combination of thoracic epidural anesthesia, prevention of hypothermia, meticulous fluid management, avoidance of drains and tubes, early ambulation, and early feeding (what was then called "fast-track surgery") dramatically reduced LOS and morbidity following major colorectal surgery (Kehlet 1997; Kehlet and Wilmore 2008). In the following decade, this led to the development of ERAS, and the ERAS® Society published procedure-specific guidelines for colorectal, gynecologic oncology, urology, hepatopancreatobiliary, bariatric, thoracic, pancreatic, orthopedic, and emergency general surgery (Nelson et al. 2023; ERAS® Society 2021).

Now we know that high-quality observational studies and meta-analyses demonstrate that high adherence to ERAS elements is associated with a stepwise reduction in complications, length of stay (LOS), and costs, with some series showing a median LOS reduction of 2–4 days, without an increase in readmissions (Thiele et al. 2015; Golder and Papalois 2021; Mithany et al. 2023). The effects of ERAS can be thought of as "flattening and shrinking" the stress curve, by decreasing the magnitude of physiological responses while increasing the baseline ability to cope through prehabilitation and improved nutrition (Kehlet and Wilmore 2008; Jain et al. 2023).

2.3 Cellular and Molecular Mechanisms of Surgical Stress

2.3.1 DAMPs, mtDAMPs and Pattern-Recognition Receptors

Surgical trauma, ischemia-reperfusion, and microbial translocation lead to the release of DAMPs (e.g., HMGB1, heat-shock proteins, extracellular matrix fragments) and mitochondrial components (mtDAMPs) such as mitochondrial DNA, cardiolipin, and N-formyl peptides (Jawa et al. 2011). These activate pattern-recognition receptors on immune and endothelial cells, such as Toll-like receptors (TLRs), NOD-like receptors (e.g., NLRP3), and the cGAS-STING pathway, resulting in NF-κB activation and transcription of pro-inflammatory cytokines and chemokines (Jawa et al. 2011; Ku et al. 2025).

mtDAMPs are powerful stimulators of neutrophils and monocytes to produce reactive oxygen species (ROS) and stimulate the formation of NETs, which can entrap microbes but also damage endothelium and other tissues. This signaling pathway connects cell damage with systemic inflammation and is enhanced when pre-existing sepsis, blood flow restriction, or organ dysfunction is present, as is often the case in emergency surgical patients and in the elderly (Ni and Zheng 2025; ERAS® Society 2021).

2.3.2 Re-progamming of Innate and Adaptive Immunity

Neutrophils rapidly infiltrate the area of surgical insult, are primed, degranulated, and release NETs, helping eliminate pathogens but potentially leading to microvascular obstruction and tissue damage when over-activated (Jawa et al. 2011; Jackson et al. 2019). Monocytes and macrophages adopt either pro-inflammatory (M1-like) or pro-resolving (M2-like) states depending on the cytokine environment, impacting wound repair and fibrosis (Jawa et al. 2011; Matsui et al. 2024). The meaning of these related inflammatory and immune markers in the perioperative setting is briefly outlined in Table 2.1.

Adaptive immune responses feature temporary lymphopenia, T-cell exhaustion, and dysfunctional NK cells in the early post-operative period, days to weeks after major surgery, which may contribute to infections and metastatic growth (Angka et al. 2017). In cancer surgery, post-operative NK cell dysfunction has been linked to metastatic progression, prompting a surge in interest in the use of perioperative measures (such as regional anesthesia, opioid-sparing pain control, immunonutrition, and potentially immunomodulatory drugs) that maintain the competence of the innate and adaptive immune responses (Market et al. 2018; Matsui et al. 2024).

Table 2.1 Selected inflammatory and immune biomarkers and their perioperative interpretation

Biomarker	Typical trajectory after major surgery	Clinical interpretation
IL-6	Rapid rise; peaks 4–24 h; magnitude ~ tissue trauma	Predicts complications, infection, and organ dysfunction
CRP	Peaks 48–72 h; resolves over days	Surrogate of global inflammatory burden
Procalcitonin	Rises with severe infection/sepsis	Differentiates sepsis from sterile inflammation
NK cell activity	Early suppression; slow recovery	Reflects anti-tumor and anti-viral immune competence
Lymphocyte count	Early lymphopenia, especially CD4+/CD8+ T cells	Marker of immunosuppressive phase and infection risk

2.4 Neuroendocrine Stress Axes

2.4.1 Sympathoadrenal Activation

Afferent stimulation from the surgical field via ascending pathways to the brainstem and hypothalamus results in sympathetic activation and release of norepinephrine and epinephrine from the adrenal medulla (Cusack and Buggy 2020; Ivascu et al. 2024). Catecholamines stimulate heart rate, contractility and systemic vascular resistance, preserving blood pressure, but also increase myocardial oxygen consumption and risk of arrhythmia, especially in patients with coronary artery disease and heart failure (Cusack and Buggy 2020; Golder and Papalois 2021).

Catecholamines also induce hepatic glycogenolysis and gluconeogenesis, suppress insulin secretion, and decrease peripheral glucose uptake, leading to hyperglycemia and insulin resistance (Ljungqvist 2010; Ku et al. 2025). Randomized controlled studies demonstrate that neuraxial or major peripheral nerve blocks that reliably block nociception significantly attenuate catecholamine responses, improve hemodynamic stability, and prevent metabolic disturbances compared to general anaesthesia (Breslow et al. 1993).

2.4.2 Hypothalamic-Pituitary-Adrenal Axis and Other Hormonal Changes

The HPA axis is stimulated via hypothalamic corticotropin-releasing hormone, which stimulates adrenocorticotropic hormone, which in turn stimulates cortisol release (Cusack and Buggy 2020; Ivascu et al. 2024). Cortisol stimulates gluconeogenesis, increases protein breakdown, increases sodium and water retention, and has immune-suppressing effects, which include T-cell suppression and changing levels of different cytokines (Jawa et al. 2011).

Cortisol levels tend to peak 24 h after major surgery, and persist longer in the setting of complications, and thoracic epidural or combined regional-general anesthesia blunts cortisol responses compared with general anesthesia alone, supporting the use of these techniques in ERAS (Breslow et al. 1993; Ivascu et al. 2024). Other hormones–such as growth hormone, glucagon, vasopressin, leptin, and ghrelin—also undergo perioperative changes, and interact with nutritional support to affect glucose, appetite, and water balance (Ljungqvist 2010; Ku et al. 2025).

2.5 Metabolic and Nutritional Stress Response

2.5.1 Insulin Resistance and Blood Glucose

Insulin resistance is a key element of the metabolic stress response, with insulin sensitivity reduced by as much as 50–90% following major abdominal surgery (Ljungqvist 2010; Ku et al. 2025). Cytokines (IL-6, TNF-α), catecholamines, cortisol, and glucagon, acting in concert to inhibit insulin receptor signaling and GLUT4 translocation in muscle and liver, lead to hyperglycemia (Jawa et al. 2011; Matsui et al. 2024).

Prospective studies demonstrate that the extent of postoperative insulin resistance is associated with operative time, blood loss, and the inflammatory response, and independently predicts wound infection, sepsis, prolonged ileus, and prolonged LOS (Ljungqvist 2010; Nur et al. 2026). ERAS interventions such as shorter fasting, carbohydrate loading, multimodal analgesia, normothermia, and early mobilization have been demonstrated to reduce insulin resistance and improve glucose control, justifying these interventions from a physiological standpoint (Kukliński et al. 2022; Ping et al. 2025; Kumar et al. 2025; Tazreean et al. 2022).

2.5.2 Hypermetabolism, Muscular Proteolysis, and Body Composition

Postoperative hypermetabolism following major surgery, trauma, and burns is associated with high resting energy expenditure, increased proteolysis and lipolysis, which enable increased gluconeogenesis, acute-phase protein production, and immune cell proliferation, but at the expense of lean mass loss (Ku et al. 2025). The elderly and frail, who may have a low baseline of muscle mass, are particularly at risk and may lose significant function even with minor surgery (Guo et al. 2023; Zeng et al. 2026).

Sarcopenia or frailty, assessed by imaging or functional tests, is an independent risk factor for postoperative complications, slow recovery, institutionalization, and death (Guo et al. 2023; Ni and Zheng 2025). This means that ERAS pathways that combine pre-and post-operative nutrition, high-protein diet, resistance training prehabilitation, and early mobilization are particularly important in these populations (Matsui et al. 2024; Sung and Oh 2026).

2.6 Endothelium, Coagulation, and Thromboinflammation

Injury from surgery activates the endothelium and coagulation, leading to a prothrombotic state that involves inflammation, now called thromboinflammation or immunothrombosis (Jawa et al. 2011; Jackson et al. 2019). Cytokines, DAMPs, and mtDAMPs up-regulate endothelial adhesion molecules, trigger release of von Willebrand factor, and increase tissue factor expression, while platelets bind

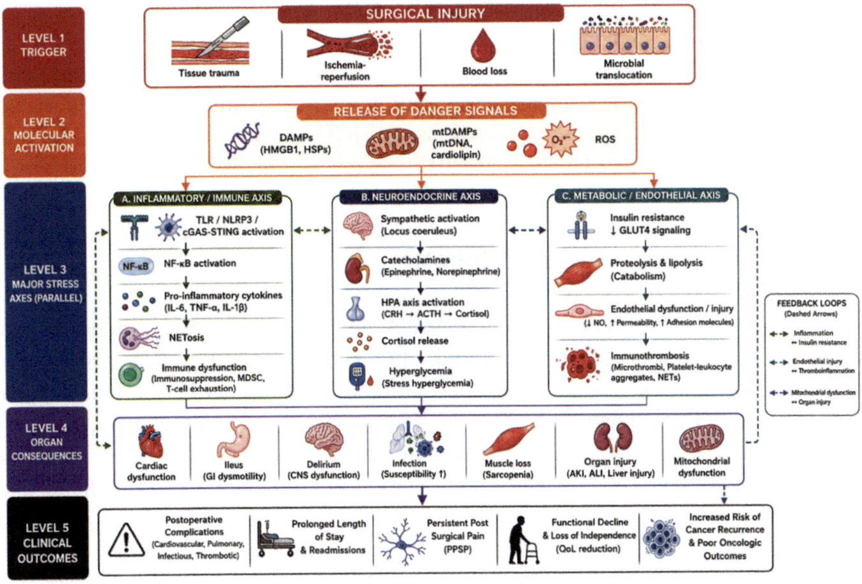

Fig. 2.1 Surgical trauma initiates interconnected inflammatory, neuroendocrine, metabolic, and thromboinflammatory pathways that drive organ dysfunction and adverse postoperative outcomes. (Figure created by the author using draw.io (diagrams.net))

to neutrophils to form aggregates and NETs, which can block the microcirculation.

This microvascular dysfunction is especially critical in end-arterial organs like the brain and splanchnic organs, where microthrombi and autoregulation failure contribute to delirium, stroke, and mesenteric ischemia. ERAS-complicit approaches, including avoiding fluid overload, maintaining normothermia and normoxia, and early mobilization and pharmacologic thromboprophylaxis, target the thromboinflammatory pathomechanism, and awareness of these processes may help to fine-tune peri-operative risk assessment (Nelson et al. 2023; Jain et al. 2023). Figure 2.1 demonstrates the interlinking pathways involved in surgical trauma (inflammatory, neuroendocrine, metabolic, and others).

2.7 Organ-System Manifestations of Surgical Stress

2.7.1 Cardiovascular and Pulmonary

Sympathoadrenal activation, hypercoagulability, and endothelial dysfunction combine to promote myocardial ischemia, arrhythmias, heart failure, and deep vein thrombosis, particularly when the cardiovascular reserve is compromised (Kehlet and Wilmore 2008; Golder and Papalois 2021). Lung complications are due to loss of functional residual capacity, atelectasis, compromised mucociliary transport, and dysfunction of the diaphragm, worsened by pain, opioids, and inactivity (Cusack and Buggy 2020; Thiele et al. 2015).

ERAS measures, including regional analgesia, lung-protective ventilation, goal-directed fluid therapy, non-invasive ventilation, and early ambulation, reduce cardiovascular and pulmonary complications and ICU and hospital length of stay in various surgical cohorts (Thiele et al. 2015; Tazreean et al. 2022).

2.7.2 Gastrointestinal and Hepatic

Postoperative ileus is caused by increased sympathetic activity, an inflammatory response in the muscularis layer, opioid administration, and bed rest, resulting in abdominal distention, nausea, vomiting, and enteral nutrition restriction (Cusack and Buggy 2020; Mithany et al. 2023). ERAS-adherent practices, such as avoiding routine nasogastric tubes, early enteral nutrition, opioid reduction, epidural or regional anesthesia (RA), and early mobilization, shorten the time to first flatus and bowel movement and LOS in both GI and non-GI surgery (Thiele et al. 2015; ERAS® Society 2021).

Hepatic surgery patients with high levels of IL-6 and liver enzymes perioperatively are at risk of liver dysfunction, providing justification for carbohydrate loading, fluid and blood transfusion management, and early enteral nutrition in ERAS liver protocols (Kofler et al. 2025; Kumar et al. 2025).

2.7.3 Neurological and Cognitive

Delirium and postoperative cognitive dysfunction (POCD) are common in older surgical patients and are associated with increased morbidity, longer LOS, institutionalization, and long-term cognitive decline (Tai et al. 2013). Systemic inflammation, endothelial dysfunction, microthrombosis, mitochondrial injury, sleep disruption, pain, and sedative and opioid exposure all contribute to neurocognitive vulnerability (Unraveling the Role of Mitochondria in POCD 2024).

ERAS elements that reduce neurocognitive complications include minimizing benzodiazepines, using multimodal opioid-sparing analgesia, maintaining circadian cues, promoting early mobilization and orientation, and integrating geriatric co-management and delirium prevention protocols (Thiele et al. 2015; Sung and Oh 2026; Zeng et al. 2026).

2.7.4 Chronic Postsurgical Pain and Long-Term Outcomes

Persistent postsurgical pain (PPSP) affects a substantial proportion of patients and is linked to nerve injury, sustained inflammation, central sensitization, and psychosocial factors (Bruce and Quinlan 2011; Kim et al. 2023; Fuller et al. 2023). Predictors include high acute postoperative pain scores, pre-existing chronic pain, anxiety, depression, and extensive tissue and nerve dissection (Rosenberger and Pogatzki-Zahn 2022; Fuller et al. 2023).

ERAS-aligned strategies—early and effective multimodal analgesia, regional blocks, minimally invasive surgery, and reduced perioperative opioid exposure—are associated with lower PPSP risk and better long-term quality of life, highlighting the continuum from acute stress control to chronic outcomes (Kim et al. 2023; Rosenberger and Pogatzki-Zahn 2022; Zeng et al. 2026).

2.8 Determinants and Modifiers of the Stress Response

The intensity and duration of the surgical stress response are influenced by:

Surgical factors: type, invasiveness (open vs. minimally invasive), duration, blood loss, contamination, and need for reoperation, with more extensive open procedures generating greater endocrine and inflammatory responses than minimally invasive approaches (Kehlet and Wilmore 2008; Jawa et al. 2011).

Urgency and sepsis: emergency and septic surgeries often occur in the context of pre-existing systemic inflammation and organ dysfunction, amplifying stress and complicating recovery (ERAS® Society 2021; Memon and Malik 2025).

Patient factors: age, frailty, sarcopenia, comorbidities (cardiovascular, pulmonary, renal, hepatic, diabetes), nutritional status, and psychological factors such as anxiety and depression (Guo et al. 2023; Ni and Zheng 2025; Sung and Oh 2026).

Perioperative care quality: anesthetic technique, analgesic strategy, fluid and hemodynamic management, infection control, glycemic control, mobilization, and nutritional support (Thiele et al. 2015; Golder and Papalois 2021; Mithany et al. 2023).

Frailty and sarcopenia in particular are powerful modifiers; elderly frail patients often exhibit an exaggerated stress response with reduced capacity to return to baseline, and combining comprehensive geriatric assessment (CGA) with ERAS has emerged as best practice in this group (Guo et al. 2023; Sung and Oh 2026; Zeng et al. 2026).

2.9 ERAS as a Physiological Intervention

ERAS pathways can be conceptualized as deliberately targeted interventions acting at three levels:

1. *Reducing primary stress input*: minimally invasive surgical techniques, regional anesthesia, normothermia, and infection prevention decrease nociception, tissue injury, and infectious burden (Kehlet and Wilmore 2008; Nelson et al. 2023).

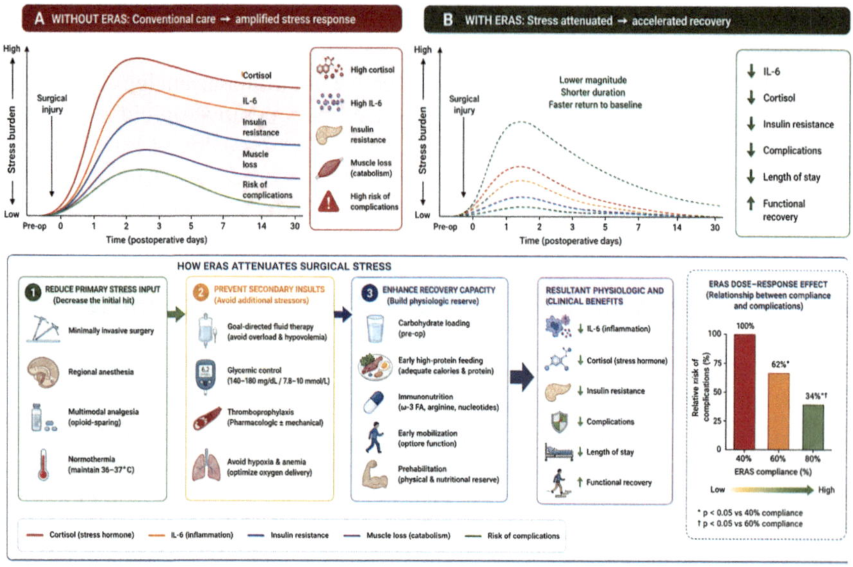

Fig. 2.2 ERAS as a physiological countermeasure: stress attenuation map. (Figure created by the author using draw.io (diagrams.net))

2. *Preventing secondary insults*: avoiding hypothermia, hypoxia, anemia, hypotension, fluid overload, and severe hyperglycemia prevents additional organ stress and inflammatory activation (Thiele et al. 2015; Jain et al. 2023).
3. *Enhancing recovery capacity*: prehabilitation, optimized nutrition, early mobilization, sleep hygiene, and psychological support improve physiological reserve and adaptive responses (Fig. 2.2) (Matsui et al. 2024; Guo et al. 2023; Sung and Oh 2026).

Multicenter data confirm that higher adherence to ERAS elements is associated with stepwise reductions in complications, LOS, and costs, with some programs showing dose–response relationships between compliance and outcomes (Thiele et al. 2015; Golder and Papalois 2021; Mithany et al. 2023). The specific role of intraoperative management in achieving these goals is outlined in Table 2.2, which details key anesthetic interventions and their principal physiological targets.

Table 2.2 Key anesthetic interventions in ERAS and their principal physiological targets

Intervention	Primary physiological targets	Expected effects on stress response
Neuraxial (epidural/spinal)	Nociceptive input, SNS outflow	↓ Catecholamines, ↓ cortisol, improved GI motility, ↓ pain
Peripheral nerve blocks	Nociception from limbs/thoracic wall	↓ Pain, ↓ opioids, earlier mobilization
Multimodal systemic analgesia	Prostaglandins, NMDA receptors, sodium channels	↓ Opioids, ↓ hyperalgesia, less ileus, better sleep
Balanced anesthetic depth	Central arousal, hemodynamic stability	Avoids sympathetic surges and hypotension
Lung-protective ventilation	Ventilator-induced lung injury, atelectasis	↓ Pulmonary complications, improved oxygenation
Goal-directed fluid therapy	Hypovolemia, hypervolemia, microcirculatory flow	Optimized perfusion, less edema, improved organ function

2.10 Anesthetic Modulation of Surgical Stress

2.10.1 Regional vs. General Anesthesia

Studies comparing general anesthesia with general plus regional anesthesia in vascular, abdominal, and orthopedic surgery show consistently lower levels of intra- and postoperative catecholamines and cortisol, improved gastrointestinal motility, less ileus, and shorter LOS with the use of neuraxial (spinal or epidural) or major peripheral nerve blocks (Breslow et al. 1993; Cusack and Buggy 2020). These physiologic changes are especially important in high-risk cardiac patients, as regional anesthesia blunts sympathetic activation and associated increases in myocardial oxygen consumption (Kehlet and Wilmore 2008; Golder and Papalois 2021).

As such, regional anesthesia is strongly encouraged in ERAS guidelines for a wide variety of surgeries, particularly thoracoabdominal and lower-limb surgery, as a stress-reducing and opioid-sparing technique (Nelson et al. 2023; ERAS® Society 2021).

2.10.2 Multimodal, Opioid-Sparing Analgesia

High-dose systemic opioids are potent analgesics but can cause ileus, nausea and vomiting, respiratory depression, immunosuppression, and delirium (Cusack and Buggy 2020). Multimodal analgesia with the use of combinations of acetaminophen, NSAIDs or COX-2 inhibitors, gabapentinoids, ketamine, IV lidocaine, and alpha-2 agonists, in addition to regional blocks, offers excellent analgesia with markedly reduced opioid use (Kim et al. 2023; Fuller et al. 2023).

Opioid-sparing approaches reduce sympathetic responses, opioid-related gastrointestinal and respiratory complications, allow earlier ambulation and nutritional support, and may prevent PPSP, and are a natural extension of ERAS protocols (Kim et al. 2023; Rosenberger and Pogatzki-Zahn 2022; Zeng et al. 2026).

2.10.3 Depth, Modality, and Mitochondrial Considerations

Depth of anesthesia is important to maintain; low anesthetic concentrations can allow sympathetic surges and myocardial ischemia in response to nociception, while deep anesthesia can lead to increased hypotension and organ under-perfusion (Ivascu et al. 2024; Jain et al. 2023). EEG and hemodynamic monitoring can guide depth and are consistent with ERAS aims of hemodynamic optimization and reducing drug use (Thiele et al. 2015; Jain et al. 2023).

Mitochondrial function is increasingly recognized as a critical factor in determining the vulnerability of organs during the perioperative period; anesthetic drugs and cardiopulmonary bypass can reduce mitochondrial respiration, induce ROS and compromise quality-control mechanisms, leading to myocardial and neural damage (Cherry 2019). Perioperative approaches to mitigate ischemia-reperfusion injury, avoid profound hypotension, maintain normoxia and euglycemia and potentially use mitochondrial-directed therapies, can be integrated into an ERAS pathway by supporting cellular energy production (Cherry 2019).

2.11 Nutritional Modulation Within ERAS

Nutrition is a vital component of the Enhanced Recovery After Surgery (ERAS) protocol, which shifts the traditional practice of starving patients before surgery to active support. Specific nutritional interventions seek to minimize surgical catabolism, maintain lean muscle, and enhance immunity. The combination of preoperative optimization, carbohydrate loading, early enteral nutrition, and immunonutrition allows active manipulation of the metabolic and inflammatory responses to surgical stress. The main nutritional interventions used in ERAS programs and their physiological and clinical impact are listed in Table 2.3.

Table 2.3 Key nutritional interventions in ERAS and their physiological and clinical effects

Intervention	Targets	Main physiological effects	Key outcome signals
Preop nutrition screening and support	Malnutrition, sarcopenia	↑ Reserves, improved immune function	↓ Complications, LOS, mortality
Fasting abbreviation	Prolonged catabolic fasting	Less insulin resistance, better comfort	Improved well-being, ↓ insulin resistance
Carbohydrate loading	Counter-regulatory hormone surge	↓ Insulin resistance, better glycemia	↓ LOS, faster functional recovery
Early enteral feeding (≤24 h)	Gut integrity, immune priming	Preserved barrier, ↓ catabolism	↓ Infections, shorter LOS
High-protein feeding	Muscle protein balance	↓ Muscle loss, improved strength	Better functional recovery, less sarcopenia
Immunonutrition	T-cell/NK function, inflammation, wound healing	Modulated cytokines, improved immune response	↓ Infectious/overall complications, fewer leaks

2.11.1 Preoperative Screening, Malnutrition, and Prehabilitation

Malnutrition and sarcopenia are prevalent in surgical patients, especially those with cancer and the elderly, and are significant predictors of complications, LOS, and death (Matsui et al. 2024; Guo et al. 2023). Regular screening using tools such as Nutritional Risk Screening (NRS-2002), Malnutrition Universal Screening Tool (MUST), and Global Leadership Initiative on Malnutrition (GLIM) criteria identifies those at risk of malnutrition who can benefit from pre-emptive nutritional support, dietary advice, and prehabilitation (Matsui et al. 2024; Sung and Oh 2026).

Multicomponent prehabilitation programs, which include high-protein diet, aerobic and resistance training, smoking and alcohol cessation, and psychological support, have been shown to increase functional capacity and decrease complications after surgery in high-risk groups (Ku et al. 2025; Sung and Oh 2026). Inclusion of these programs in ERAS pathways boosts pre-operative physiological capacity (Kehlet and Wilmore 2008).

2.11.2 Shortening the Fasting Time and Carbohydrate Loading

Historical "nil per os from midnight" increases catabolism, thirst, and discomfort, and induces insulin resistance (Ljungqvist 2010; Nur et al. 2026). ERAS guidelines recommend solids until 6 h and clear liquids until 2 h before surgery in most elective surgeries, and 50–100 g of carbohydrate 2–3 h prior to anesthesia (Kukliński et al. 2022; ERAS® Society 2021).

RCTs and meta-analyses demonstrate that carbohydrate loading reduces insulin resistance, increases patient satisfaction, and may reduce LOS, particularly for major abdominal surgery (Kukliński et al. 2022; Ping et al. 2025; Sebestyén et al. 2025). A study in living donor hepatectomy showed carbohydrate beverages decrease perioperative insulin resistance and speed up functional recovery of the remnant liver (Kumar et al. 2025).

2.11.3 Early Enteral Nutrition and Protein

Early enteral feeding (within 24 h) is safe in most non-GI and GI surgeries, and reduces infectious complications, duration of ileus, and LOS when compared with the traditional prolonged fasting approach (Thiele et al. 2015; ERAS® Society 2021). ERAS pathways target 1.2–1.5 g/kg/day of protein with higher targets for sarcopenic or critically ill patients to be delivered as high-protein oral supplements or enteral nutrition (Matsui et al. 2024; Ku et al. 2025; Zeng et al. 2026).

When combined with early mobilization and physiotherapy focused on resistance training, sufficient protein intake helps maintain muscle protein synthesis, prevents loss of lean muscle mass, and enhances muscle mass and quality (Tazreean et al. 2022).

2.11.4 Perioperative Immunonutrition

Perioperative immunonutrition (e.g., formulas enriched in arginine, omega-3 fatty acids, and nucleotides) has been extensively studied in gastrointestinal and head-and-neck cancer surgery, with several randomized controlled trials and meta-analyses that show that immunonutrition reduces infectious and other complications, especially in malnourished patients (Matsui et al. 2024). The formulations also seem to maintain body weight and potentially shorten LOS (Matsui et al. 2024).

The mechanisms of action for omega-3 fatty acids include altered eicosanoid and pro-resolving mediator production, arginine supports nitric oxide formation, T-cell activation, and wound repair, and nucleotides to support rapidly proliferating immune and gut epithelial cells (Matsui et al. 2024; Ku et al. 2025). Perioperative immunonutrition is often recommended in high-risk patients within ERAS protocols, as part of a multimodal approach to modulate the immune system (e.g., regional anesthesia, opioid-sparing analgesics).

2.12 Early Mobilization and Functional Recovery

Early mobilization is a key component of ERAS that directly counteracts the harmful effects of bed rest on thrombosis, insulin resistance, muscle catabolism, atelectasis, and delirium (Tazreean et al. 2022). Observational and randomized studies show that systematic early mobilization programs, which aim to achieve certain milestones such as sitting out of bed and ambulation on day 0 or 1, enhance walking ability, decrease complications, and reduce time in hospital following colorectal, orthopedic, and abdominal surgery (Tazreean et al. 2022; Mithany et al. 2023).

In critical care, goal-directed early mobilization decreases ICU-acquired weakness, duration on ventilator, delirium, and long-term functional disability. Early mobilization is critical in regaining functionality and independence when combined with high-protein nutrition and prehabilitation (Matsui et al. 2024; Guo et al. 2023).

2.13 Implementation Science: Barriers and Facilitators

Even with high-quality evidence, ERAS uptake varies, and there are many barriers to individual, team, and organizational implementation. Barriers include reluctance to change, lack of awareness or training, fear of additional workload, limited resources, lack of integrated care pathways, and lack of local ERAS champions.

Effective ERAS processes incorporate multidisciplinary involvement, ERAS coordinator (usually a specialist nurse), ongoing education and audit, electronic order sets, and local modification of protocols to resource limitations (Enhanced

Recovery After Surgery (ERAS®): Barriers and Solutions 2022). Staged adoption of ERAS in low- and middle-income countries involving initial high-value and low-cost interventions (e.g., patient education, early mobilization, multimodal analgesia, early feeding) has been successful (Memon and Malik 2025).

2.13.1 Toward Precision ERAS

Next-generation ERAS will likely involve "precision ERAS," with interventions tailored to dynamic monitoring of stress and recovery (Ku et al. 2025; Jain et al. 2023). Repeated measurement of IL-6, CRP, cortisol, procalcitonin, glucose, mitochondrial damage-associated molecular patterns (mtDAMPs), and metabolomic signatures may allow for earlier identification of risk phenotypes and escalation of analgesia, nutrition, activity, and surveillance (Laishram et al. 2024; Kofler et al. 2025).

Wearable devices and mobile apps can track steps, sleep quality, heart rate variability, and patient-reported outcomes in the recovery phase after surgery, enabling remote monitoring and leveraging these data to inform rehabilitation strategies (Tazreean et al. 2022; Zhang et al. 2025; Mithany et al. 2023). Coupling these data with comprehensive geriatric assessment, frailty/sarcopenia, and other age-related metrics will be vital for ERAS in older patients (Guo et al. 2023; Sung and Oh 2026; Zeng et al. 2026).

2.14 Conclusion

The surgical stress response is a multi-faceted composite of neuroendocrine, inflammatory, immune re-programming, metabolic and mitochondrial, endothelial, thromboinflammation, and organ-system responses. This response is adaptive, but when expressed in an unmodulated fashion in the elderly, frail, and multimorbid, it results in complications, extended LOS, long-term disability, and oncologic outcomes.

ERAS pathways translate a physiologic model of surgical stress into integrated, multidisciplinary care bundle approaches that reduce stress inputs, avoid secondary insults, and improve recovery potential, with anesthesia and nutrition in its DNA. Multimodal and regional anesthesia reduce nociceptive input, catecholamine and cortisol peaks, opioid use, and immune suppression, while rigorous perioperative nutrition strategies, including preoperative screening and prehabilitation, carbohydrate loading, early high-protein feeding, and immunonutrition, affect metabolic, immune, and mitochondrial processes to promote healing and recovery.

Coupled with early mobility, geriatric and frailty-oriented approaches and implementation strategies, ERAS pathways reliably lower complications and LOS, and enhance patient-reported outcomes, across elective and urgent surgical populations. Going forward, the use of stress and recovery biomarkers, frailty and sarcopenia measures, mitochondrial science and digital health technologies to "precision ERAS" will allow further personalization of anesthetic and nutritional strategies to individual patient physiology, and unlock the full potential of ERAS to revolutionize surgery.

References

Angka L, Khan ST, Kilgour MK, Xu R, Kennedy MA, Auer RC. Dysfunctional natural killer cells in the aftermath of cancer surgery. Int J Mol Sci. 2017;18(8):1787. https://doi.org/10.3390/ijms18081787.

Breslow MJ, Parker SD, Frank SM, Norris EJ, Yates H, Raff H, Rock P, Christopherson R, Rosenfeld BA, Beattie C. Determinants of catecholamine and cortisol responses to lower extremity revascularization. The PIRAT Study Group. Anesthesiology. 1993;79(6):1202–9. https://doi.org/10.1097/00000542-199312000-00010.

Bruce J, Quinlan J. Chronic Post-Surgical Pain. Revs in Pain. 2011;5(3):23–9. https://doi.org/10.1177/204946371100500306.

Cherry AD. Mitochondrial dysfunction in cardiac surgery. Anesthesiol Clin. 2019;37(4):769–85. https://doi.org/10.1016/j.anclin.2019.08.003.

Cusack B, Buggy DJ. Anaesthesia, analgesia, and the surgical stress response. BJA Educ. 2020;20(9):321–8. https://doi.org/10.1016/j.bjae.2020.04.006.

ERAS® Society. (2021). ERAS® Society guidelines and resources. https://erassociety.org.

Fuller AM, Bharde S, Sikandar S. The mechanisms and management of persistent postsurgical pain. Front Pain Res (Lausanne). 2023;4:1154597. https://doi.org/10.3389/fpain.2023.1154597.

Golder HJ, Papalois V. Enhanced recovery after surgery: history, key advancements and developments in transplant surgery. J Clin Med. 2021;10(8):1634. https://doi.org/10.3390/jcm10081634.

Guo K, Wang X, Lu X, Yang Y, Lu W, Wang S, Tang X, Wu Y, Xu Y, Chen Q, Liu S. Effects of sarcopenia and frailty on postoperative recovery in elderly patients: a prospective cohort study. J Cachexia Sarcopenia Muscle. 2023;14(6):2642–52. https://doi.org/10.1002/jcsm.13337.

Ivascu R, Torsin LI, Hostiuc L, Nitipir C, Corneci D, Dutu M. The surgical stress response and anesthesia: a narrative review. J Clin Med. 2024;13(10):3017. https://doi.org/10.3390/jcm13103017.

Jackson SP, Darbousset R, Schoenwaelder SM. Thromboinflammation: challenges of therapeutically targeting coagulation and other host defense mechanisms. Blood. 2019;133(9):906–18. https://doi.org/10.1182/blood-2018-11-882993.

Jain SN, Lamture Y, Krishna M. Enhanced recovery after surgery: exploring the advances and strategies. Cureus. 2023;15(10):e47237. https://doi.org/10.7759/cureus.47237.

Jawa RS, Anillo S, Huntoon K, Baumann H, Kulaylat M. Interleukin-6 in surgery, trauma, and critical care part II: clinical implications. J Intensive Care Med. 2011;26(2):73–87. https://doi.org/10.1177/0885066610384188.

Kehlet H. Multimodal approach to control postoperative pathophysiology and rehabilitation. Br J Anaesth. 1997;78(5):606–17. https://doi.org/10.1093/bja/78.5.606.

Kehlet H, Wilmore DW. Evidence-based surgical care and the evolution of fast-track surgery. Ann Surg. 2008;248(2):189–98. https://doi.org/10.1097/SLA.0b013e31817f2c1a.

Kim BR, Yoon SH, Lee HJ. Practical strategies for the prevention and management of chronic postsurgical pain. Korean J Pain. 2023;36(2):149–62. https://doi.org/10.3344/kjp.23080.

Kofler A, Trattner M, Mairinger V, Urban I, Søreide K, Stättner S, Primavesi F. The role of perioperative interleukin-6 serum levels on liver dysfunction and infectious complications after hepatectomy—a systematic review. Cancer. 2025;17(19):3120. https://doi.org/10.3390/cancers17193120.

Ku D, Bartelt J, Feeley J, Perez-Guzman MC, Guerrero-Arroyo L, Abraham A, Kollipara S, Gonzalez N, Usman S, Huneault HE, Corujo-Rodriguez A, Davis GM, Kibbey RG, Jones DP, Ziegler TR, Halkos M, Quyyumi AA, Smith MR, Li J, Pasquel FJ. Metabolic trajectories during surgical stress in patients undergoing cardiac surgery. bioRxiv. 2025; https://doi.org/10.1101/2025.09.16.676529.

Kukliński J, Steckiewicz KP, Owczuk R. Perioperative carbohydrate loading in patients undergoing one-day surgery. A systematic review of randomized controlled trials. Wideochir Inne Tech Maloinwazyjne. 2022;17(3):457–66. https://doi.org/10.5114/wiitm.2022.116750.

Kumar M, Patil NS, Mohapatra N, Yadav A, Sindwani G, Dhingra U, Thomas S, Pamecha V. Preoperative carbohydrate loading reduces perioperative insulin resistance and hastens functional recovery of remnant liver after living donor hepatectomy: an open-label randomized controlled trial. Hepatol Int. 2025;19(5):1151–61. https://doi.org/10.1007/s12072-025-10831-5.

Laishram K, Borgohain B, Laishram A, Khonglah TG, Ruram AA, Debbarma S. Serum IL-6 as a surrogate biomarker of post-operative complications in invasive orthopaedic surgeries: a prospective observational study. Indian J Orthop. 2024;58(8):1153–8. https://doi.org/10.1007/s43465-024-01195-3.

Ljungqvist O. Insulin resistance and outcomes in surgery. J Clin Endocrinol Metab. 2010;95(9):4217–9. https://doi.org/10.1210/jc.2010-1525.

Market M, Baxter KE, Angka L, Kennedy MA, Auer RC. The potential for cancer immunotherapy in targeting surgery-induced natural killer cell dysfunction. Cancer. 2018;11(1):2. https://doi.org/10.3390/cancers11010002.

Matsui R, Sagawa M, Inaki N, Fukunaga T, Nunobe S. Impact of perioperative immunonutrition on postoperative outcomes in patients with upper gastrointestinal cancer: a systematic review and meta-analysis of randomized controlled trials. Nutrients. 2024;16(5):577. https://doi.org/10.3390/nu16050577.

Memon MM, Malik FR. Enhanced recovery after surgery (ERAS) guidelines in emergency general surgery: a prospective evaluation of feasibility and clinical outcomes in a developing country. Med Forum Mon. 2025;36(8):3–7. https://doi.org/10.60110/medforum.360801.

Mithany RH, Daniel N, Shahid MH, Aslam S, Abdelmaseeh M, Gerges F, Gill MU, Abdallah SB, Hannan A, Saeed MT, Manasseh M, Mohamed MS. Revolutionizing surgical care: the power of enhanced recovery after surgery (ERAS). Cureus. 2023;15(11):e48795. https://doi.org/10.7759/cureus.48795.

Nelson G, Fotopoulou C, Taylor J, Glaser G, Bakkum-Gamez J, Meyer LA, Stone R, Mena G, Elias KM, Altman AD, Bisch SP, Ramirez PT, Dowdy SC. Enhanced recovery after surgery (ERAS®) society guidelines for gynecologic oncology: addressing implementation challenges – 2023 update. Gynecol Oncol. 2023;173:58–67. https://doi.org/10.1016/j.ygyno.2023.04.009.

Ni F, Zheng L. Impact of sarcopenia and frailty on outcomes of patients with sepsis or septic shock: a systematic review and meta-analysis. Front Nutr. 2025;12:1679632. https://doi.org/10.3389/fnut.2025.1679632.

Nur RF, Synthana MR, Kurnia Y, Rudiarto KM, Alicia RJ, Kurniawaty J, Pratomo BY, Deviatika FE. The effect of preoperative oral carbohydrate loading on insulin resistance in adult patients undergoing on-pump cardiac surgery: a randomized controlled trial. Ann Card Anaesth. 2026;29(2):228–36. https://doi.org/10.4103/aca.aca_313_25.

Ping W, Jingbo Z, Shanshan W, Zihao D, Wanchen Y, Jiayi L, Jiayu W, Hui M. Different regimens of preoperative carbohydrate loading on insulin resistance: a network meta-analysis. Clin Nutr ESPEN. 2025;66:142–50. https://doi.org/10.1016/j.clnesp.2025.01.035.

Rosenberger DC, Pogatzki-Zahn EM. Chronic post-surgical pain – update on incidence, risk factors and preventive treatment options. BJA Educ. 2022;22(5):190–6. https://doi.org/10.1016/j.bjae.2021.11.008.

Sebestyén AR, Turan C, Szemere A, Virág M, Ocskay K, Dembrovszky F, Szabó L, Hegyi P, Engh MA, Molnár Z. Preoperative carbohydrate loading reduces length of stay after major elective, non-cardiac surgery when compared to fasting: a systematic review and meta-analysis. Sci Rep. 2025;15(1):19119. https://doi.org/10.1038/s41598-025-00767-z.

Sung TY, Oh CS. Frailty assessment in perioperative geriatric patients: a narrative review. Anesth Pain Med. 2026;21(1):51–66. https://doi.org/10.17085/apm.25480.
Tai LH, de Souza CT, Bélanger S, Ly L, Alkayyal AA, Zhang J, Rintoul JL, Ananth AA, Lam T, Breitbach CJ, Auer RC. Preventing postoperative metastatic disease by inhibiting surgery-induced dysfunction in natural killer cells. Cancer Res. 2013;73(1):97–107. https://doi.org/10.1158/0008-5472.CAN-12-1993.
Tazreean R, Nelson G, Twomey R. Early mobilization in enhanced recovery after surgery pathways: current evidence and recent advancements. J Comp Eff Res. 2022;11(2):121–9. https://doi.org/10.2217/cer-2021-0258.
Thiele RH, Rea KM, Turrentine FE, Friel CM, Hassinger TE, McMurry TL, Goudreau BJ, Umapathi BA, Kron IL, Sawyer RG, Hedrick TL. Standardization of care: impact of an enhanced recovery protocol on length of stay, complications, and direct costs after colorectal surgery. J Am Coll Surg. 2015;220(4):430–43. https://doi.org/10.1016/j.jamcollsurg.2014.12.042.
Zeng J, Yang T, Li J. Chronic post-surgical pain in older adults: mechanisms, assessment, and management strategies. Front Med. 2026;12:1719477. https://doi.org/10.3389/fmed.2025.1719477.
Zhang W, Yu P, Yu M, Mi J. Effect of early goal directed mobilization on clinical outcomes in mechanically ventilated ICU patients. Sci Rep. 2025;15(1):45399. https://doi.org/10.1038/s41598-025-28991-7.

Role of Anesthesia in Enhanced Recovery After Surgery

3

Sourabh Jakhar, Paramveer Singh, Asha Yadav, and Ankit

Abstract

The ERAS pathways represent a comprehensive, evidence-based approach to pre-operative and intra/post-operative care aimed at reducing surgical stress response, preserving physiological function, and facilitating recovery. The current chapter will discuss the key role played by anesthesiologists in the application of ERAS protocols by shifting their attention not only to hypnosis but also to influencing neuroendocrine, metabolic, and immune disturbances arising from surgery. The physiologic basis for surgical stress will allow for the discussion of mechanisms, such as sympathetic stimulation, insulin resistance, and immunosuppression, that can be controlled by an appropriate anesthetic management and timing interventions, for instance, carbohydrate intake before surgery. Of special interest is the transition from opioid-dominated care to OFA approaches.

The chapter explains how the use of regional anesthesia and systemic multimodal analgesia together, which includes spinal or epidural anesthesia as well as peripheral nerve blocks, ensures better pain control, with a lower incidence of side effects such as PONV, ileus, and delayed ambulation. In addition, this chapter considers the current controversy in the medical community regarding the use

S. Jakhar (✉)
Department of Anesthesiology, Pt NRS Govt Medical College, Rohtak, India

P. Singh
Department of Anesthesiology, Max Superspeciality Hospital, Bathinda, India

A. Yadav
Department of Anesthesiology and Critical Care, AIIMS Jodhpur, Jodhpur, India

Ankit
Department of Anesthesiology, Pt. BD Sharma PGIMS, Rohtak, India

P. K. Bhattacharyya et al. (eds.), *Integrated Anesthesia and Nutrition Approaches to Enhanced Recovery after Surgery*,
https://doi.org/10.1007/978-981-92-3294-9_3

of inhalational agents versus propofol-based TIVA, especially with regard to their differing effects on immune function. Suggested practical implementation strategies include the use of goal-directed fluid therapy, strict temperature control, and constant collaboration among all disciplines from the preoperative phase through the end of the early postoperative period. Finally, the chapter confirms the critical importance of good compliance with ERAS-based anesthetic protocols in achieving better results, including decreased morbidity, faster discharge from the hospital, and improved recovery; this makes the modern anesthesiologist a true perioperative specialist.

Keywords

Enhanced Recovery After Surgery (ERAS) · Surgical stress response · Multimodal analgesia · Regional anesthesia · Opioid-sparing anesthesia

3.1 Introduction

The enhanced recovery after surgery (ERAS) protocol refers to perioperative multimodal regimens based on scientific evidence, with the aim of minimizing the stress response, maintaining physiological function, and hastening recovery (Ljungqvist et al. 2017; Grant and Engelman 2025). In the ERAS protocols, anesthesia does not simply refer to the procedure that results in patient unconsciousness but also plays a major role in modulating neuroendocrine, metabolic, and immunological responses during surgery (Kurz et al. 1996; Scott et al. 2015). Through the selection of proper anesthetics and pain control regimens, the anesthesiologist can directly impact the outcome of the surgical patient.

3.1.1 Historical Evolution of ERAS and Fast-Track Surgery

The idea of fast-track surgery, or rapid recovery, was developed by Henrik Kehlet, who believed that postoperative organ dysfunction and extended convalescence were primarily iatrogenic and, hence, preventable (Kehlet 1997; Kehlet and Wilmore 2008). Initial fast-track procedures included minimally invasive approaches, optimal regional anesthesiology, early ambulation, and nutrition therapy to minimize postoperative catabolism and complications. Later clinical trials and meta-analyses confirmed that fast-track protocols shortened hospitalization periods by about 30–50% and decreased morbidity associated with colorectal and other major operations (Fearon et al. 2005; Zhuang et al. 2013).

Later on, the ERAS Society codified these principles into guidelines for procedures, starting with colorectal surgery and extending to several other specialities (Gustafsson et al. 2019; Ljungqvist et al. 2017). In the guidelines, there is clarity about the involvement of anesthesiologists in aspects such as anesthetic technique, multimodal pain control, fluid administration, thermal regulation, and postoperative monitoring.

3.1.2 Conceptual Framework and Role of Anesthesia in ERAS

A typical ERAS pathway includes 15 to 25 interrelated measures that cover the pre-operative, operative, and post-operative periods (Ljungqvist et al. 2017). Some of these measures require anesthetic care directly, including fasting and carbohydrate loading, avoiding the use of long-acting sedatives, choice between general and regional anesthesia, perioperative fluid management, vasopressor administration, pain relief, and prevention of PONV (Scott et al. 2015; Miller et al. 2014), as shown in Fig. 3.1. There is a strong association between high adherence to anesthetic and analgesic components and positive patient outcomes and reduced length of stay, indicating the crucial role of anesthesiology in the successful implementation of ERAS (Gustafsson et al. 2011; Varadhan et al. 2010).

Anesthetic procedures have been seen from a mechanistic point of view to alter the surgery-related stress response via changes in afferent pain input, neuroendocrine stimulation, release of pro-inflammatory mediators, and the immune system (Kehlet 1997; Ivascu et al. 2024). It is thus relevant for this chapter to discuss how certain anesthetic options can lead to decreased stress responses, altered metabolism, and enhanced patient outcomes.

3.1.3 Scope and Objectives

Objectives of this chapter include the elucidation of the physiology of the surgical stress response and its impact on recovery after surgery. This chapter will discuss various methods of anesthesia, which will minimize the surgical stress response, especially regional anesthesia and multimodal analgesia. Anesthesia and its effects on metabolism, immunology, and oncology will also be addressed in this chapter. Lastly, useful models, tables, and diagrams are provided here to facilitate ERAS-friendly anesthesia.

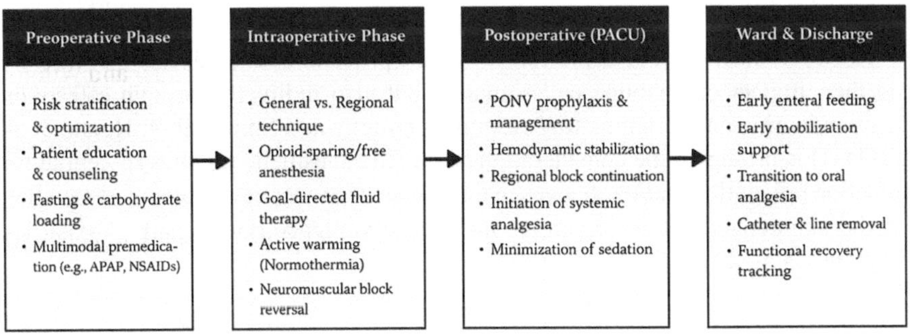

Fig. 3.1 Anesthetic touchpoints along an ERAS pathway. (Created by author using MS Word 2021)

3.2 Pathophysiology of Surgical Stress and Recovery

3.2.1 Neuroendocrine and Metabolic Responses

Surgery produces nociceptive impulses, sympathetic nerve activation, and HPA axis activation, resulting in increased levels of catecholamines, cortisol, glucagon, and growth hormone (Kehlet 1997; Desborough 2000). The hormonal changes facilitate the process of gluconeogenesis, insulin resistance, proteolysis, and lipolysis; they are referred to as the surgical stress response syndrome. Chronic or excessive levels of stress lead to various health conditions like tachycardia, hypertension, hypercoagulability, myocardial ischemia, ileus, and poor wound healing (Desborough 2000; Kehlet and Wilmore 2008).

One of the best means for reducing this reaction is regional neural blockades, which decrease afferent transmission of nociceptive stimuli into the brain and reduce sympathetic responses (Kehlet 1997; Ivascu et al. 2024). For instance, thoracic epidural blockade has been reported to decrease ileus, pulmonary problems, and risks of thrombosis and embolism, which provides an excellent clinical example of stress reduction (Block et al. 2003; Guay et al. 2016).

3.2.2 Inflammatory and Immune Responses

Injury causes an acute inflammatory reaction involving the production of cytokines like interleukin-6, interleukin-1β, and tumor necrosis factor-alpha, after which there is a counter-regulatory anti-inflammatory response (Sista et al. 2013; Ivascu et al. 2024). Although an acute inflammatory reaction is important for wound healing and defense against infections, when this becomes uncontrolled or excessive, it results in systemic inflammatory response syndrome, multiorgan dysfunction, and increased susceptibility to infection (Desborough 2000; Sista et al. 2013). On the other hand, a surgical procedure that involves general anesthesia leads to perioperative lymphopenia, decreased NK cell function, and T cell response suppression, thereby causing an immunocompromised state (Hogan et al. 2011; Sessler 2016).

However, the impact of anesthesia drugs and procedures extends not only directly via their impact on immune cell signaling but also indirectly through effects on neuroendocrine and inflammatory responses (Buggy and Smith 1999; Hogan et al. 2011). This prompted the consideration of specific anesthetic regimes' potential for infection prevention and/or changes in the course of cancer development, depending on the maintenance of perioperative immunosurveillance (Gottschalk et al. 2010; Wigmore et al. 2016).

3.2.3 Concept of Stress-Minimized Anesthesia

Kehlet formulated the "stress-free anesthesia and surgery" approach, where optimized regional analgesia and balanced anesthesia counteract the negative effects of stress, without interfering with necessary processes for maintaining homeostasis (Kehlet 1997; Kehlet and Wilmore 2008). Current ERAS pathways implement this approach by using neuraxial or regional blocks, fast-acting general anesthesia, multimodal systemic analgesia, normothermia, early feeding, and early ambulation as a strategy to minimize the negative effects of neuroendocrine and metabolic disturbance (Ljungqvist et al. 2017; Scott et al. 2015). It should be emphasized that the goal is to minimize the negative effects of stress, rather than eliminate all stresses, since this may lead to catabolism, insulin resistance, and immune suppression (Desborough 2000; Kehlet and Wilmore 2008). The mechanisms involved, along with corresponding interventions, are shown in Table 3.1 and Fig. 3.2.

Table 3.1 Components of the surgical stress response and anesthetic modifiers

Component	Clinical manifestations	Anesthetic modifiers
Sympathetic activation	Tachycardia, hypertension, hypercoagulability	Regional blocks, adequate depth of anesthesia, beta-blockade, opioid-sparing and analgesia (Kehlet 1997; Ivascu et al. 2024)
HPA axis activation	Elevated cortisol, hyperglycemia, and insulin resistance	Thoracic epidural, balanced general anesthesia, perioperative glucocorticoids, and early nutrition (Desborough 2000; Kehlet and Wilmore 2008)
Inflammatory response	Elevated IL-6, CRP, SIRS	Minimally invasive surgery, regional techniques, lidocaine infusions, and normothermia (Sista et al. 2013; Kaye et al. 2019)
Immune suppression	Lymphopenia, reduced NK cell activity	Regional anesthesia, opioid minimization, propofol-based TIVA, and normothermia (Buggy and Smith 1999; Hogan et al. 2011)

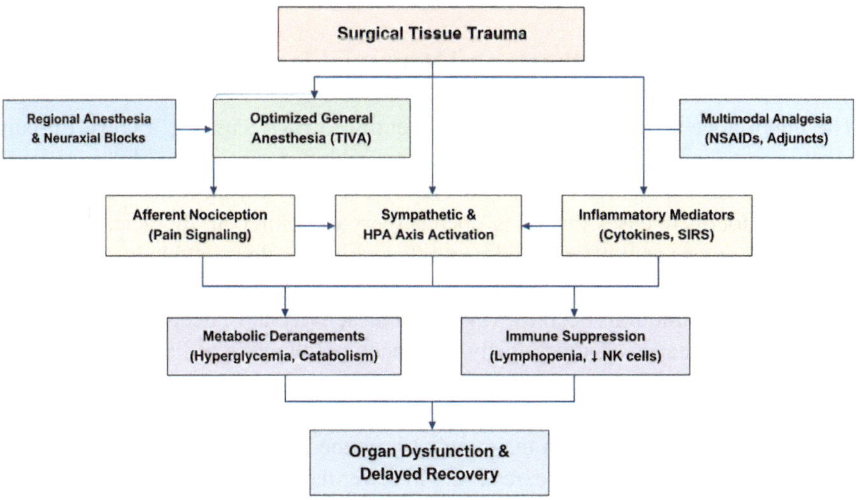

Fig. 3.2 Overview of surgical stress and anesthetic modulation. (Created by author using MS PowerPoint 2021)

3.3 Anesthetic Techniques Within ERAS Pathways

3.3.1 General Anesthesia: Volatile Agents Versus Total Intravenous Anesthesia

Although general anesthesia is still predominantly the preferred method for most procedures performed according to ERAS principles, there are controversies regarding the use of volatile drugs in comparison to propofol-based TIVA as the maintenance anesthetics (Golder and Papalois 2021; Kurz et al. 1996). Indeed, volatile anesthetics, including sevoflurane and desflurane, induce reliable sedation and maintain cardiovascular stability but have been shown to cause immunosuppression and activate the hypoxia-inducible factor system, potentially contributing to tumor development (Loop et al. 2005; Wigmore et al. 2016). On the other hand, propofol is an anti-inflammatory drug that displays antioxidative properties, maintains NK cell function, and improves perioperative cancer cell survival rate (Gottschalk et al. 2010; Wigmore et al. 2016).

However, a significant retrospective cohort study revealed better outcomes regarding survival in patients undergoing propofol-based total intravenous anesthesia (TIVA) for cancer surgery when compared to volatile anesthesia despite potential confounders and biases (Wigmore et al. 2016). Several more recent studies of both narrative and systematic review nature did not provide consistent results and stressed the importance of lacking evidence to justify the requirement of using TIVA in all cases, exclusively based on oncologic considerations (Golder and Papalois 2021; Iqbalbhai et al. 2025). Despite that, TIVA remains more preferable than other types of anesthesia in ERAS for the reasons stated above (Scott et al. 2015; Miller et al. 2014).

3.3.2 Regional Anesthesia and Neuraxial Techniques

The importance of regional anesthesia is central to ERAS as it is a powerful pain reliever and decreases the afferent input responsible for causing the stress response (Kaye et al. 2019; Kehlet 1997). Thoracic epidural anesthesia is advised by many ERAS protocols in cases involving open surgery of colorectal, thoracic, and major abdominal organs as it offers good pain relief, prevents ileus, and helps pulmonary mechanics (Gustafsson et al. 2019; Guay et al. 2016). A combination of local anesthetic-opioid in epidurals decreases sympathetic activity and catecholamines, causes less insulin resistance perioperatively, and increases the time of first flatus and defecation (Kehlet 1997; Block et al. 2003).

The use of general and regional anesthesia techniques together has been demonstrated to be more effective in maintaining immune function after surgery than the use of general anesthesia alone, resulting in fewer reductions in the number of CD4 and NK cells and lower levels of catecholamines and cortisol (Hogan et al. 2011;

Sessler 2016). For oncological surgeries, regional anesthesia techniques could potentially decrease the incidence of cancer recurrence by minimizing the use of opioids and preserving cell-mediated immunity (Gottschalk et al. 2010; Iqbalbhai et al. 2025).

3.3.3 Peripheral Nerve and Fascial Plane Blocks, Local Infiltration, and Wound Catheters

Interference by the peripheral nerves, as well as blocks in the interfascial planes, has gained significance and become part of the ERAS pathway, particularly with minimally invasive surgeries (Kaye et al. 2019; Scott et al. 2015). Some such blocks include transverse abdominis plane blocks (TAP), rectus sheath block, paravertebral blocks, and erector spinae plane blocks, which provide good somatic anesthesia while having minimal effect on the motor function. In laparoscopic surgery involving the colon, rectum, and gynecology, TAP blocks have been shown to decrease the amount of pain experienced by patients (Kaye et al. 2019; Kehlet and Wilmore 2008).

Local infusion analgesia and continuous catheter infusions provide the benefit of delivering local anesthetics directly to the surgical site, providing excellent pain relief without significant systemic opioid consumption (Peng et al. 2020; Holm et al. 2010). Local infusion analgesia has been shown to improve patient mobility following surgery and lead to shorter hospital stays than systemic opioids used for pain management in joint replacement surgery (Kaye et al. 2019; Ljungqvist et al. 2017).

3.3.4 Depth of Anesthesia, Neuromuscular Blockade, and Emergence

According to ERAS, the key is to ensure that there is no over-sedation and incomplete neuromuscular blockage since both are linked to delayed emergence and adverse outcomes (Golder and Papalois 2021; Miller et al. 2014). The balanced anesthetic approach requires that the smallest possible amount of hypnotics and analgesics be used according to clinical indicators and EEG-based depth of anesthesia monitors (Golder and Papalois 2021; Sessler 2016).

Quantitative neuromuscular blockade and proper reversal become important because residual blockade increases the likelihood of hypoventilation, airway obstruction, aspiration, and delay in mobilization (Miller et al. 2014; Scott et al. 2015). All these factors are consistent with the objectives of ERAS since they will enable patients to gain rapid recovery, early neurologic examination, and involvement in physiotherapy.

3.3.5 Fluid Management and Hemodynamic Optimization

Fluid management is a critical component for optimizing tissue oxygen delivery, edema development, and bowel activity, thus constituting one of the essential roles played by anesthetists in ERAS (Miller et al. 2014; Thacker et al. 2016). Historically, liberal fluid therapy protocols have been associated with the development of interstitial edema, delayed wound healing, and ileus, whereas overly conservative protocols have been prone to causing hypoperfusion and renal complications. Goal-directed fluid management (GDFT) through dynamic parameters of stroke volume or cardiac output can help personalize fluid and vasoactive medication delivery without fluid excess (Thacker et al. 2016; Miller et al. 2014).

According to ERAS protocols, balanced solutions should be used, sodium and chloride loading must be minimized, and the use of IV fluids should be stopped early when enteral feeding has been started (Gustafsson et al. 2019; Ljungqvist et al. 2017). Vasopressor medications should be used in preference to volume expansion to achieve hypotensive states, especially for cases receiving neuraxial or regional anesthesia (Thacker et al. 2016; Scott et al. 2015). This relationship among anesthesia, fluids, and patient outcome is illustrated in Fig. 3.3.

3.3.6 Temperature Management, Oxygenation, and Transfusion Strategies

Normothermia is part of the traditional ERAS approach and helps prevent coagulopathy, surgical site infections, and cardiovascular complications (Sessler 2016; Kurz et al. 1996). Warming interventions, including forced-air warming systems and heated intravenous solutions, must be implemented during surgery and immediately after the procedure, especially for lengthy or open surgeries (Miller et al. 2014; Gustafsson et al. 2019).

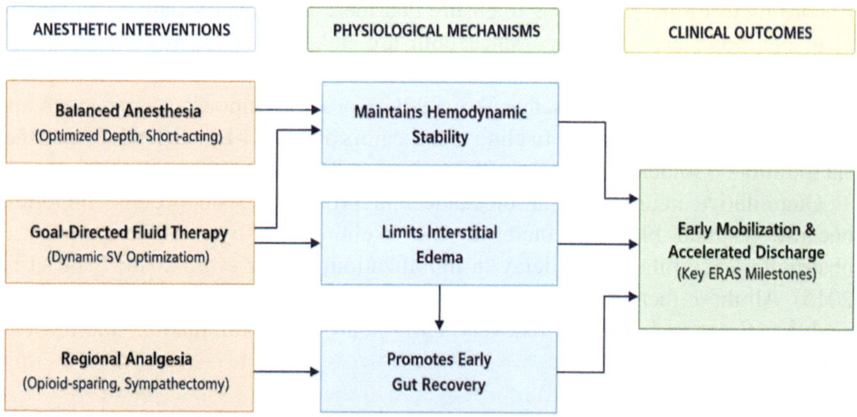

Fig. 3.3 Interaction of anesthetic technique, fluid therapy, and recovery. (Created by author using MS PowerPoint 2021)

Oxygen supplementation is optimized to achieve appropriate saturation levels without prolonged periods of hyperoxia, since hyperoxia could induce oxidative stress, and there is no clear evidence that hyperoxia helps in preventing surgical site infections (Sessler 2016; Chen et al. 2024). Allogenic blood exposure can be reduced by employing restrictive transfusion techniques, which have been shown to affect immunomodulation, leading to poor oncologic results (Gustafsson et al. 2019; Hogan et al. 2011).

3.4 Multimodal Analgesia and Opioid-Sparing Strategies

3.4.1 Rationale and Evidence Base

Multimodal analgesia utilizes a combination of pain medications and strategies with diverse mechanisms of action to ensure synergy in pain relief while decreasing the utilization of opioids and their side effects (Beverly et al. 2017; Kaye et al. 2019). The multimodal systemic and regional anesthesia strategy has been considered an essential component of the ERAS guidelines across multiple medical specialties to facilitate early mobility, breathing, and nutrition (Gustafsson et al. 2019; Ljungqvist et al. 2017). In the case of systematic reviews, evidence has demonstrated that standardized multimodal ERAS protocol decreases pain scores, opioid usage, PONV, ileus, and hospital stay (Scott et al. 2015; Beverly et al. 2017).

The ongoing opioid epidemic, coupled with the awareness of opioid-related side effects such as respiratory depression, PONV, ileus, urinary retention, delirium, and long-term opioid usage, has also contributed to the implementation of opioid-sparing and opioid-free anesthesia techniques (Leech et al. 2021; Oderda et al. 2013). The use of these techniques is consistent with ERAS principles that emphasize the quick restoration of gut functions and early mobility.

3.4.2 Systemic Non-opioid Analgesic Agents

In order to effectively minimize the dependence on opioids and ensure effective pain management, the emphasis of the ERAS pathway is on the systematic use of non-opioid medication for pain relief. This not only provides a synergistic effect in the treatment but also eliminates the risks of side effects that can come from higher dosages of opioids. The key systemic components of multimodal analgesia, used in the various nociceptive pathways, are shown in Table 3.2.

3.4.3 Opioid-Sparing and Opioid-Free Anesthesia

The former utilizes regional approaches along with non-opioid medications and intraoperative opioids with low dose and fast onset, while the latter strives to make the anesthetic process free from any use of opioids (Leech et al. 2021; Xiong et al.

Table 3.2 Systemic components of multimodal analgesia in ERAS

Drug class	Mechanism and benefits	ERAS-specific considerations
Acetaminophen	Central analgesic, antipyretic, opioid-sparing	Scheduled dosing starting preoperatively; monitor hepatic function (Beverly et al. 2017)
NSAIDs/COX-2 inhibitors	Peripheral anti-inflammatory, reduce prostaglandin synthesis and opioid need	Useful unless contraindicated; caution in renal impairment, bleeding risk, and some colorectal anastomoses (Beverly et al. 2017; Kaye et al. 2019)
Gabapentinoids	Modulate calcium channels, reduce central sensitization	Modest opioid-sparing; risk of sedation and dizziness; many ERAS guidelines recommend limited or single low-dose administration (Scott et al. 2015)
Ketamine (low dose)	NMDA receptor antagonism, antihyperalgesic	Particularly useful in opioid-tolerant patients; monitor for psychotomimetic effects (Beverly et al. 2017; Kaye et al. 2019)
Lidocaine infusion	Anti-inflammatory and antihyperalgesic; promotes bowel function	Evidence strongest in major abdominal surgery; monitor for toxicity (Kaye et al. 2019; Thacker et al. 2016)
Alpha-2 agonists (dexmedetomidine, clonidine)	Sedative, analgesic, sympatholytic	Reduce opioid needs and PONV; risk of bradycardia and hypotension (Leech et al. 2021)
Dexamethasone	Anti-inflammatory, antiemetic	Single perioperative dose reduces PONV and pain; consider glycemic effects (Gustafsson et al. 2019; Sista et al. 2013)

2025). In ERAS pathways, both retrospective and prospective analyses have proved the reduction of postoperative opioid intake, PONV, ileus, and hospital stay with preserved pain management (Bourazani et al. 2026; Scott et al. 2015). Randomized experiments performed for laparoscopic cholecystectomy and bariatric surgery have found that patients receiving OFA or an opioid-sparing technique achieve higher recovery scores than those with opioid-based anesthetic procedures (Leech et al. 2021; Xiong et al. 2025).

Current narrative reviews warn about the need for stringent patient selection and the monitoring of bradycardia and hypotension associated with high doses of alpha-2 agonists during OFA, but conclude that when incorporated into ERAS pathways, it can effectively expedite recovery goals (Leech et al. 2021; Xiong et al. 2025).

3.4.4 Impact on Functional Recovery and Persistent Pain

Multimodal analgesia not only helps in decreasing postoperative pain but also improves functional outcomes like time to walking, time to passage of flatus or stool, and discharge (Scott et al. 2015; Ljungqvist et al. 2017). Patients following

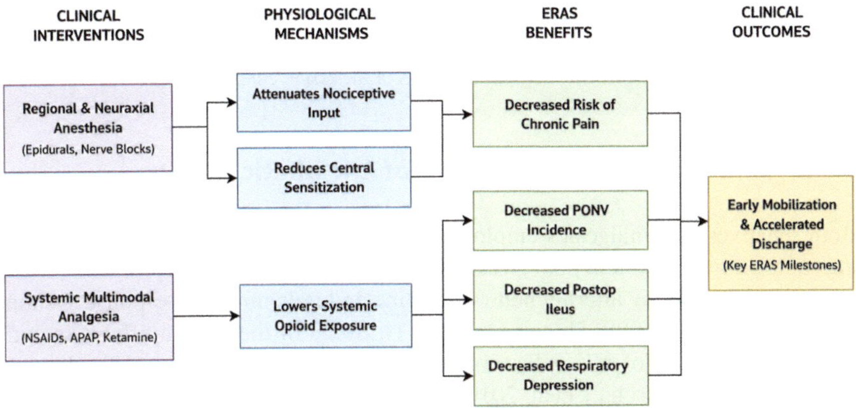

Fig. 3.4 Mechanistic pathways linking regional anesthesia and multimodal analgesia to enhanced recovery. (Created by author using MS PowerPoint 2021)

an ERAS protocol often exhibit high patient satisfaction along with faster return to normalcy compared to patients receiving conventional therapy, mainly because of pain relief and fewer side effects of opioids (Grant and Engelman 2025; Thacker et al. 2016). Multimodal therapy also decreases the risk of the development of chronic pain after surgery through decreased intensity of postoperative pain and prevention of central sensitization. This issue is still under study because of conflicting evidence (Kaye et al. 2019; Hogan et al. 2011). The underlying mechanisms by which regional and multimodal analgesia lead to better outcomes are shown in Fig. 3.4.

3.5 Anesthesia, Metabolism, and Immune Function

3.5.1 Insulin Resistance and Metabolic Modulation

Major Surgical procedures cause insulin resistance, which may last for several days and cause hyperglycemia, enhanced protein breakdown, and poor wound healing (Ljungqvist et al. 2017; Sista et al. 2013). Insulin resistance is proportional to the degree of injury caused by the operation and worsened by prolonged fasting, lack of physical activity, and unresolved pain (Desborough 2000; Kehlet and Wilmore 2008). Anesthesia techniques that limit the secretion of stress hormones, such as regional anesthesia and adequate analgesia, help decrease insulin resistance and metabolic processes after surgery (Kehlet 1997; Thacker et al. 2016).

Carbohydrate loading before surgery and minimal fasting are common ERAS practices performed in conjunction with anesthesia to enhance insulin sensitivity in perioperative care and improve the patient's well-being (Gustafsson et al. 2019; Ljungqvist et al. 2017). The consumption of clear carbohydrate beverages up to 2–4 h before anesthesia is safe and will reduce thirst, anxiety, and insulin resistance, if appropriate candidates are chosen (Ljungqvist et al. 2017; Scott et al. 2015). Postoperative early enteral feeding assisted by pain control and PONV management decreases the metabolic rate and enhances immunity (Gustafsson et al. 2019; Sista et al. 2013).

3.5.2 Immunomodulatory Effects of Anesthetic Agents

Both sedatives and analgesics employed in general anesthesia influence the workings of the immune system both directly through their action on receptors in immune cells and indirectly by altering neuroendocrine and inflammatory response systems (Buggy and Smith 1999; Hogan et al. 2011). Some of the known effects include decreased activities of NK cells, compromised proliferation rates in T-cells, and cytokine levels (Gottschalk et al. 2010; Wigmore et al. 2016). On the other hand, the use of propofol for induction anesthesia maintains or increases immune activities, acting as an anti-inflammatory agent through the inhibition of cyclooxygenase activity and reducing oxidative stress (Buggy and Smith 1999; Golder and Papalois 2021).

The use of regional anesthesia and analgesia helps preserve the immune system due to lower neuroendocrine stress and opioid use (Hogan et al. 2011; Sessler 2016). Various clinical trials involving gastrointestinal surgery have shown improved preservation of lymphocyte subpopulations and NK cell levels when general anesthesia is used in combination with either epidural or nerve block anesthesia (Hogan et al. 2011; Guay et al. 2016). The maintenance of normothermia, conservative transfusions, and early ambulation as recommended in the ERAS protocol also help achieve this goal (Gustafsson et al. 2019; Chen et al. 2024).

3.5.3 Oncologic Implications and Long-Term Outcomes

Increasing awareness suggests that the perioperative phase is the critical stage when factors like surgical interventions, stress, inflammation, and immunosuppression could help disseminate tumor cells (Gottschalk et al. 2010; Sessler 2016). Various investigations indicate that general anesthetics and opioids could stimulate angiogenesis, interfere with NK cells, and assist in the growth of tumor cells, while anesthetic strategies like propofol-based total intravenous anesthesia and regional anesthesia may protect the immune system and reduce pro-tumor factors (Gottschalk et al. 2010; Wigmore et al. 2016).

While retrospective studies have shown a link between TIVA or regional anesthesia and better disease-free or overall survival in various cancers, these findings are conflicting and susceptible to bias (Iqbalbhai et al. 2025; Golder and Papalois 2021). More recent systematic reviews have suggested that while there is biological plausibility, the available data are not strong enough to mandate particular anesthetic modalities to affect tumor recurrence, and there are ongoing large randomized controlled trials (Iqbalbhai et al. 2025; Chen et al. 2024). Under the ERAS framework, it is acceptable to use principles of immunoprotection, such as stress reduction, opioid-sparing pain relief, temperature maintenance, and blood conservation, while tailoring the anesthetic technique to each patient and tumor (Gustafsson et al. 2019; Grant and Engelman 2025).

3.6 Perioperative Phases and Practical Implementation

3.6.1 Preoperative Assessment and Optimization

ERAS assessment prior to surgery concentrates on risk assessment, patient education, and optimal management of associated diseases such as anemia, malnutrition, and cardiopulmonary disorders (Gustafsson et al. 2019; Scott et al. 2015). Airway evaluation, cardiopulmonary function, frailty, and functional assessment are the responsibilities of anesthetists who plan and organize interventions such as smoking, alcohol abstinence, correction of anemia, and exercise programs for selected patients at higher risk (Ljungqvist et al. 2017; Thacker et al. 2016).

The education of patients plays an important role in setting patient expectations for pain, mobility, and discharge. This will promote adherence to mobilization and nutritional regimens after surgery (Fearon et al. 2005; Grant and Engelman 2025). The anesthesiologist should provide a detailed explanation for the need for multimodal pain therapy, early mobilization, and low opioid dosing.

3.6.2 Intraoperative Anesthetic Management in ERAS: A Practical Schema

The implementation of ERAS strategies in practice involves the transformation of general recommendations in perioperative care into specific anesthetic protocols. The application of such protocols ensures consistency within each phase from before the operation to after the operation. An example of a complete anesthetic protocol for open colorectal surgery, showcasing the integration of each of the ERAS strategies mentioned above, is shown in Table 3.3.

3.6.3 Postoperative Care, Mobilization, and Discharge Readiness

Postanesthetic care in the context of ERAS includes continuous pain relief, prevention of PONV, hemodynamic stabilization, and rapid switching to oral medication after parenteral administration (Scott et al. 2015; Miller et al. 2014). Early mobilization, preferably starting on the same day of the procedure, requires adequate regional or local pain relief without excessive sedation (Fearon et al. 2005; Grant and Engelman 2025). Prompt removal of urinary catheters and lines prevents infections and promotes mobility, while specific discharge criteria, including pain relief, mobility, and oral intake, make the discharge process safe but fast (Gustafsson et al. 2019).

Table 3.3 Example ERAS-consistent anesthetic protocol for open colorectal surgery

Phase	Intervention	Key details
Preoperative	Fasting and carbohydrate loading	Clear carbohydrate drink up to 2–4 h pre-induction in low-risk patients (Ljungqvist et al. 2017)
	Multimodal premedication	Oral acetaminophen and NSAID if not contraindicated; avoidance of long-acting sedatives (Beverly et al. 2017)
Intraoperative	Regional technique	Thoracic epidural initiation before incision; alternative TAP block for minimally invasive procedures (Gustafsson et al. 2019)
	General anesthesia	Propofol-based TIVA or low-dose volatile with depth titration; opioid-sparing regimen (Golder and Papalois 2021)
	Fluid management	GDFT using stroke-volume optimization; balanced crystalloids, judicious vasopressor use (Thacker et al. 2016)
	Temperature and PONV	Active warming; PONV prophylaxis with dexamethasone and 5-HT3 antagonist (Gustafsson et al. 2019)
Postoperative	Analgesia	Continuation of epidural or wound catheter; scheduled acetaminophen and NSAID; rescue short-acting opioids (Beverly et al. 2017)
	Early mobilization and feeding	Sit out of bed and begin oral intake on day of surgery if feasible; physiotherapy involvement (Fearon et al. 2005)

3.6.4 Special Populations and Procedure-Specific Considerations

The elderly and the weak stand to gain a lot from the use of ERAS; however, such patients can easily develop hypotension, delirium, and respiratory depression, making it necessary to have caution in anesthesia depth, hemodynamic targets, and sparing opioids (Scott et al. 2015; Thacker et al. 2016). The obese patients and those suffering from OSA must be accorded special attention when it comes to their airways, ventilation, and post-op respiratory monitoring (Leech et al. 2021).

Anesthesiologist-specific ERAS guidelines (e.g., for colorectal surgery, pancreatitis, esophagectomy, hip and knee arthroplasty, and gynecological oncology) offer precise anesthesia recommendations that need to be implemented based on the local conditions (Gustafsson et al. 2019; Nygren et al. 2012). The anesthesiologists need to study the above literature and get actively involved in the relevant ERAS specialty groups. Overall, the adaptation to all these different patient groups would necessitate the implementation of an integrated standard-based approach throughout the whole process of surgical intervention. Important anesthesia contributions to the ERAS processes at each of the stages are summarized in Table 3.4.

Table 3.4 Summary of key anesthetic contributions to ERAS by perioperative phase

Phase	Anesthetic contributions
Preoperative	Risk stratification, optimization of comorbidities, patient education, fasting and carbohydrate protocols, multimodal premedication (Gustafsson et al. 2019; Ljungqvist et al. 2017)
Intraoperative	Choice of general vs regional anesthesia, multimodal analgesia, opioid-sparing strategies, GDFT, normothermia, PONV prophylaxis, depth and neuromuscular monitoring (Scott et al. 2015; Miller et al. 2014)
Postoperative	Continuation of multimodal analgesia, PONV management, hemodynamic and respiratory optimization, early mobilization and nutrition support, planning for transition to home (Fearon et al. 2005; Gustafsson et al. 2019)

3.7 Implementation, Audit, and Quality Improvement

3.7.1 ERAS Compliance and Outcomes

Several clinical studies have demonstrated a significant reduction in complications, LOS, and costs in patients with higher compliance with the ERAS components (Gustafsson et al. 2011; Varadhan et al. 2010). The anesthetic and analgesic components account for some of the heaviest-weighted measures in terms of compliance as they play a critical role in achieving the mobilization and nutrition of the patient (Ljungqvist et al. 2017; Scott et al. 2015). Regular monitoring of anesthetic practice is crucial in the context of maintaining the long-term benefits of the ERAS program.

3.7.2 Multidisciplinary Collaboration and Pathways

The effective adoption of ERAS necessitates coordinated efforts among anesthetists, surgeons, nurses, physical therapists, dieticians, and healthcare facility administrators (Fearon et al. 2005; Grant and Engelman 2025). Anesthetists are generally regarded as ERAS advocates, overseeing perioperative committees, preparing standard order sets, and educating others about multimodal anesthesia and fluid therapy (Scott et al. 2015). Incorporating ERAS guidelines into electronic medical records and care pathways aids in achieving consistency and compliance.

3.7.3 Barriers and Opportunities in Diverse Practice Settings

Some barriers for the use of ERAS in healthcare practice are limited resources for regional anesthesia, lack of availability for monitoring tools, safety of using NSAIDs, and reluctance toward change in the hospital environment (Ljungqvist et al. 2017; Thacker et al. 2016). For low-income regions, simplified bundles of ERAS, concentrating on cost-effective measures like education, mobilization, multimodal analgesia, and normothermia, can bring considerable advantages despite limited monitoring and regional techniques' unavailability (Gustafsson et al. 2019; Nygren et al. 2012).

Continuous learning, localized guideline implementation, and lessons from audit cycles play an important role in surmounting these obstacles and sustaining the interest of multidisciplinary teams (Scott et al. 2015; Grant and Engelman 2025).

3.8 Future Directions and Conclusions

3.8.1 Emerging Themes and Research Priorities

The future areas of interest in the research of anesthesia in ERAS would include precision perioperative medicine where the anesthesia and pain protocols are customized according to the patients' genetic, metabolic, and immunological status; large scale randomized trials to determine the efficacy of different anesthetic methods and their effect on cancer recurrence rates; and digital health technology to monitor recovery remotely (Iqbalbhai et al. 2025; Chen et al. 2024). There is a need for further studies on establishing effective protocols for OFA procedures, optimizing multimodal analgesia, and evaluating the effects of ERAS on chronic pain management (Leech et al. 2021; Kaye et al. 2019).

3.8.2 Key Messages for Clinical Practice

Anesthesia is crucial for ERAS protocols as anesthesia and analgesic management influence the surgical stress reaction, metabolism, and immune system (Kehlet 1997; Ljungqvist et al. 2017). Regional anesthesia and multimodal analgesia are essential components that decrease pain, opioid consumption, and organ dysfunction, leading to early mobility, nutritional intake, and discharge from hospital (Beverly et al. 2017; Scott et al. 2015).

Through adherence to ERAS concepts, anesthesiologists shift from being mere operating room technicians to perioperative physicians who oversee physiological optimization throughout the surgery timeline, thereby ensuring safer surgery, enhanced patient satisfaction, and improved health care system efficiency (Grant and Engelman 2025; Gustafsson et al. 2019).

References

Beverly A, Kaye AD, Ljungqvist O, Urman RD. Essential elements of multimodal analgesia in Enhanced Recovery After Surgery (ERAS) guidelines. Anesthesiol Clin. 2017;35(2):e115–43. https://doi.org/10.1016/j.anclin.2017.01.018.

Block BM, Liu SS, Rowlingson AJ, Cowan AR, Cowan JA Jr, Wu CL. Efficacy of postoperative epidural analgesia: a meta-analysis. JAMA. 2003;290(18):2455–63. https://doi.org/10.1001/jama.290.18.2455.

Bourazani M, Fyrfiris N, Galanis P, Maglari C, Anagnostopoulos A, Papatheodorou DC, Kelesi M, Poulopoulou S. Effect of opioid-sparing multimodal anesthesia within an Enhanced Recovery After Surgery (ERAS) protocol on postoperative recovery in gynecologic oncology surgery: a randomized clinical study. Cureus. 2026;18(3):e104812. https://doi.org/10.7759/cureus.104812.

Buggy DJ, Smith G. Epidural anaesthesia and analgesia: better outcome after major surgery? Growing evidence suggests so. BMJ (Clin Res Ed). 1999;319(7209):530–1. https://doi.org/10.1136/bmj.319.7209.530.

Chen Y, Kang J, Wang Y, Pan X. Effects of anesthesia and other perioperative factors on immune function: a narrative review. Signa Vitae. 2024;20(9):1–15. https://doi.org/10.22514/sv.2024.105.

Desborough JP. The stress response to trauma and surgery. Br J Anaesth. 2000;85(1):109–17. https://doi.org/10.1093/bja/85.1.109.

Fearon KCH, Ljungqvist O, Von Meyenfeldt M, Revhaug A, Dejong CHC, Lassen K, Nygren J, Hausel J, Soop M, Andersen J, Kehlet H. Enhanced recovery after surgery: a consensus review of clinical care for patients undergoing colonic resection. Clin Nutr. 2005;24(3):466–77. https://doi.org/10.1016/j.clnu.2005.02.002.

Golder HJ, Papalois V. Enhanced recovery after surgery: history, key advancements and developments in transplant surgery. J Clin Med. 2021;10(8):1634. https://doi.org/10.3390/jcm10081634.

Gottschalk A, Sharma S, Ford J, Durieux ME, Tiouririne M. Review article: the role of the perioperative period in recurrence after cancer surgery. Anesth Analg. 2010;110(6):1636–43. https://doi.org/10.1213/ANE.0b013e3181de0ab6.

Grant MC, Engelman DT. Enhanced recovery after surgery: overarching themes of the ERAS® society guidelines & consensus statements for adult specialty surgery. Perioper Med (Lond). 2025;14:120. https://doi.org/10.1186/s13741-025-00590-0.

Guay J, Nishimori M, Kopp SL. Epidural local anesthetics versus opioid-based analgesic regimens for postoperative gastrointestinal paralysis, vomiting, and pain after abdominal surgery: a Cochrane review. Anesth Analg. 2016;123(6):1591–602. https://doi.org/10.1213/ANE.0000000000001628.

Gustafsson UO, Hausel J, Thorell A, Ljungqvist O, Soop M, Nygren J, Enhanced Recovery After Surgery Study Group. Adherence to the enhanced recovery after surgery protocol and outcomes after colorectal cancer surgery. Arch Surg. 2011;146(5):571–7. https://doi.org/10.1001/archsurg.2010.309.

Gustafsson UO, Scott MJ, Hubner M, Nygren J, Demartines N, Francis N, Rockall TA, Young-Fadok TM, Hill AG, Soop M, de Boer HD, Urman RD, Chang GJ, Fichera A, Kessler H, Grass F, Whang EE, Fawcett WJ, Carli F, Lobo DN, Rollins KE, Balfour A, Baldini G, Riedel B, Ljungqvist O. Guidelines for perioperative care in elective colorectal surgery: Enhanced Recovery After Surgery (ERAS®) Society recommendations: 2018. World J Surg. 2019;43:659–95. https://doi.org/10.1007/s00268-018-4844-y.

Hogan BV, Peter MB, Shenoy HG, Horgan K, Hughes TA. Surgery induced immunosuppression. Surgeon. 2011;9(1):38–43. https://doi.org/10.1016/j.surge.2010.07.011.

Holm B, Kristensen MT, Bencke J, Husted H, Kehlet H, Bandholm T. Loss of knee-extension strength is related to knee swelling after total knee arthroplasty. Arch Phys Med Rehabil. 2010;91(11):1770–6. https://doi.org/10.1016/j.apmr.2010.07.229.

Iqbalbhai SA, Haizal Dixit R, Patel SA. Systematic review: the impact of anaesthesia on cancer recurrence and outcomes. J Contemp Clin Pract. 2025;11(4):243–50. https://doi.org/10.61336/jccp/25-04-40.

Ivascu R, Torsin LI, Hostiuc L, Nitipir C, Corneci D, Dutu M. The surgical stress response and anesthesia: a narrative review. J Clin Med. 2024;13(10):3017. https://doi.org/10.3390/jcm13103017.

Kaye AD, Urman RD, Rappaport Y, Siddaiah H, Cornett EM, Belani K, Salinas OJ, Fox CJ. Multimodal analgesia as an essential part of enhanced recovery protocols in the ambulatory settings. J Anaesthesiol Clin Pharmacol. 2019;35(Suppl 1):S40–5. https://doi.org/10.4103/joacp.JOACP_51_18.

Kehlet H. Multimodal approach to control postoperative pathophysiology and rehabilitation. Br J Anaesth. 1997;78(5):606–17. https://doi.org/10.1093/bja/78.5.606.

Kehlet H, Wilmore DW. Evidence-based surgical care and the evolution of fast-track surgery. Ann Surg. 2008;248(2):189–98. https://doi.org/10.1097/SLA.0b013e31817f2c1a.

Kurz A, Sessler DI, Lenhardt R. Perioperative normothermia to reduce the incidence of surgical-wound infection and shorten hospitalization. N Engl J Med. 1996;334(19):1209–15. https://doi.org/10.1056/NEJM199605093341901.

Leech J, Oswalt K, Tucci MA, Alam Mendez OA, Hierlmeier BJ. Opioid sparing anesthesia and enhanced recovery after surgery protocol for pancreaticoduodenectomy. Cureus. 2021;13(11):e19558. https://doi.org/10.7759/cureus.19558.

Ljungqvist O, Scott M, Fearon KC. Enhanced recovery after surgery: a review. JAMA Surg. 2017;152(3):292–8. https://doi.org/10.1001/jamasurg.2016.4952.

Loop T, Dovi-Akue D, Frick M, Roesslein M, Egger L, Humar M, Hoetzel A, Schmidt R, Borner C, Pahl HL, Geiger KK, Pannen BH. Volatile anesthetics induce caspase-dependent, mitochondria-mediated apoptosis in human T lymphocytes in vitro. Anesthesiology. 2005;102(6):1147–57. https://doi.org/10.1097/00000542-200506000-00014.

Miller TE, Thacker JK, White WD, Mantyh C, Migaly J, Jin J, Roche AM, Eisenstein EL, Edwards R, Anstrom KJ, Moon RE, Gan TJ, Enhanced Recovery Study Group. Reduced length of hospital stay in colorectal surgery after implementation of an enhanced recovery protocol. Anesth Analg. 2014;118(5):1052–61. https://doi.org/10.1213/ANE.0000000000000206.

Nygren J, Thacker J, Carli F, Fearon KCH, Norderval S, Lobo DN, Ljungqvist O, Soop M, Ramirez J, Enhanced Recovery After Surgery Society. Guidelines for perioperative care in elective rectal/pelvic surgery: Enhanced Recovery After Surgery (ERAS®) Society recommendations. Clin Nutr. 2012;31(6):801–16. https://doi.org/10.1016/j.clnu.2012.08.012.

Oderda GM, Gan TJ, Johnson BH, Robinson SB. Effect of opioid-related adverse events on outcomes in selected surgical patients. J Pain Palliat Care Pharmacother. 2013;27(1):62–70. https://doi.org/10.3109/15360288.2012.751956.

Peng XQ, Fei ZG, Sun CG, Zhou QJ. Efficacy and safety of local infiltration analgesia for pain management in total knee and hip arthroplasty: a meta-analysis of randomized controlled trial. Medicine. 2020;99(22):e20640. https://doi.org/10.1097/MD.0000000000020640.

Scott MJ, Baldini G, Fearon KCH, Feldheiser A, Feldman LS, Gan TJ, Ljungqvist O, Lobo DN, Rockall TA, Schricker T, Carli F. Enhanced Recovery After Surgery (ERAS) for gastrointestinal surgery, part 1: pathophysiological considerations. Acta Anaesthesiol Scand. 2015;59(10):1212–31. https://doi.org/10.1111/aas.12601.

Sessler DI. Perioperative thermoregulation and heat balance. Lancet. 2016;387(10038):2655–64. https://doi.org/10.1016/S0140-6736(15)00981-2.

Sista F, Schietroma M, Santis GD, Mattei A, Cecilia EM, Piccione F, Leardi S, Carlei F, Amicucci G. Systemic inflammation and immune response after laparotomy vs laparoscopy in patients with acute cholecystitis, complicated by peritonitis. World J Gastrointest Surg. 2013;5(4):73–82. https://doi.org/10.4240/wjgs.v5.i4.73.

Thacker JK, Mountford WK, Ernst FR, Krukas MR, Mythen MM. Perioperative fluid utilization variability and association with outcomes: considerations for enhanced recovery efforts in sample US surgical populations. Ann Surg. 2016;263(3):502–10. https://doi.org/10.1097/SLA.0000000000001402.

Varadhan KK, Neal KR, Dejong CH, Fearon KC, Ljungqvist O, Lobo DN. The enhanced recovery after surgery (ERAS) pathway for patients undergoing major elective open colorectal surgery: a meta-analysis of randomized controlled trials. Clin Nutr. 2010;29(4):434–40. https://doi.org/10.1016/j.clnu.2010.01.004.

Wigmore TJ, Mohammed K, Jhanji S. Long-term survival for patients undergoing volatile versus IV anesthesia for cancer surgery: a retrospective analysis. Anesthesiology. 2016;124(1):69–79. https://doi.org/10.1097/ALN.0000000000000936.

Xiong M, Liu Y, Liang Y, Wang H, Zhang L, Zhang Z, Fang M. Opioid-free versus opioid-sparing anesthesia for postoperative pain and early recovery after laparoscopic cholecystectomy: a randomized controlled trial. J Pain Res. 2025;18:2137–46. https://doi.org/10.2147/JPR.S506147.

Zhuang CL, Ye XZ, Zhang XD, Chen BC, Yu Z. Enhanced recovery after surgery programs versus traditional care for colorectal surgery: a meta-analysis of randomized controlled trials. Dis Colon Rectum. 2013;56(5):667–78. https://doi.org/10.1097/DCR.0b013e3182812842.

Perioperative Nutritional Assessment and Rehabilitation

4

Luxita Sharma, Gunjan, Keshav Singh, and Dhananjay Sharma

Abstract

Perioperative nutritional assessment and rehabilitation play a critical role in improving surgical outcomes and reducing postoperative complications. Patients undergoing surgery often experience metabolic stress, which increases nutritional demands and can worsen pre-existing malnutrition. Therefore, early identification of nutritional risk is essential for effective perioperative care. This chapter highlights the importance of systematic nutritional assessment before surgery and the implementation of targeted nutritional rehabilitation strategies. Various validated screening and assessment tools are discussed to help clinicians identify patients at risk of malnutrition and determine the severity of nutritional deficits. The chapter also explores how poor nutritional status can negatively affect wound healing, immune response, and overall recovery following surgery. Emphasis is placed on the development of individualized nutritional intervention plans, including dietary counseling, oral nutritional supplementation, and, when necessary, enteral or parenteral nutrition. Additionally, the role of a multidisciplinary team in optimizing perioperative nutrition is examined, highlighting collaboration between surgeons, dietitians, anesthesiologists, and nursing staff. By addressing nutritional deficiencies prior to surgery and maintaining adequate nutritional support throughout the perioperative period, healthcare providers can significantly enhance patient recovery, reduce hospital stays, and improve overall surgical success rates. This chapter

L. Sharma · Gunjan · D. Sharma (✉)
Department of Dietetics and Applied Nutrition, Amity Medical School, Amity University Haryana, Manesar, Gurugram, Haryana, India
e-mail: lshrama@ggn.amity.edu

K. Singh
Department of Public Health and Hospital Administration, Amity Medical School, Amity University Haryana, Manesar, Gurugram, Haryana, India

P. K. Bhattacharyya et al. (eds.), *Integrated Anesthesia and Nutrition Approaches to Enhanced Recovery after Surgery*,
https://doi.org/10.1007/978-981-92-3294-9_4

underscores the importance of integrating nutritional assessment and rehabilitation as a standard component of modern perioperative care.

Keywords

Perioperative · Nutritional assessment · Rehabilitation · Dietitians · Nutritional deficiencies

4.1 Introduction to Perioperative Nutrition

Perioperative nutrition focuses on optimizing a patient's nutritional status before, during, and after surgery to improve recovery and reduce complications. It involves nutritional assessment, risk identification, and tailored interventions such as enteral or parenteral support. Proper perioperative nutrition enhances immune function, promotes wound healing, and contributes to better surgical outcomes and shorter hospital stays (Groh-Wargo and Barr 2022; Braunschweig et al. 2001). Modern surgery has shifted its focus from only procedures to patient safety, patient recovery, and a range of factors. In this shift, the major focus is on the required physiological resources and considering the complex metabolic processes of the surgery. Rehabilitation and nutritional status assessments are two key components of the approach, which connect patients' physiological and nutritional status to surgical outcomes (Ljungqvist et al. 2017).

In the past, nutrition acted as a reactive measure, only used when severe weight loss or complications were faced by a patient during a surgery. As per the new guidelines, including Enhanced Recovery After Surgery (ERAS), for "metabolic preparations," nutrition is viewed as a proactive step. In addition, malnutrition is now a main concern rather than just a secondary issue in the traditional approach (Jain et al. 2023). It can lead to many problems such as physiological failures, making patients more prone to infections, hindering tissue regeneration, and putting various body systems at risk during surgery (Weimann et al. 2017). Surgeries stimulate the release of cytokines and catabolic hormones, which ultimately lead to hypermetabolism. A patient with malnutrition loses lean mass very quickly, which results in weak diaphragm muscles, slower wound healing, and lower cardiac output. Therefore, to identify if the patient needs nutritional support, the nutritional assessment is mandatory (Singer et al. 2019; Munoz et al. 2020).

4.1.1 Importance of Nutritional Status in Surgical Patients

In modern medicine, parenteral nutrition plays a crucial role in managing nutritional status, particularly in critical situations where it is more accessible; however, under normal conditions, enteral nutrition is generally preferred as the first line of support (Berlana 2022). Since the practice of surgery began, the early recovery and complications related to the postoperative situations. The two most fundamental pillars that allow us to shift the focus to the improvement of perioperative nutritional management and the procedure of surgical techniques. Even after the huge advancements in these two fields, the rationalization of postoperative recovery (especially in surgery of digestive or oncological pathways and elderly patients suffering from malnutrition) is slow (Martínez-Ortega et al. 2022). Perioperative malnutrition emerges as a huge challenge, as it is not easy to diagnose, define, and treat. Even after all these challenges, a concerning predictor of poor postoperative outcomes is suboptimal nutritional conditions. Postoperative morbidity, mortality, readmission rates, and length of stay (LOS) are most common in surgical malnourished patients (Wischmeyer et al. 2018).

The International Nutrition Society underscores the urgency of enhancing perioperative nutrition diagnostics and improving practices (Weimann et al. 2006). But even after that, limited guidelines from surgical and perioperative societies exist on the optimal status and for screening of the surgical patient for malnutrition in the perioperative stage. The connection between nutrition and healing depends on the body's metabolic reactions to surgical stress (Smith Jr et al. 2020). Delayed wound healing and aggravated inflammatory reactions are two indicators of poor nutritional conditions. It has been seen that individuals having adequate nutritional reserves recover faster, have fewer issues and are able to withstand the physiological demands of surgery. Even after surgical practices and preoperative care practices improvement, nearly 40% of the patients of general surgery are at risk of malnutrition (Kutnik et al. 2023; Munoz et al. 2020). Figure 4.1 presents a perioperative nutrition management algorithm, starting with nutritional risk assessment and guiding interventions based on risk level. It shows the preference for enteral nutrition

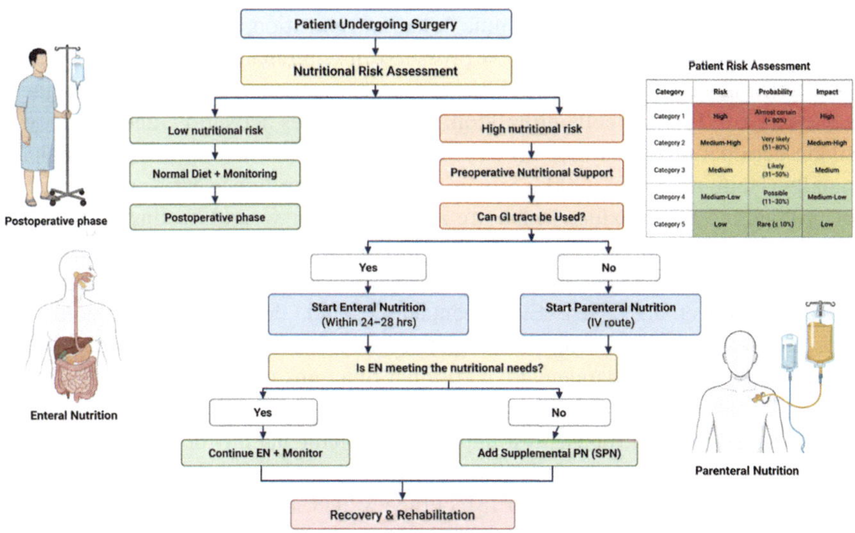

Fig. 4.1 Management of a patient undergoing surgery. (Created by author using MS PowerPoint 2021)

when the GI tract is functional, with parenteral nutrition as an alternative or supplement if needs are not met. The approach emphasizes continuous monitoring and progression toward recovery and rehabilitation.

4.1.1.1 Nutritional Support in Metabolism

In the recovery of postoperative patients, nutritional support plays a crucial role. Sufficient nutrition promotes tissue repair and cell metabolism; it provides energy and nutrients to the body; it also reduces the risk of infection and increases the immune function. Additionally, wound healing, regeneration, and repair of tissues are the processes that depend upon adequate protein status (Singer et al. 2019; Munoz et al. 2020). Additionally, at the time of postoperative recovery, a majority of patients have insufficient protein and macronutrient intake due to anorexia, surgical stress, and improper function of the digestive tract, affect the recovery process and wound healing (Shim et al. 2013).

To promote tissue healing and repair, and help patients cope with stress after surgeries by providing adequate protein, trace elements, vitamins, and calories. A crucial part of nutritional support in postoperative patients is adequate fluid management, which can enhance the elimination of metabolic waste and help in maintaining the electrolyte balance in the body, which ultimately reduces the postoperative complications (Singer et al. 2019). Nutritional support in perioperative patients not only enhances healing but also reduces complications and enhances the quality of life and recovery quality in patients, specifically those at risk of pressure ulcers. To promote or maximize patient's recovery, a personalized nutrition plan is needed according to the individual's requirements.

4.1.1.2 Role of Nutrition in EN and ONS Formulations

Adequate nutrition supports immune function. Nutrition, such as omega-3 fatty acids, antioxidants, and arginine, is provided in combination with major EN and ONS formulas for patients over 25 years as a risk reduction therapy. As arginine is necessary for T-helper cells promotion, T lymphocytes activation, and phagocytosis, in perioperative conditions (i.e., surgical stress), essential arginine is depleted rapidly (Helminen, et al., 2007; Singer et al. 2019). Arginine serves as a precursor of proline and nitric oxide, which are responsible for wound healing and anastomotic integrity. Proline promotes collagen deposition during healing, and nitric oxide, on the other hand, increases oxygenation and vasodilation (Debats et al. 2009; Munoz et al. 2020). Eicosapentaenoic acid, docosahexaenoic acid, and omega-3 fatty acids exert anti-inflammatory effects. Generation of resolvins and reduction of oxidative damage are additional functions of these nutritional supplements (Debats et al. 2009).

Most studies have focused on applying supplementation for 5 days preoperatively and 7 days postoperatively. Studies that use single immunonutrients have not shown the same benefit. For better IMN efficacy, it is suggested that complete nutritional support and a combination of different nutritional components be provided. A study at the Cochrane library analysis shows that with the help of preoperative IMN, we can reduce infection-related complications in patients related to any surgery. (Xu et al. 2006). Some studies suggest that high-risk GI surgery patients benefited positively because of the higher risk of perioperative complications.

4.1.2 Impact of Malnutrition on Surgical Outcomes

While there is increasing attention being paid to precision medicine and modern surgical techniques, the biological essence of a patient sometimes seems forgotten. One of the most critical and, at the same time, easily adjustable risks is malnutrition. It can be described as a situation when insufficient nutrient intake or inadequate metabolism of those nutrients alters body composition and reduces the physiological and psychological capacities of a person. As per research, malnutrition impacts 30–50% of all patients undergoing surgical intervention (Singer et al. 2019).

4.1.2.1 The Pathophysiology of Surgical Malnutrition

A surgical procedure elicits a complex metabolic stress response consisting of two phases, which are called "ebb" and "flow." During both stages, a person experiences hypermetabolism and catabolism to use energy stored in the organism and aid in recovery. When a person is in good health, such energy resources are plentiful. But during malnutrition, these sources become depleted. Inflammation, on the other hand, worsens the catabolic process by triggering muscle proteolysis in order to supply amino acids for the synthesis of acute-phase proteins, as well as immune defence mechanisms such as cell signaling through pro-inflammatory cytokines IL-1, IL-6, and TNF-alpha. Without sufficient external nutrition, this catabolism will result in significant frailty, which predicts surgical failure (Weimann et al. 2017).

4.1.2.2 The Triad of Adverse Outcomes

Nutrient deficiency in perioperative medicine is manifested most clearly by this triad of complications, which affect not only the safety but also the post-operative course of the patient. First of all, it should be mentioned that malnutrition is a leading risk factor for developing infections, delays in wound healing, and increased hospital stays (Munoz et al. 2020).

4.1.2.3 Increased Risk of Infection

Malnutrition often leads to a secondary deficiency of the body's immune system. Malnutrition results in lymphoid atrophy and weakening of innate and adaptive immunity systems. For example, protein and micronutrient deficiency causes defects in T-lymphocyte functions, decreased phagocytosis, and inhibition of cytokine production. Thus, under these conditions, patients develop a high susceptibility to Surgical Site Infections, pneumonia, and sepsis. The literature indexed in PubMed shows that even moderate malnutrition doubles the risk of postoperative sepsis in gastrointestinal surgery (Gianotti et al. 2018).

4.1.2.4 Delayed Wound Healing

The healing of wounds is a process that involves a lot of energy and needs certain nutrients for the formation of collagen and remodeling of tissues. However, for patients who suffer from protein-energy malnutrition, the inflammatory stage takes a long time, whereas the proliferation stage is underdeveloped because of the shortage of certain amino acids such as Arginine and Proline (Chaudhary et al. 2025).

4.1.2.5 Prolonged Hospitalization and Economic Burden

As highlighted above, the consequences will eventually create a domino effect for healthcare utilization. Infections or wound complications, which occur among patients, necessitate intensive treatment and the use of extensive antibiotic regimens. Studies have found that patients who suffer from malnutrition spend two to six additional days in hospitals when compared to those with proper nutrition (Ljungqvist et al. 2017). This translates to a considerable loss from the public health point of view. In light of this, the importance of addressing the issue of preoperative malnutrition, the need to screen patients using standardized tools becomes necessary. The Nutritional Risk Screening (NRS-2002) is one such method that may be used for this purpose. Following diagnosis, the patient requires prehabilitation or optimal preoperative nutrition. The use of immunonutrition, which is rich in arginine and omega-3 fatty acids, modulates the body's immune response, improving the activation of T-lymphocytes (Ljungqvist et al. 2017; Pannirselvam et al. 2025).

4.2 Nutritional Risk Screening and Assessment

The screening of nutritional risks is one of the key elements of perioperative care since the early detection of malnutrition has been demonstrated to enhance the clinical outcomes of surgical patients (Weimann et al. 2017). The European Society of Clinical Nutrition and Metabolism (ESPEN) clinical guidelines directly indicate that all hospitalized patients, even surgical patients, should be subjected to nutritional screening during the admission process to identify at-risk patients and begin to intervene as soon as possible (Weimann et al. 2017).

The Global Leadership Initiative on Malnutrition (GLIM) also stresses that both phenotypic (weight loss, low body mass index, and reduced muscle mass) and etiologic (reduced food intake and inflammation) criteria should be used in the diagnosis of malnutrition (Cederholm et al. 2019). This paradigm indicates evidence that inflammation and disease burden have a tremendous impact on nutritional status in surgical groups (Cederholm et al. 2019). Poor nutritional status has been linked to higher morbidity of complications, such as infections and longer hospital stay, in critically ill and surgical patients, which explains the significance of conducting screening and assessment (Singer et al. 2019).

4.2.1 Nutritional Screening Tools

The use of validated screening tools should be considered the standard practice since they offer standardized and reproducible ways of identifying patients at nutritional risk (Weimann et al. 2017). Among them, the most popular resources to use in the process of perioperative practice are NRS-2002, MUST, and SGA. The habitual use of these tools has been found to enhance early malnutrition identification and guide acceptable nutritional intervention, which has been linked to enhanced clinical results (Cederholm et al. 2019). Besides, global guidelines underline that screening must be conducted at the time of admission and throughout the clinical course because the state of nutrition can quickly get worse in patients undergoing surgery (Singer et al. 2019). The regular use of validated tools will also improve the communication between healthcare providers and promote the use of evidence-based decision-making in perioperative care (Weimann et al. 2017).

4.2.1.1 Nutritional Risk Screening (NRS-2002)

The Nutritional Risk Screening 2002 (NRS-2002) instrument is particularly suggested by ESPEN to be used with hospitalized patients due to the consideration of both the nutritional condition and severity of the disease (Weimann et al. 2017). The scoring system considers such parameters as recent weight loss, decreased diet intake, body mass index, and the severity of illness, indicating more metabolic demand (Weimann et al. 2017).

Clinical study evidence shows that patients who are at risk based on the NRS-2002 are predisposed to postoperative complications and prolonged hospitalization compared to patients without nutritional risk (Garth et al. 2019). This predictive validity makes it acceptable to use it routinely in surgical populations. Furthermore, as a tool, NRS-2002 is the most appropriate to use with perioperative patients, whose surgical stress adds to the metabolic demands (Singer et al. 2019).

4.2.1.2 Malnutrition Universal Screening Tool (MUST)

The MUST is popular because of its simplicity and its ability to be implemented in the hospital and community. It evaluates the nutritional risk using three criteria, which include body mass index, percentage of unintentional weight loss, and the presence of acute disease that is impacting nutritional intake (Barker et al. 2011). Studies have demonstrated that MUST is useful in recognizing patients who have a risk of malnutrition, and it has clinical outcomes in terms of length of hospital stay and the rate of complications (Barker et al. 2011). It is simple to screen and, thus, is especially applicable to preoperative outpatient clinics. Moreover, the GLIM framework allows adhering to the use of validated screening instruments like MUST that is the initial step prior to the official diagnosis of malnutrition (Cederholm et al. 2019).

4.2.1.3 Subjective Global Assessment (SGA)

SGA is a popular clinical instrument used to assess the nutritional status in patients, especially in surgical and oncology settings (Correia and Waitzberg 2016). It also includes the history of the patient (such as weight loss, nutrition, and GI symptoms), and physical examination (such as muscle wasting and fat loss) (Correia and Waitzberg 2016).

Research has shown that SGA classification is associated with the postoperative outcomes, such as complication rates and mortality, suggesting its clinical applicability to surgical populations (Correia and Waitzberg 2016). In contrast to strictly quantitative measures, SGA offers a holistic clinical approach that includes both functional and physical components of malnutrition that are not always represented by laboratory values only (Cederholm et al. 2019). Table 4.1 explains the comparison of common nutritional screening tools used for surgical patients.

4.2.2 Clinical and Biochemical Indicators

After screening, extensive nutritional screening implies the assessment of anthropometric, dietary, biochemical, and clinical signs and determination of the severity and etiology of malnutrition (Weimann et al. 2017). The rationale behind the use of this multidimensional approach is that no one parameter is enough to determine cases of malnutrition (Cederholm et al. 2019). Body mass index and weight loss are anthropometric measurements that can be used to provide information on body composition changes, whereas dietary assessment can be used to determine poor nutrient intake (Thompson and Subar 2017). Other supporting evidence is provided by biochemical markers, such as serum proteins and inflammatory indicators, but should be viewed with caution because of the impact of inflammation caused by the disease (Shenkin 2016). These findings are further complemented by clinical assessment, which is used to detect any physical symptoms and functional deterioration that come with malnutrition (White et al. 2012).

4.2.2.1 Anthropometric Indicators

One of the most frequently used indicators of nutritional status is body mass index (BMI); nevertheless, it does not consider alterations in body composition (muscle loss) (Cederholm et al. 2019). One of the major diagnostic criteria of malnutrition is unintentional weight loss, and GLIM recognizes the considerable weight loss as one of the key phenotypic signs linked with adverse outcomes (Cederholm et al. 2019). Muscle mass assessment has become more and more important, with sarcopenia proving to be a predictor of postoperative complications, extended hospital stay, and death in surgical patients (Cruz-Jentoft et al. 2019a, b).

4.2.2.2 Dietary Intake Assessment

Dietary intake should be assessed to help ascertain whether patients are attaining their nutritional needs or not. One of the etiologic criteria of malnutrition according to GLIM is reduced food intake (Cederholm et al. 2019). The dietary intake and deficiencies should be assessed with the help of standardized methods of dietary assessment, which include the use of dietary recalls and food frequency questionnaires (Thompson and Subar 2017). Poor appetite and insufficient consumption are

Table 4.1 Comparison of common nutritional screening tools used for surgical patients

Tool	Components assessed	Scoring/classification	Clinical use	Strengths	Limitations	References
NRS-2002 (Nutritional Risk Screening)	BMI, recent weight loss, reduced dietary intake, disease severity	Score ≥3 indicates nutritional risk	Recommended for hospitalized and surgical patients	Evidence-based, validated in hospital settings, guideline-supported	Requires clinical judgment for disease severity	Weimann et al. (2017)
MUST (Malnutrition Universal Screening Tool)	BMI, unintentional weight loss, acute disease effect	Low (0), medium (1), high (≥2) risk	Community and hospital screening	Simple, rapid, easy to use	Less sensitive in acute inflammatory conditions	Cederholm et al. (2019)
SGA (Subjective Global Assessment)	Weight change, dietary consumption, gastrointestinal symptoms, functional capacity, physical examination	Well nourished (A), moderate (B), severe (C) malnutrition	Clinical and perioperative nutritional assessment	Comprehensive and clinically relevant	Subjective; depends on clinician expertise	White et al. (2012)
GLIM Criteria	Phenotypic + etiologic	Diagnosis requires ≥1 phenotypic + ≥1 etiologic criterion	Global diagnostic framework for malnutrition	Standardized, internationally accepted criteria	Requires prior screening tool for diagnosis	Cederholm et al. (2019)

common phenomena in surgical patients because of disease-specific reasons and psychological stress, which leads to a decrease in nutrition (Weimann et al. 2017).

4.2.2.3 Biochemical Indicators

Biochemical markers are informative in nutritional evaluation and have to be analyzed with caution because of the effects of inflammation (Singer et al. 2019). Traditionally, serum albumin is considered to be an indicator of nutritional status, but it is currently understood as a negative acute-phase reactant that falls in line with inflammation instead of being a response to nutritional intake alone (Shenkin 2016). Prealbumin has a lower half-life and thus is more sensitive to changes in the nutritional intake, but also is influenced by inflammatory processes, which reduces its specificity (Shenkin 2016).

C-reactive protein (CRP) is a biochemical used to determine the presence of inflammation and can be used to interpret other biochemical markers (Singer et al. 2019). The increase in CRP levels is a sign of systemic inflammation, which is an important etiologic factor in malnutrition (Cederholm et al. 2019). Clinical significance of electrolyte imbalances is also evident because imbalances in sodium, potassium, and magnesium levels may influence the stability and outcomes during perioperative (Weimann et al. 2017).

4.2.2.4 Clinical Indicators

Clinical assessment is an important aspect of nutritional assessment. The physical symptoms that are identified as signs of malnutrition include wasting of the muscle, fat loss, and edema (White et al. 2012). Functional evaluation, which incorporates muscle strength assessments, like handgrip strength, has been identified as correlated with nutritional status and a predictor of clinical outcome (Norman et al. 2019). Comorbidity is very important in nutritional status. Cancer and other diseases are related to metabolic changes and systemic inflammation that cause malnutrition and cachexia associated with the disease (Fearon et al. 2016).

4.2.2.5 Integrated Approach

The latest recommendations presuppose that there is no single parameter that can be used to diagnose malnutrition, and a multiplex of screening tools with clinical, anthropometric, dietary, and biochemical indicators is necessary (Cederholm et al. 2019). With such an integrated approach, nutritional risk may be accurately identified, malnutrition classified, and specific measures to enhance the perioperative outcomes may be implemented (Weimann et al. 2017).

4.3 Preoperative Nutritional Optimization

Nutritional optimization is an important aspect of perioperative care that focuses on enhancing outcomes of surgery by rectifying nutritional deficiencies present preoperatively. There is clinical evidence proving that patients who undergo preoperative nutritional support have fewer postoperative complications, wounds heal better, and they spend shorter periods in the hospital (Weimann et al. 2017). According to international recommendations by the European Society of Clinical Nutrition and Metabolism (ESPEN), patients who are found to be malnourished or at nutritional risk should be given nutritional support at least 7–14 days before a major surgery, despite the fact that this may require a delay of surgery (Weimann et al. 2017). This is supported by the evidence that nutritional intervention before surgery leads to better metabolic reserves and increases the body's ability to endure surgical stress (Weimann et al. 2017).

Malnutrition harms immune function, muscle mass, and tissue-repairing mechanisms, all of which are crucial to postoperative recovery (Correia and Waitzberg 2016). Thus, preoperative optimization measures aim at enhancing energy and protein consumption, micronutrient deficiencies, and metabolic disturbances associated with the disease (Cederholm et al. 2019). Evidence from recent systematic reviews has revealed a remarkable decrease in postoperative complications and infections with preoperative nutritional interventions, especially in high-risk surgical patients (Sowerbutts et al. 2024). These results demonstrate the significance of including nutritional care in the process of everyday surgical planning.

4.3.1 Dietary Counseling and Nutritional Planning

Dietary counseling is an essential element of preoperative nutritional optimization and is a personalized evaluation and advice to enhance dietary consumption and rectify nutritional imbalances. There is some evidence that individualized nutrition interventions are more successful than broad-based dietary guidance to enhance patient outcomes (Weimann et al. 2017). Dietary counseling starts with an overall examination of the patient's present dietary consumption, nutritional needs, and obstacles to proper nutrition. Decreased appetite, gastrointestinal symptoms, and psychological stress are the factors that are usually resolved as contributing to the insufficient intake in patients in the post-surgical period (Thompson and Subar 2017). Individualized dietary interventions can go a long way in helping to address these factors and enhance nutritional status before surgery (Weimann et al. 2017).

According to clinical guidelines, the range of energy needs of surgical patients should typically be 25–30 kcal/kg/day with an addition of 1.2–2.0 g/kg/day of protein intake to help patients who are at risk of malnutrition recover tissues and maintain immune functions (Weimann et al. 2017; Deutz et al. 2014). These guidelines are upheld by the research that has shown that proper protein consumption is crucial in muscle mass maintenance and sarcopenia prevention (Deutz et al. 2014). Dietary counseling also aims at enhancing the quality of the nutrient intake. Immune functioning and wound healing require sufficient intake of micronutrients like vitamins A, C, and E; trace elements like zinc and selenium (Calder 2020). Lack of these nutrients has been linked to poor healing and high chances of developing postoperative complications (Calder 2020).

Besides the adequacy of nutrients, meal timing and frequency are also of concern. Patients with decreased appetite are likely to be advised to use small, frequent meals, which may enhance the total caloric intake and alleviate gastrointestinal discomfort (Weimann et al. 2017). Dietary counseling also involves behavioral interventions and educational interventions. Structured nutritional education and counseling have been shown to increase adherence to dietary recommendations and better clinical results in patients in comparison with those who are provided with standard care (Sowerbutts et al. 2024).

Additionally, dietary counseling also contributes to perioperative preparation (Enhanced Recovery After Surgery (ERAS) which suggests that patients should be prepared by minimizing preoperative fasting and promoting carbohydrate consumption until the time of surgery (Ljungqvist et al. 2017; Jain et al. 2023). Appropriate counseling ensures that patients understand and follow these guidelines, thereby maximizing the metabolic status prior to surgery. Dietary counseling needs to be more personalized to consider disease-specific metabolic alterations and functional restrictions and be applied to high-risk groups such as elderly patients and cancer patients (Cruz-Jentoft et al. 2019a, b; Fearon et al. 2016). The example of cancer patients is one where patients undergo cachexia, which causes an increased energy and protein demand and special nutritional approaches (Fearon et al. 2016). In sum, dietary counseling is an evidence-based and cost-effective approach to enhancing nutritional status before surgery. Its success relies on a timely intervention, personalized intervention planning, and ongoing evaluation (Weimann et al. 2017).

4.3.2 Oral Nutritional Supplements (ONS)

ONS plays a significant role in preoperative care to enhance energy and protein intake in patients with a lack of ability to achieve their nutritional needs through diet. They are normally high-energy products that are fortified with nutrients such as protein, vitamins, and minerals and, therefore, can be used to effectively address nutritional deficiencies (Weimann et al. 2017). Randomized controlled trials and systematic reviews evidence shows that ONS can significantly enhance nutritional intake and decrease postoperative complications in surgical patients (Sowerbutts et al. 2024). Specifically, preoperative nutrition has been demonstrated to reduce the rate of infection and the length of hospitalization of malnourished patients with major surgery (Sowerbutts et al. 2024).

ONS are particularly useful when patients have decreased appetite or higher metabolic requirements, and their ability to obtain adequate intake with a normal diet only might be problematic (Cederholm et al. 2019). ONS assists in enhancing the overall nutrition level and metabolic response to surgical stress by offering a concentrated source of nutrients (Weimann et al. 2017). Protein supplements are of great importance in maintaining muscle mass and avoiding sarcopenia. Protein supplementation has been reported to enhance muscle protein synthesis and minimize the potential complications of postoperative decreases in muscle (Deutz et al. 2014).

Most of the ONS formulations, in addition to the macronutrients, are fortified with micronutrients and bioactive compounds that improve immune activity and healing. As an illustration, omega-3 fatty acid-containing, arginine-containing, and nucleotide-containing supplements have been demonstrated to have an anti-inflammatory effect and lead to better clinical outcomes in surgical patients (Calder 2020). When ONS is administered and how long it is administered are other factors. It is advised that patients at nutritional risk should start the supplementation at least 714 days before surgery to realize any significant changes in nutritional status (Weimann et al. 2017).

An important predictor of the success of ONS is compliance with it. Research has indicated that taste, gastrointestinal tolerance, and patient education are some of the factors that affect patient compliance with supplementation regimens (Sowerbutts et al. 2024). Hence, it is necessary to make sure that the correct choice of products is made by healthcare workers, and they counsel on adherence. ONS are, in general, well tolerated and possess a good safety profile, making them a viable choice of preoperative nutritional support. Nevertheless, they are to be incorporated in the overall plan of nutrition that also involves dietary counseling and frequent follow-ups (Weimann et al. 2017). To conclude, oral nutritional supplementation is an evidence-based intervention that is at the center of preoperative nutritional optimization. Properly used, it can dramatically change nutritional status, decrease complications, and improve recovery of surgical patients (Sowerbutts et al. 2024). Table 4.2 elaborates the anthropometric and biochemical indicators for preoperative nutritional assessment.

Table 4.2 Anthropometric and biochemical indicators for preoperative nutritional assessment

Indicator type	Parameter	Description/ clinical significance	Limitations	Reference
Anthropometric	Body mass index (BMI)	Assesses body weight relative to height; identifies undernutrition (<18.5 kg/m^2) and obesity	Does not reflect body composition or muscle mass	Weimann et al. (2017)
Anthropometric	Unintentional weight loss	>5% loss in 6 months or > 10% over a longer period indicates malnutrition risk	Requires accurate patient history	Cederholm et al. (2019)
Anthropometric	Muscle mass (Sarcopenia)	Reduction in skeletal muscle mass linked to poor surgical outcomes and increased complications	Requires imaging (CT, DEXA) or specialized tools	Cruz-Jentoft et al. (2019a, 2019b)

(Continued)

Table 4.2 (Continued)

Indicator type	Parameter	Description/clinical significance	Limitations	Reference
Anthropometric	Mid-upper arm circumference (MUAC)	Reflects muscle and fat stores; useful when weight/height unavailable	Less precise compared to imaging methods	Cederholm et al. (2019)
Biochemical	Serum albumin	Low levels associated with poor surgical outcomes and increased morbidity	Influenced by inflammation, not a specific nutrition marker	Shenkin (2016)
Biochemical	Prealbumin (transthyretin)	Short half-life; reflects recent nutritional changes	Affected by acute-phase response and illness	Shenkin (2016)
Biochemical	Hemoglobin	Indicates anemia; low levels impair oxygen delivery and recovery	Not specific to nutritional status alone	Weimann et al. (2017)
Biochemical	C-reactive protein (CRP)	Marker of inflammation; helps interpret other biochemical markers	Does not indicate nutrition directly	Cederholm et al. (2019)
Biochemical	Electrolytes (Na^+, K^+, Mg^{2+})	Reflect metabolic balance; abnormalities affect perioperative stability	Influenced by hydration and disease state	Singer et al. (2019)

4.4 Nutritional Rehabilitation Strategies

The required components of the modern surgical treatment are nutrition and rehabilitation evaluation in the perioperative phase, and special consideration is given to better avenues to recovery. Malnutrition is not noticeable most of the time, and it leads to postoperative complications, increased level of infection, delayed wound healing, and prolonged hospital stay. Perioperative practices used today before and after surgery involve a strict level of nutritional screening (through devices like MUST and NRS-2002), metabolic analysis, and individualized nutrition planning (Martínez-Ortega et al. 2022). Recent studies have demonstrated that early nutritional risk identification and immediate intervention (prehabilitation and postoperative recovery) can have a substantial positive impact, especially in high-risk populations such as cancer, gastrointestinal surgery, and patients with acute illnesses (Ambulkar et al. 2025; Bozzetti 2002).

The existing trends imply the use of a comprehensive approach encompassing premature enteral nutrition, a selective approach that proposes parenteral supplements, immunonutrition therapy (arginine and omega-3 fatty acids), and personalized nutrition with reference to metabolic monitoring. Early feeding within 24–48 h and a decrease in lengthy fasting are promoted by the employment of recovery enhancement after surgical (ERAS) methods (Li et al. 2024; Pannirselvam et al. 2025).

4.4.1 Enteral Nutrition Support

Enteral nutrition (EN) refers to the provision of food to the gastrointestinal system via tube (nasogastric, Naso-jejunal, gastrostomy, or jejunostomy) or oral (with oral nutritional supplements). If the gut is functioning, EN is the preferred and physiologically superior method of nutritional support in the perioperative setting. The rationale is that using the functional gut helps maintain intestinal integrity and immune function (Adeyinka et al. 2026).

Enteral feeding has a major physiological benefit owing to its ability to preserve the integrity and barrier coverage of the gut mucosal lining, without bacterial transmission or systemic infection. EN also helps gut-associated lymphoid tissue (GALT), which enhances immune response and minimizes inflammatory effects. The effects are particularly prominent in surgical patients who experience immunosuppression due to stress (Szefel et al. 2015). Figure 4.2 outlines the surgical

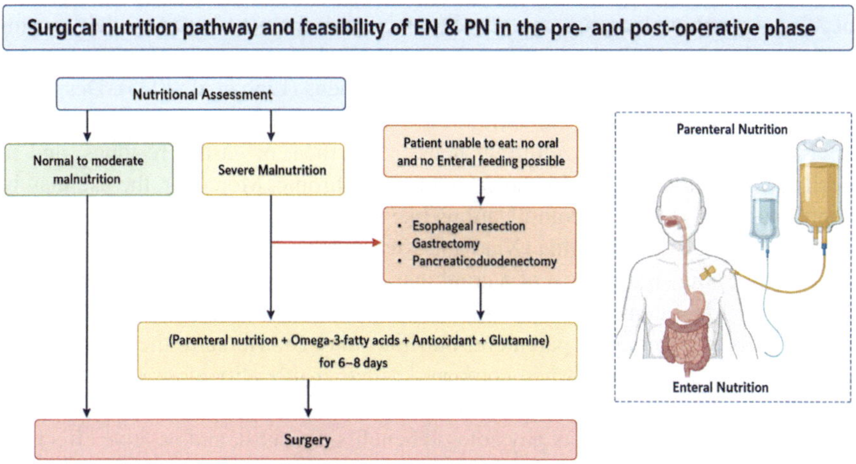

Fig. 4.2 Surgical nutrition pathway and feasibility of EN and PN in surgery. (Created by author using MS PowerPoint 2021)

nutrition pathway, emphasizing nutritional assessment and the selection of enteral or parenteral nutrition based on patient condition. It shows that parenteral nutrition is used when oral or enteral feeding is not feasible, especially in severe malnutrition or major surgeries. The goal is to optimize nutritional status before surgery to improve outcomes.

The implementation of early enteral nutrition (EEN) has currently become a novel form of treatment in the perioperative context, which can be provided as soon as 24–48 h post-surgery. Studies have shown that EEN enhances wound healing, reduces postoperative infections, and decreases issues like anastomotic leak and delayed stomach discharge. Additionally, EN has been reported to achieve shorter hospitalization and higher patient satisfaction in other surgical units as compared to parenteral nutrition (Shi et al. 2025).

The recent trends in research have been directed toward the timing, formulation, and administration of enteral nutrition. Among the significant advances is a contrast between continuous and intermittent feeding. Constant nutrition provides a steady source of nutrition and is applicable in critically ill/hemodynamically compromised patients, but intermittent nutrition is similar to normal physiological processes and can enhance gastrointestinal transit and metabolic homeostasis. Recent studies indicate that intermittent eating can reduce the risk of infection and improve the performance of the gut in some people (Zhou and Zhou 2025).

Another significant improvement is the use of immunonutrition and specific formulations. The benefits of nutritional preparations enriched with arginine, glutamine, and fatty acids like omega-3, and with nucleotides were promising regarding the reduction of postoperative complications and management of inflammation. These equations are highly applicable during cancer and huge gastrointestinal surgeries (Kaźmierczak-Siedlecka et al. 2020; Pannirselvam et al. 2025).

The belief in specialized enteral feeding is also gaining popularity. In the systems, to regulate the administration of calories and proteins, through the integration of AI and machine learning, systems like the reinforcement-based model learning are being developed. Such techniques have recorded a better survival and nutritional outcome compared to the already practiced regimens (Liao et al. 2025). Despite its benefits, enteral feeding has its limitations. One of them is feeding intolerance that is characterized by either vomiting, nausea, diarrhea, or gastric residues, and its occurrence varies between 50 and 60 when it is chronic. Moreover, the use may be contraindicated in case of complications like intestinal blockage, acute ischemia of the ileus, or high output fistula (Xiao and Xu 2023).

The emerging significance of a combination of enteral and parenteral treatment is also noted in recent studies. In all cases where EN is inadequate to meet nutritional needs, supplemental parenteral nutrition may contribute to the improvement of recovery and outcomes when compared to either modality alone (Papanikolaou et al. 2025). To sum up, enteral nutrition is still at the center of preoperative nutritional recovery because of its physiologic benefits, low cost, and positive effects on clinical outcomes. Recent research is dedicated to maximizing timing, dose, and altered feeding to enhance human safety and effectiveness in operative patients (Weng et al. 2025).

4.4.2 Parenteral Nutrition Support

Parenteral nutrition (PN) is the administration of nutrients, such as amino acids, glucose, lipids, electrolytes, vitamins, and trace minerals, bypassing the gastrointestinal tract. It is an important therapeutic method of perioperative treatment when enteral nutrition cannot be used or is insufficient to meet metabolic requirements (Hamdan and Puckett 2026). PN is required in patients with dysfunctional or inaccessible gastrointestinal tracts, which include severe malabsorption, intestinal obstruction, small bowel syndrome, or surgical ileus. It is also indicated to be used in extremely malnourished patients who cannot receive enteral nutrition, particularly in the preoperative phase, to improve nutritional status and surgical outcomes (Berlana 2022).

PN in the past has been associated with increased risks such as liver dysfunction, metabolic issues, and infections. Nevertheless, the developments in subsequent manufacturing processes, catheter care, and monitoring have led to immense improvement in its safety profile. To reduce the challenges, the latest PN practices incorporate close attention to metabolic monitoring, careful patient selection, and avoiding overfeeding (Arenas Villafranca et al. 2017). Studies on PN during perioperative situations are ongoing. By the existing standards, patients who cannot meet their nutritional requirements through enteral mechanisms must commence PN within 3–7 days. Whereas delayed PN is often best in healthy individuals to avoid such complications as hyperglycemia and infections, early PN could be beneficial in patients with severe malnutrition (Lakananurak and Gramlich 2020).

As a result of a comparative study of recent research, PN can be associated with elevated levels of issues in certain population groups, such as infections and metabolic issues, although it provides adequate nutritional intake at an equivalent level to EN. Nevertheless, the clinical setting, the present state of the patient, and the safety of PN usage influence these outcomes significantly (Wischmeyer et al. 2024). The idea of supplementary parenteral nutrition (SPN) is a major development in current perioperative nutrition. PN is not the option when the enteral feeding is shown to be unable to meet the calorie and protein needs; it is the alternative option to replace the enteral feeding. Studies show that this hybrid approach improves postoperative recovery and nutritional adequacy, especially in critically ill and high-risk surgical patients (Alsharif et al. 2020).

Another new area is the improvement of the PN formulations. One example of improvements is the use of lipid emulsions with the improvement of omega-3 fatty acids, which have anti-inflammatory properties and can contribute to the reduction of infections and hospitalization. Additionally, hyperglycemia, as one of the predictive factors of an adverse outcome, should be tightly controlled (glucose) during PN delivery (Haines et al. 2023). There is also a transformation in the way of providing PN due to technological innovations. High-tech infusion pump technology, computer prescription systems, and metabolic monitoring devices enable the creation of a more precise and individualized supply of nutrients. In order to be able to dynamically switch the PN regimens, research is looking into the possibility of adding biomarker and real-time metabolic information (Villena Gonzales et al. 2019).

PN is a process that risks doing its part despite its usefulness, such as bloodstream infections related to the use of the catheter, electrolyte alterations, and hepatic problems such as cholestasis or steatosis. These hazards need to be mitigated using strict aseptic care, frequent observation, and multidisciplinary care involving doctors, intensivists, and nutritionists (Park et al. 2025). Scientifically, the parenteral vs enteral feeding debate is emerging as a more sophisticated concept of the fact that the choice is complementary and not binary. Rather than promoting the need to conform to a single solution, the studies are starting to focus on individualized treatment depending on the factors of health, the fears associated with the operation, and the susceptibility to becoming fat or skinny, among other things (Park et al. 2025).

In this context, parenteral nutrition is an essential aspect of the nutritional rehabilitation in a perioperative process, such as in patients who are unable to experience enteral nutrition. Its use as secondary treatment has changed due to the advancement of standard practice and research; it has become a tactical part of the individualized nutrition treatment that is frequently, but not always, combined with enteral nutrition in a manner that should allow obtaining the most particular benefits. Table 4.3 explains the comparison of enteral vs parenteral nutrition support.

Table 4.3 Comparison table of enteral vs parenteral nutrition support

Feature	Enteral nutrition (EN)	Parenteral nutrition (PN)
Definition	Nutrients delivered through the GI tract (McClave et al. 2016)	Nutrients delivered intravenously (Singer et al. 2019)
Route of administration	Oral, NG, NJ, gastrostomy, jejunostomy (Weimann et al. 2017)	Peripheral or central venous catheter (Singer et al. 2019)
Physiological basis	Uses natural digestion & absorption (Weimann et al. 2017)	Direct delivery into the bloodstream (Singer et al. 2019)
Indication	Functional GI tract (McClave et al. 2016)	Non-functional GI tract (Singer et al. 2019)
Examples of use	ICU, postoperative, cancer patients (Weimann et al. 2017)	Ileus, obstruction, malabsorption (Singer et al. 2019)
Timing in surgery	Early (24–48 h) preferred (Weimann et al. 2017)	After 3–7 days, if EN is not feasible (McClave et al. 2016)
Effect on gut integrity	Maintains mucosa, prevents translocation (McClave et al. 2016)	May cause mucosal atrophy (Singer et al. 2019)
Immune function	Supports gut immunity (Calder 2020)	No direct immune benefit (Casaer and Van den Berghe 2014)
Risk of infection	Lower risk (Weimann et al. 2017)	Higher (catheter infections) (Casaer and Van den Berghe 2014)

(Continued)

Table 4.3 (Continued)

Feature	Enteral nutrition (EN)	Parenteral nutrition (PN)
Metabolic complications	Mild (diarrhea, intolerance) (McClave et al. 2016)	Higher (hyperglycemia, liver dysfunction) (Singer et al. 2019)
Cost	Economical (Weimann et al. 2017)	Expensive (Singer et al. 2019)
Ease of use	Relatively simple (McClave et al. 2016)	Requires expertise (Singer et al. 2019)
Tolerance issues	GI intolerance possible (McClave et al. 2016)	Better metabolic tolerance if monitored (Singer et al. 2019)
Special formulations	Immunonutrition (arginine, omega-3) (Calder 2020; Pannirselvam et al. 2025)	Customized PN admixtures (Singer et al. 2019)
Recent trends	Early feeding, personalization (Weimann et al. 2017)	Supplemental PN, AI-based delivery (Singer et al. 2019)
Combination approach	EN first-line (McClave et al. 2016)	SPN if EN insufficient (Singer et al. 2019)
Clinical outcomes	↓ infection, ↓ hospital stay (Weimann et al. 2017)	Useful in critical cases (Casaer and Van den Berghe 2014)
Contraindications	Ileus, obstruction (McClave et al. 2016)	Severe instability (relative) (Singer et al. 2019)

4.5 Multidisciplinary Approach in Perioperative Nutrition

The orientation of surgical practice has changed drastically, moving from technical success to optimal physiology. Indeed, within this development, the multidisciplinary approach towards perioperative nutrition has become a crucial element of high-level care. Unlike the former perception of nutritional therapy as a supplementary measure, today it is considered as a key factor influencing the modulation of a patient's physiological state in the period following the surgery (Weimann et al. 2021).

Specifically, the stress associated with surgery affects a patient through numerous metabolic disturbances, such as systemic inflammation, release of catecholamines, and insulin resistance. This results in the depletion of skeletal muscle tissue and weakened immunity, which is strongly linked to the risk of developing various complications and associated adverse outcomes, including prolonged hospital stay and mortality (Ljungqvist et al. 2017). To address this "storm of metabolism," there is a need for coordinated actions that go beyond individual specialists' expertise. A multidisciplinary team consists of members who represent various disciplines, such as surgery, anesthesia, dietary therapy, and nursing, and whose actions are based on providing a "continuum of care" starting from the first appointment until a patient achieves complete functional restoration (Martínez-Ortega et al. 2022).

With the fragmentation of traditional boundaries of hospital care addressed through the multi-drug therapy, the approach guarantees that nutritional screening is conducted universally, and the measures taken are preventive and not reactive. The following section outlines the duties of such healthcare workers and the strict monitoring mechanisms required for achieving nutritional objectives.

4.5.1 Role of Healthcare Professionals

As stated above, perioperative nutritional rehabilitation involves an interdisciplinary teamwork effort. Every healthcare discipline plays an important role in achieving the nutritional aims of surgery, which are evidence-based and focused on fulfilling the unique metabolic requirements of the patient (Martínez-Ortega et al. 2022). Figure 4.3 illustrates the multidisciplinary perioperative medical team involved in patient care, including surgeons, doctors, dietitians, microbiologists, and laboratory staff. It highlights collaborative efforts in monitoring, treatment, and nutritional management. Such teamwork ensures comprehensive care and improved surgical outcomes.

The Surgeons

Surgeons frequently play the role of the "team captain" in the early phases of the perioperative period. Their main task is the early detection of nutritional risks. It is recommended that nutritional screening be conducted at the patient's first visit to the hospital several weeks before surgery (Gillis and Wischmeyer 2019).

It is the clinical opinion of the surgeon that determines the timing of the surgery. In cases where patients have been marked as having severe nutritional risk, i.e., losing more than 10% of their weight in the last 6 months, a BMI of less than 18.5 kg/m^2, or serum albumin levels of less than 3.0 g/dL, the surgeon must delay the procedure for 7–14 days (Weimann et al. 2021). Additionally, surgeons' choices in the operating room, including placing feeding on patients with high-risk upper gastrointestinal conditions, determine the feasibility of early enteral feeding after surgery (Gianotti et al. 2018).

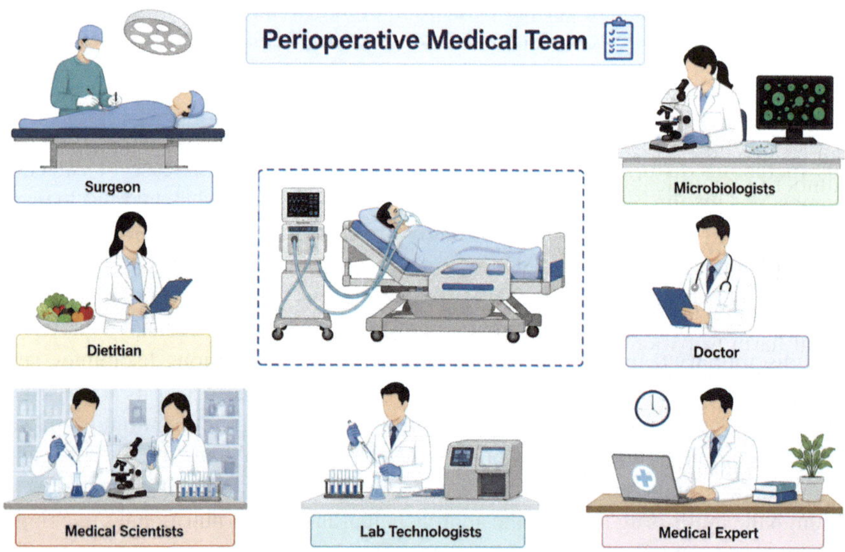

Fig. 4.3 The role of healthcare professionals in higher-risk patients. (Created using PowerPoint 2021)

The Clinical Dietitian

The key technical specialist for medical nutritional therapy will be the dietitian. While the responsibility for risk detection falls on the surgeon, the task of making an in-depth assessment to create a highly personalized nutritional plan lies with the dietitian. Calorie and protein needs in patients are determined based on validated techniques, such as the Subjective Global Assessment (SGA) or the Nutritional Risk Screening 2002 (NRS-2002) (Ljungqvist et al. 2017).

An important task assigned to the dietitian as part of the MDT is handling patients with "hidden" types of malnutrition, for instance, patients suffering from sarcopenic obesity. In these patients, a high BMI level hides a dramatic decrease in lean body mass, the primary cause of poor results after surgery (Prado, et al., 2020; Pedersen et al. 2017). It is the dietitian who determines the form (oral, enteral, parenteral), and, importantly, the content of the diet that will include arginine, omega-3 fatty acids, and nucleotides to reduce inflammation (Wischmeyer et al. 2018).

The Anesthesiologists

The participation of the anesthesiologist in the nutritional MDT team has been transformed entirely through the adoption of the ERAS (Enhanced Recovery After Surgery) process. The major goal of the anesthesiologist in this context is that of controlling the metabolic stress of surgery and preventing insulin resistance within the patient (Martínez-Ortega et al. 2022; Jain et al. 2023).

The anesthesiologist assists in the "carbohydrate loading" of the patient. They encourage the consumption of carbohydrate drinks 2 h before the initiation of anesthesia in order to move the patient out of a state of metabolism focused on fat burning into one that encourages protein synthesis (Gillis and Wischmeyer 2019). Furthermore, through the use of opioids in anesthesia and effective fluid management, the anesthesiologists work to prevent gut edema and ileus, thus "clearing the way" for early oral intake (Ljungqvist et al. 2017).

The Nursing Staff

Nurses are responsible for the implementation of the MDT nutrition intervention protocol. Since nurses are at the bedside throughout the day and night, they can monitor how much the patients actually consume compared to what they should consume. Nurses are also the ones who can detect gastrointestinal intolerance issues, like nausea and distension, that would call for a modification in the nutrition regimen. Apart from providing clinical assistance to patients, nurses will also act as the educators of patients and their families. Nurses can offer the emotional support needed to motivate patients to start moving and eating. Nurses will also handle all the technical requirements for enteral and parenteral feeding systems. According to literature, nursing-driven nutritional protocols can significantly reduce the occurrence of post-operative infection (Teixeira et al. 2025; Serin and Şanlıer 2018).

4.5.2 Monitoring and Follow-Up

The continuous assessment of nutritional status enhances recovery and patient outcomes. The perioperative nutritional process is a continuous process that calls for close monitoring at three different stages: acute inpatient monitoring, transitional monitoring, and outpatient rehabilitation.

Acute Inpatient Monitoring

During the initial phase following surgery, the team's goal is to safely increase nutritional intake. In terms of monitoring, the focus is on metabolic balance and tolerance of the alimentary tract. An important issue, especially for those who are severely undernourished, is the management of refeeding syndrome. This is a condition in which electrolyte imbalances, such as phosphate, potassium, and magnesium, occur due to the transition from catabolism to anabolism (Weimann et al. 2021). The electrolytes must be measured daily when feeding high-risk patients.

Moreover, the MDT should track the effectiveness of the treatment regimen. Although the serum albumin test can be applied, it is affected by inflammation and changes in fluid balance. The better assessment would come from the prealbumin level and other clinical parameters, like resuming gut activity and increased muscle tone (Martínez-Ortega et al. 2022).

Transitional and Post-Discharge Monitoring

The post-discharge phase is often associated with a "nutrition gap," as individuals experience difficulties providing themselves with sufficient nutrition, especially because of their fatigue, changed appetite, and the side effects of the medications prescribed to them. According to Gillis and Wischmeyer 2019, patients undergoing major surgeries are likely to lose considerable amounts of weight during the first 30 days after discharge. A solution to this involves scheduling proper follow-up procedures. Most patients are advised to take oral nutritional supplements (ONS) after being discharged from the hospital for 4–8 weeks, as a way of ensuring that there is closure in terms of filling the gap in their nutritional requirements. Body mass monitoring, wound healing progression, and functional assessments can be conducted in the process using indicators such as six minutes' walk or handgrip strength (Pedersen et al. 2017).

Long-Term Rehabilitation and Quality of Life Improvements

In patients who undergo major surgery such as gastrectomies and esophagectomies, lifelong monitoring of nutrition becomes necessary because these patients remain vulnerable to nutrient deficiency problems involving vitamins B12, iron, and calcium deficiency due to poor absorption (Gianotti et al. 2018). Lifelong monitoring helps ensure that the results of the surgery improve the QoL of the patient. Ensuring a continuous cycle of assessment and treatment allows for the prevention of chronic cachexia development and the ability to withstand other treatments, such as chemo or radiation, in the future.

4.6 Conclusion

Perioperative nutritional assessment and rehabilitation are vital for improving surgical outcomes and minimizing postoperative complications. Surgical procedures trigger metabolic stress, increasing nutritional requirements and potentially worsening existing malnutrition. Early identification of patients at nutritional risk is therefore essential. Using validated screening and assessment tools helps clinicians evaluate nutritional status and identify deficiencies accurately. Poor nutrition can impair wound healing, weaken immune response, and delay recovery. To address this, individualized nutritional plans should be developed, including dietary advice, oral supplements, and, when necessary, enteral or parenteral nutrition. A multidisciplinary team approach involving surgeons, dietitians, anesthesiologists, and nurses plays a key role in delivering effective care. By correcting nutritional deficits before surgery and ensuring continuous support throughout the perioperative period, patient recovery can be improved, hospital stays shortened, and complications reduced. Thus, integrating nutritional assessment and rehabilitation into standard perioperative care is essential for achieving better clinical outcomes.

References

Adeyinka A, Rouster AS, Valentine M. Enteral feeding. 2022 Dec 26. In: StatPearls [Internet]. Treasure Island (FL): StatPearls Publishing; 2026. PMID: 30422471. https://pubmed.ncbi.nlm.nih.gov/30422471/.

Alsharif DJ, Alsharif FJ, Aljuraiban GS, Abulmeaty MM. Effect of supplemental parenteral nutrition versus enteral nutrition alone on clinical outcomes in critically ill adult patients: a systematic review and meta-analysis of randomized controlled trials. Nutrients. 2020;12(10):2968. https://doi.org/10.3390/nu12102968.

Ambulkar R, Kunte A, Solanki SL, Thakkar V, Deshmukh B, Rana PS. Impact of prehabilitation in major gastrointestinal oncological surgery: a systematic review. J Gastrointest Cancer. 2025;56(1):133. https://doi.org/10.1007/s12029-025-01196-x.

Arenas Villafranca JJ, Nieto Guindo M, Álvaro Sanz E, Moreno Santamaria M, Garrido Siles M, Abilés J. Effects of cyclic parenteral nutrition on parenteral-associated liver dysfunction parameters. Nutr J. 2017;16(1):66. https://doi.org/10.1186/s12937-017-0289-7.

Barker LA, Gout BS, Crowe TC. Hospital malnutrition: prevalence, identification and impact on patients and the healthcare system. Int J Environ Res Public Health. 2011;8(2):514–27. https://doi.org/10.3390/ijerph8020514.

Berlana D. Parenteral nutrition overview. Nutrients. 2022;14(21):4480. https://doi.org/10.3390/nu14214480.

Bozzetti F. Perioperative nutrition of patients with gastrointestinal cancer. Br J Surg. 2002;89(10):1201–2. https://doi.org/10.1046/j.1365-2168.2002.02176.x.

Braunschweig CL, Levy P, Sheean PM, Wang X. Enteral compared with parenteral nutrition: a meta-analysis. Am J Clin Nutr. 2001;74(4):534–42. https://doi.org/10.1093/ajcn/74.4.534.

Calder PC. Nutrition, immunity and COVID-19. BMJ Nutr Prev Health. 2020;3(1):74. https://doi.org/10.1136/bmjnph-2020-000085.

Casaer MP, Van den Berghe G. Nutrition in the acute phase of critical illness. N Engl J Med. 2014;370(13):1227–36. https://doi.org/10.1056/nejmra1304623.

Cederholm T, Jensen GL, Correia MITD, Gonzalez MC, Fukushima R, Higashiguchi T, Barazzoni R, Blaauw R, Coats A, Crivelli A, Evans DC, Gramlich L, Fuchs-Tarlovsky V, Keller H, Llido

L, Malone A, Mogensen KM, Morley JE, Muscaritoli M, et al. GLIM criteria for the diagnosis of malnutrition: a consensus report. Clin Nutr. 2019;38(1):1–9. https://doi.org/10.1016/j.clnu.2018.08.002.

Chaudhary A, Reddy BR, Rao GV, Raveendran S, Mandal S, Radhakrishna P, Dhar P, Krishnamurthy A, Doctor N, Shaikh I, Deora A. Consensus-based recommendations for optimizing perioperative nutritional support and muscle health in major surgery in India. Front Nutr. 2025;12:1538161. https://doi.org/10.3389/fnut.2025.1538161.

Correia MITD, Waitzberg DL. The impact of malnutrition on morbidity, mortality, length of hospital stay and costs evaluated through a multivariate model analysis. Clin Nutr. 2016;35(2):247–52.

Cruz-Jentoft AJ, Bahat G, Bauer J, Boirie Y, Bruyère O, Cederholm T, Cooper C, Landi F, Rolland Y, Sayer AA, Schneider SM, Sieber CC, Topinková E, Vandewoude M, Visser M. Sarcopenia: revised European consensus on definition and diagnosis. Age Ageing. 2019a;48(1):16–31. https://doi.org/10.1093/ageing/afy169.

Cruz-Jentoft AJ, Bahat G, Bauer J, Boirie Y, Bruyère O, Cederholm T, et al. Sarcopenia: revised European consensus on definition and diagnosis. Age Ageing. 2019b;48(1):16–31. https://doi.org/10.1093/ageing/afy169.

Debats IB, Wolfs TG, Gotoh T, Cleutjens JP, Peutz-Kootstra CJ, van der Hulst RR. Role of arginine in superficial wound healing in man. Nitric Oxide Biol Chem. 2009;21(3–4):175–83. https://doi.org/10.1016/j.niox.2009.07.006.

Deutz NEP, Bauer JM, Barazzoni R, Biolo G, Boirie Y, Bosy-Westphal A, Cederholm T, Cruz-Jentoft A, Krznariç Z, Nair KS, Singer P, Calder PC. Protein intake and exercise for optimal muscle function with aging: recommendations from the ESPEN Expert Group. Clin Nutr. 2014;33(6):929–36. https://doi.org/10.1016/j.clnu.2014.04.007.

Fearon K, Arends J, Baracos V. Understanding the mechanisms and treatment options in cancer cachexia. Lancet Oncol. 2016;17(2):e72–83. https://doi.org/10.1016/S1470-2045(15)00542-6.

Garth AK, Newsome CM, Simmance N, Crowe TC. Nutritional status, nutrition practices and postoperative complications in patients undergoing gastrointestinal surgery. J Parenter Enter Nutr. 2019;43(1):83–90. https://doi.org/10.1002/jpen.1454.

Gianotti L, Besselink MG, Sandini M, Hackert T, Conlon K, Gerritsen A, Griffin O, Fingerhut A, Probst P, Abu Hilal M, Marchegiani G, Nappo G, Zerbi A, Amodio A, Perinel J, Adham M, Raimondo M, Asbun HJ, Sato A, Takaori K, et al. Nutritional support and therapy in pancreatic surgery: a position paper of the International Study Group on Pancreatic Surgery (ISGPS). Surgery. 2018;164(5):1035–48. https://doi.org/10.1016/j.surg.2018.05.040.

Gillis C, Wischmeyer PE. Pre-operative nutrition and the elective surgical patient: why, how and what? Anaesthesia. 2019;74(Suppl 1):27–35. https://doi.org/10.1111/anae.14506.

Groh-Wargo S, Barr SM. Parenteral nutrition. Clin Perinatol. 2022;49(2):355–79. https://doi.org/10.1016/j.clp.2022.02.002.

Haines K, Grisel B, Gorenshtein L, Wischmeyer PE. Lipid emulsions in parenteral nutrition: does it matter? Curr Opin Crit Care. 2023;29(4):293–9. https://doi.org/10.1097/MCC.0000000000001058.

Hamdan M, Puckett Y. Total parenteral nutrition. 2023 Jul 4. In: StatPearls [Internet]. Treasure Island (FL): StatPearls Publishing; 2026. PMID: 32644462. https://www.ncbi.nlm.nih.gov/books/NBK559036/.

Helminen H, Raitanen M, Kellosalo J. Immunonutrition in elective gastrointestinal surgery patients. Scand J Surg. 2007;96(1):46–50. https://doi.org/10.1177/145749690709600109.

Jain SN, Lamture Y, Krishna M. Enhanced recovery after surgery: exploring the advances and strategies. Cureus. 2023;15(10):e47237. https://doi.org/10.7759/cureus.47237.

Kaźmierczak-Siedlecka K, Daca A, Folwarski M, Makarewicz W, Lebiedzińska A. Immunonutritional support as an important part of multidisciplinary anti-cancer therapy. Central Eur J Immunol. 2020;45(4):454–60. https://doi.org/10.5114/ceji.2020.103339.

Kutnik P, Wichowska O, Sysiak-Sławecka J, Szczukocka M, Rypulak E, Piwowarczyk P, Borys M, Czuczwar M. Malnutrition risk in elective surgery patients and effectiveness of preoperative nutritional interventions at a pre-anaesthetic clinic: a 4-year apart, single-centre, obser-

vational study. Anaesthesiol Intensive Ther. 2023;55(3):179–85. https://doi.org/10.5114/ait.2023.130632.
Lakananurak N, Gramlich L. The role of preoperative parenteral nutrition. Nutrients. 2020;12(5):1320. https://doi.org/10.3390/nu12051320.
Li J, Xiang QL, Zhu JX, Zhang YX, Li SQ. Comparison of enteral immunonutrition and enteral nutrition in patients undergoing gastric cancer surgery: a systematic review and meta-analysis of randomized, controlled trials. J Int Med Res. 2024;52(1):03000605231220870. https://doi.org/10.1177/03000605231220870.
Liao X, Li C, Liu Q, Xia W, Liu Z, Zhu J, et al. Machine learning-based predictive model for enteral nutrition-associated diarrhea in ICU patients and its nursing applications. Front Nutr. 2025;12:1584717. https://doi.org/10.3389/fnut.2025.1584717.
Ljungqvist O, Scott M, Fearon KC. Enhanced recovery after surgery: a review. JAMA Surg. 2017;152(3):292–8. https://doi.org/10.1001/jamasurg.2016.4952.
Martínez-Ortega AJ, Piñar-Gutiérrez A, Serrano-Aguayo P, González-Navarro I, Remón-Ruíz PJ, Pereira-Cunill JL, García-Luna PP. Perioperative nutritional support: a review of current literature. Nutrients. 2022;14(8):1601. https://doi.org/10.3390/nu14081601.
McClave SA, Taylor BE, Martindale RG, Warren MM, Johnson DR, Braunschweig C, et al. Guidelines for the provision and assessment of nutrition support therapy in the adult critically ill patient: Society of Critical Care Medicine (SCCM) and American Society for Parenteral and Enteral Nutrition (ASPEN). JPEN J Parenter Enteral Nutr. 2016;40(2):159–211. https://doi.org/10.1177/0148607115621863.
Munoz N, Posthauer ME, Cereda E, Schols JMGA, Haesler E. The role of nutrition for pressure injury prevention and healing: the 2019 international clinical practice guideline recommendations. Adv Skin Wound Care. 2020;33(3):123–36. https://doi.org/10.1097/01.ASW.0000653144.90739.ad.
Norman K, Haß U, Pirlich M. Malnutrition in older adults—recent advances and remaining challenges. Clin Nutr. 2019;38(1):27–32. https://doi.org/10.1016/j.clnu.2018.08.008.
Pannirselvam M, Zakaria Z, Wong MP, Abdul Satar MHS, Jusoh NS, Zakaria AD, Othman MF. Effects of preoperative immunonutrition vs standard oral nutrition in patients undergoing colorectal surgery: a randomized controlled trial. World J Gastrointes Surg. 2025;17(9):108127. https://doi.org/10.4240/wjgs.v17.i9.108127.
Papanikolaou P, Theodoridis X, Papaemmanouil A, Papageorgiou NN, Tsankof A, Haidich AB, et al. Enteral nutrition versus a combination of enteral and parenteral nutrition in critically ill adult patients in the intensive care unit: an overview of systematic reviews and meta-analysis. J Clin Med. 2025;14(3):991. https://doi.org/10.3390/jcm14030991.
Park JW, Maeng SA, Kim SG, Kim YS, Yoo JJ. Parenteral nutrition-induced liver function complications: incidence, risk factors, and prognosis. J Clin Med. 2025;14(4):1220. https://doi.org/10.3390/jcm14041220.
Pedersen JL, Pedersen PU, Damsgaard EM. Nutritional follow-up after discharge prevents readmission to hospital-a randomized clinical trial. J Nutr Health Aging. 2017;21(1):75–82. https://doi.org/10.1007/s12603-016-0745-7.
Prado CM, Purcell SA, Laviano A. Nutrition interventions to treat low muscle mass in cancer. J Cachexia Sarcopenia Muscle. 2020;11(2):366–80. https://doi.org/10.1002/jcsm.12525.
Serin Y, Şanlıer N. Emotional eating, the factors that affect food intake, and basic approaches to nursing care of patients with eating disorders. J Psychiatr Nurs/Hemşireleri Derneği. 2018;9(2) https://doi.org/10.14744/phd.2018.23600.
Shenkin A. Serum prealbumin: is it a marker of nutritional status or of risk of malnutrition? Clin Nutr. 2016;35(5):1097–104. https://doi.org/10.1016/j.clnu.2015.06.010.
Shi B, Shen L, Xu Z, Yu B, Yang X, Yang H, Chen C. Early nurse-initiated enteral nutrition and its impact on postoperative recovery and complication rates: a meta-analysis of surgical patient outcomes. Front Nutr. 2025;12:1671718. https://doi.org/10.3389/fnut.2025.1671718.
Shim H, Cheong JH, Lee KY, Lee H, Lee JG, Noh SH. Perioperative nutritional status changes in gastrointestinal cancer patients. Yonsei Med J. 2013;54(6):1370–6. https://doi.org/10.3349/ymj.2013.54.6.1370.

Singer P, Blaser AR, Berger MM, Alhazzani W, Calder PC, Casaer MP, Hiesmayr M, Mayer K, Montejo JC, Pichard C, Preiser JC, van Zanten ARH, Oczkowski S, Szczeklik W, Bischoff SC. ESPEN guideline on clinical nutrition in the intensive care unit. Clin Nutr. 2019;38(1):48–79. https://doi.org/10.1016/j.clnu.2018.08.037.

Smith TW Jr, Wang X, Singer MA, Godellas CV, Vaince FT. Enhanced recovery after surgery: a clinical review of implementation across multiple surgical subspecialties. Am J Surg. 2020;219(3):530–4. https://doi.org/10.1016/j.amjsurg.2019.11.009.

Sowerbutts AM, et al. Preoperative nutrition support for patients undergoing gastrointestinal surgery. Cochrane Database Syst Rev. 2024; https://doi.org/10.1002/14651858.CD008879.pub3.

Szefel J, Kruszewski WJ, Buczek T. Enteral feeding and its impact on the gut immune system and intestinal mucosal barrier. Gastroenterol Rev/Przegląd Gastroenterologiczny. 2015;10(2):71–7. https://doi.org/10.5114/pg.2015.48997.

Teixeira J, Reis N, Chawłowska E, Rocha P, Czech-Szczapa B, Godinho AC, et al. Current approaches on nurse-performed interventions to prevent healthcare-acquired infections: an umbrella review. Microorganisms. 2025;13(2):463. https://doi.org/10.3390/microorganisms13020463.

Thompson FE, Subar AF. Dietary assessment methodology. Nutr Clin Pract. 2017;32(1):49–69. https://doi.org/10.1177/0884533617693285.

Villena Gonzales W, Mobashsher AT, Abbosh A. The progress of glucose monitoring—a review of invasive to minimally and non-invasive techniques, devices and sensors. Sensors. 2019;19(4):800. https://doi.org/10.3390/s19040800.

Weimann A, Braga M, Harsanyi L, Laviano A, Ljungqvist O, Soeters P, DGEM (German Society for Nutritional Medicine), Jauch KW, Kemen M, Hiesmayr JM, Horbach T, Kuse ER, Vestweber KH, ESPEN (European Society for Parenteral and Enteral Nutrition). ESPEN guidelines on enteral nutrition: surgery including organ transplantation. Clin Nutr (Edinburgh, Scotland). 2006;25(2):224–44. https://doi.org/10.1016/j.clnu.2006.01.015.

Weimann A, Braga M, Carli F, Higashiguchi T, Hübner M, Klek S, Laviano A, Ljungqvist O, Lobo DN, Martindale R, Waitzberg DL, Singer P. ESPEN guideline: clinical nutrition in surgery. Clin Nutr. 2017;36(3):623–50. https://doi.org/10.1016/j.clnu.2017.02.013.

Weimann A, Braga M, Carli F, Higashiguchi T, Hübner M, Klek S, Laviano A, Ljungqvist O, Lobo DN, Martindale RG, Waitzberg D, Bischoff SC, Singer P. ESPEN practical guideline: clinical nutrition in surgery. Clin Nutr (Edinburgh, Scotland). 2021;40(7):4745–61. https://doi.org/10.1016/j.clnu.2021.03.031.

Weng PH, Du Y, Yuan F. Early postoperative enteral nutrition and its impact on postoperative recovery in gastrointestinal tumor surgery. Front Oncol. 2025;15:1649306. https://doi.org/10.3389/fonc.2025.1649306.

White JV, Guenter P, Jensen G, Malone A, Schofield M. Consensus statement: characteristics recommended for the identification and documentation of adult malnutrition. J Parenter Enter Nutr. 2012;36(3):275–83. https://doi.org/10.1177/0148607112440285.

Wischmeyer PE, Carli F, Evans DC, Guilbert S, Kozar R, Pryor A, Thiele RH, Everett S, Grocott M, Gan TJ, Shaw AD, Thacker JKM, Miller TE, Hedrick TL, McEvoy MD, Mythen MG, Bergamaschi R, Gupta R, Holubar SD, Senagore AJ, et al. American Society for Enhanced Recovery and Perioperative Quality Initiative Joint Consensus Statement on nutrition screening and therapy within a surgical enhanced recovery pathway. Anesth Analg. 2018;126(6):1883–95. https://doi.org/10.1213/ANE.0000000000002743.

Wischmeyer PE, Klek S, Berger MM, Berlana D, Gray B, Ybarra J, Ayers P. Parenteral nutrition in clinical practice: international challenges and strategies. Am J Health Syst Pharm. 2024;81(Supplement_3):S89–S101. https://doi.org/10.1093/ajhp/zxae079.

Xiao Y, Xu L. Prevalence and risk factors of enteral feeding intolerance in critically ill patients and the effectiveness of preventive treatments: a prospective study. Saudi J Med Med Sci. 2023;11(2):135–42. https://doi.org/10.4103/sjmms.sjmms_384_22.

Xu J, Zhong Y, Jing D, Wu Z. Preoperative enteral immunonutrition improves postoperative outcome in patients with gastrointestinal cancer. World J Surg. 2006;30(7):1284–9. https://doi.org/10.1007/s00268-005-0756-8.

Zhou Z, Zhou J. Intermittent vs. continuous: a comparative narrative review of enteral and parenteral nutrition support strategies in the perioperative setting. Eur J Clin Nutr. 2025:1–6. https://doi.org/10.1038/s41430-025-01669-z.

Perioperative Fasting Guidelines and Metabolic Optimization

5

Mamta Sharma

Abstract

The management of perioperative fasting has undergone significant modification since the introduction of the enhanced recovery after surgery protocol, which uses scientifically backed methods aimed at reducing surgery-induced stress and enhancing postoperative results. The conventional practice that calls for long periods of fasting before surgery has been gradually superseded by modern guidelines based on physiological principles that allow patients to consume clear fluids within 2 h and solids within 6 h before undergoing anesthesia. This is backed by scientific literature showing increased patient satisfaction, decreased instances of dehydration, and prevention of perioperative insulin resistance without increasing the likelihood of pulmonary aspiration.

Apart from modified fasting times, the use of pre-operative carbohydrate loading is another essential procedure that is intended to maximize metabolic state, maintain lean muscle tissue, and improve post-operative recovery. The metabolic effects of prolonged fasting, such as elevated catabolic reactions and disturbances in glucose metabolism, highlight the necessity for updated fasting guidelines.

The chapter will give an extensive discussion on the physiological fundamentals of fasting, the historical development of guidelines regarding fasting, and contemporary ERAS recommendations. It will also examine the metabolic consequences of fasting, review the scientific literature on the risks of aspiration, and consider issues regarding the implementation of fasting strategies among various patient cohorts, particularly those at high risk.

In summary, optimized fasting techniques incorporated into ERAS pathways are an essential part of perioperative management that helps achieve better results from the perspective of medical, patient, and efficiency factors.

M. Sharma (✉)
Pt. B. D. Sharma University of Health Sciences, Rohtak, Haryana, India

P. K. Bhattacharyya et al. (eds.), *Integrated Anesthesia and Nutrition Approaches to Enhanced Recovery after Surgery*,
https://doi.org/10.1007/978-981-92-3294-9_5

Keywords

Preoperative fasting · Perioperative fasting · Fasting guidelines · Carbohydrate loading · Insulin resistance · Metabolic optimization · Pulmonary aspiration risk · Surgical stress response

5.1 Introduction

The perioperative practice has greatly evolved due to the implementation of ERAS Society protocols, which are designed using an evidence-based patient-centric approach to optimize surgical procedures and enhance recovery time (Ljungqvist et al. 2017). While there are several steps in the process that ERAS pathways encompass, preoperative fasting and nutritional care during perioperative periods are still critical aspects of treatment. In general, patients were told to fast from midnight before surgery. Even though such an approach used to be regarded as a reasonable way to manage surgical schedules, it often leads to unnecessary fasting times, especially when surgeries are performed in a busy setting (Panjiar et al. 2019).

It is evident that the practice of extended fasting does not offer any further benefits in preventing aspiration pneumonia in most patients. Rather, it brings about various unwanted physical and clinical responses (Gebremedhn and Nagaratnam 2014).

With the advancement of knowledge about the physiology of the stomach and the dynamic nature of stomach emptying, there is now a revolution in fasting guidelines. These new fasting guidelines have been formulated to strike a balance between the safety of patients and their comfort level as well as metabolic stability (Ljungqvist et al. 2017; Joshi et al. 2023).

In addition to adjusting the duration of fasting before surgery, the concept of metabolic optimization is given significant weight in ERAS guidelines. Specifically, preoperative carbohydrate loading has come to be recognized as an important way of preventing perioperative insulin resistance and depletion of glycogen reserves. This can prevent the metabolic stress response that would otherwise be triggered by surgery.

The existence of strong guidelines does not negate the prevalence of the old-fashioned methods of fasting in clinical practice. Inadequate awareness, organizational difficulties, and other factors often lead to failure to comply with the new guidelines. It proves once again the importance of following evidence-based guidelines of fasting among anesthesiologists and other medical professionals (Panjiar et al. 2019; Hamid 2014).

It is necessary to acknowledge that the approach to fasting cannot be universal for each patient. Fasting in individualized cases is vital for patients with diabetes mellitus, obesity, pregnancy, and other diseases characterized by delayed gastric emptying (Hausel et al. 2001; Bopp et al. 2011).

This chapter intends to cover all the aspects related to perioperative fasting from an ERAS standpoint such as the physiological background of fasting, development of fasting recommendations, metabolic consequences, risk of aspiration, and techniques to implement fasting.

5.2 Physiology of Fasting and Metabolic Response

Preoperative fasting (POF) has traditionally been considered a key part of the perioperative management process with the primary objective of reducing the incidence of pulmonary aspiration in patients undergoing anesthesia. The traditional approach, which has existed for more than a century, consists of preventing the consumption of solid and liquid food for a specific period before surgery (Joshi et al. 2023; Hamid 2014). Although widely used, the physiologic effects of preoperative fasting do not limit themselves to reducing gastric content, but include a wide range of metabolic and hormonal adjustments.

In terms of physiologic consequences, fasting triggers an energy-preserving metabolic adjustment in the body under fasting conditions. This response is achieved through the interaction between various hormones, such as insulin, glucagon, cortisol, and catecholamines, that contribute to the regulation of metabolism and energy levels (Ljungqvist et al. 2002; Carli 2015). However, it is noteworthy that the intensity and pattern of the response vary according to several factors, including the fasting period, nutrition, medical conditions, and age.

The fasting-induced metabolic changes within the perioperative setting also occur along with the stress responses related to the surgical procedure. These physiological responses are associated with sympathetic activity, and they include hormonal alterations that can lead to insulin resistance, increased protein breakdown, and the development of a catabolic state (Desborough 2000). It should be noted, however, that while these physiological trends are possible, they are not necessarily expected in all patients.

It is essential to comprehend these principles in order to ensure adequate perioperative care, where unnecessary or prolonged fasting may contribute to metabolic problems and negatively impact postoperative recovery. The metabolic changes are shown schematically in Fig. 5.1.

5.2.1 Metabolic Changes During Fasting

The absorptive stage is achieved after the intake of nutrients, in which the glucose produced from carbohydrates in food acts as the main source of energy. In this stage, there is a secretion of insulin to facilitate glucose uptake in peripheral tissue, formation of glycogen in the liver and muscles, and prevention of lipolysis and gluconeogenesis. This stage is defined as a catabolic process of energy production (Ljungqvist et al. 2002).

There is a shift towards the post-absorptive stage as soon as one starts fasting. The process happens after several hours when one stops eating. Endogenous glucose production takes place in order to maintain euglycemia; the process takes place

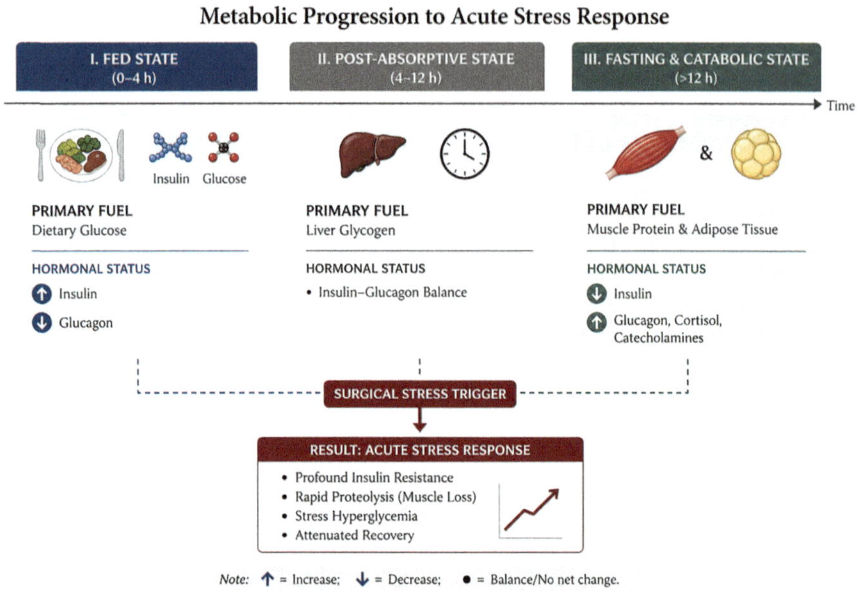

Fig. 5.1 Timeline of metabolic adaptation: from the absorptive phase to early starvation and the impact of surgical stress. (Created by author using draw.io (diagrams.net))

with glycogenolysis being the main process occurring in the liver. The shift from the absorptive stage to post absorptive is facilitated by a decrease in the level of insulin and increase in the levels of glucagon and catecholamines. But there are certain determinants that influence the stage, such as nutritional state, metabolic rate, recent diet, and other disorders (Gillis et al. 2015).

Further fasting leads to hepatic depletion of glycogen stores, with gluconeogenesis playing a dominant role in the regulation of blood glucose levels. It makes use of amino acids, lactate, and glycerol as substrates, pointing out the activation of endogenous energy stores. At the same time, there is a gradual shift to lipid metabolism in which fat cells undergo increased lipolysis, releasing fatty acids, which function as an energy source for peripheral cells. The breakdown of protein from muscle cells also occurs due to increased proteolysis, allowing amino acid utilization by gluconeogenesis (Desborough 2000; Puthucheary et al. 2013; Schricker & Lattermann 2015).

These metabolic changes, when viewed together, can be regarded as a physiological mechanism designed to achieve metabolic balance when nutrient intake is decreased. It should be noted that the extent, development, and manifestations of the described changes show a marked degree of variability between different patients. This fact is especially important when considering the influence of these mechanisms in the perioperative period, when patient age, body type, and preexisting medical conditions play a role in the process. Variability in metabolic responses to fasting can be seen in patients with various health problems, such as diabetes, obesity, malnutrition, or hormonal disorders.

Moreover, for a patient undergoing surgery, the process of metabolism during the fast usually goes hand-in-hand with the neuroendocrine stress response, increasing the level of insulin resistance, proteolysis, and metabolic catabolism (Desborough 2000).

Overall, even if such measures are physiologic adaptations that ensure energy homeostasis, the differences observed in their occurrence and interactions with perioperative stress illustrate the need for personalized fasting approaches. Clinical relevance of such changes will be further discussed in the next sections.

5.2.2 Neuroendocrine Response to Fasting

Fasting triggers a series of neuroendocrine responses designed to maintain metabolic stability in the face of no external nutrient supply. The neuroendocrine responses involve decreased levels of insulin in the blood with increased concentrations of counteracting hormones such as glucagon, cortisol, and catecholamines. The physiological processes that occur as a result of these hormone levels support the metabolic conversion from anabolism to catabolism in order to provide a constant source of energy substrates for the organs (Ljungqvist et al. 2002).

Insulin production inhibition in the fasting condition results in a decrease in glucose uptake in the periphery with the stimulation of glucose production in the liver via the breakdown of glycogen and gluconeogenesis. Increased glucagon concentrations cause glucose production, whereas catecholamines induce lipolysis and the release of fatty acids. In addition, cortisol promotes gluconeogenesis and proteolysis to regulate circulating glucose concentration, especially for glucose-dependent organs like the brain (Desborough 2000). This type of reaction constitutes a highly controlled biological adaptation, the degree of which is determined by variables including fasting time, nutritional condition, and metabolic differences between individuals.

The ability to control this neuroendocrine response has been shown to affect perioperative metabolism in both experimental and clinical settings.

Significantly, there is significant interindividual variation in the neuroendocrine response to fasting. Factors such as age, nutritional state prior to fasting, presence of co-morbid conditions like diabetes mellitus, and body composition play a role in how pronounced these changes can be. They can be accentuated in certain high-risk groups like the elderly, malnourished, and endocrinological/metabolic patients.

The significance of these changes in relation to clinical practice will be explored in the following sections.

5.2.3 Insulin Response and Glucose Regulation

As a result of perioperative fasting, there is a relative lowering of circulating insulin concentrations along with elevated levels of counter-regulatory hormones such as glucagon, cortisol, and catecholamines. Such changes lead to the disruption of glucose regulation due to decreased insulin-stimulated glucose transport into tissues and increased production of endogenous glucose mainly via glycogenolysis and gluconeogenesis in the liver (Ljungqvist et al. 2002).

It is worth mentioning that the changes in glucose regulation should not be considered in isolation from the overall response of the neuroendocrine system to fasting and surgical stress but rather as part of a wider process. It is associated with the effects of a complex network of hormones and inflammatory mediators that lead to lowered insulin sensitivity and elevated levels of glucose in circulation (Desborough 2000). Such metabolic changes occur as an adaptive mechanism designed to provide sufficient energy during conditions of physiological stress.

Physiologically, these adjustments facilitate the uninterrupted availability of glucose to important organs like the brain, which have a glucose demand that cannot be compromised. However, these adjustments are strictly controlled and dependent on several factors, including the metabolic state, degree of fasting, and level of surgical stress (Gillis et al. 2015).

According to evidence provided by clinical trials, perioperative glucose metabolism has been shown to greatly affect results. This includes results indicating that perioperative glucose administration leads to reduced insulin resistance after operations (Ljungqvist et al. 2017), and another where preoperative carbohydrate feeding leads to an improved insulin effect and metabolic response after surgery (Hausel et al. 2001).

The distinction between these initial adaptive mechanisms and the marked insulin resistance seen during long-term fasting and major stress situations, such as surgery, will be considered in further detail below. Understanding the mechanisms involved can help inform optimal metabolic management of patients undergoing surgeries under the ERAS pathway (Ljungqvist et al. 2017).

5.2.4 Fluid and Hemodynamic Changes

Fasting is linked to decreased oral intake of fluids, thus leading to some reduction in intravascular volume and hypovolemia. Though clinically insignificant in healthy persons, these parameters should be considered in a clinical setting, especially when considering the effect on perioperative management (Jacob and Chappell 2012).

In clinical practice, it has been shown that prolonged fasting results in increased sensitivity to changes in blood pressure following administration of anesthesia. Nonetheless, it is crucial to point out that perioperative hypotension is a phenomenon characterized by several predisposing conditions. These include, apart from effects caused by fasting, the mode of anesthesia administration, the use of vasoactive drugs, cardiovascular function, and bleeding (Desborough 2000; Carli 2015).

Physiologically speaking, small volumes of intravascular fluid loss could affect preload and cardiac output, especially in patients whose physiologic reserves are minimal. This is even more critical in vulnerable patient groups, such as elderly patients, patients with cardiac disease, or dehydrated patients. It is important to consider these issues when assessing patients preoperatively.

5.3 Evolution of Fasting Practices

There have been a number of changes in preoperative fasting, influenced by developments in the field of gastric physiology, anesthesia, and metabolism. The initial recommendations for fasting prior to surgery arose out of fear of pulmonary aspiration, which was first systematically documented by Curtis Lester Mendelson in 1946. These guidelines led to the implementation of the "nothing by mouth after midnight" strategy, which was seen as being effective enough to make sure that the stomach was empty before anesthesia induction (Mendelson 1946).

While widely accepted for many years, the traditional practice did not rely on scientific findings but only on assumptions. With time, some studies came to question the need for long periods of fasting, noting that the process of gastric clearance of liquids took less time than was initially presumed, meaning that fasting beyond a certain point did not offer any further advantage (Brady et al. 2003).

With the accumulating evidence, there began to be a move towards a more personalized and physiological approach to fasting. The importance of understanding the metabolic impact of long-term fasting and the significance of perioperative optimization for faster recovery was another factor that contributed to the shift. With this, modern approaches to perioperative management shifted from fixed fasting rules based on time to a more flexible, evidence-informed approach.

This would eventually lead to the formulation of current fasting recommendations within ERAS protocols and anesthesia associations, which will be presented in the next part of this paper.

5.3.1 Traditional Practice: "Nil Per Oral After Midnight"

The concept of recommending patients to be nil per oral (NPO) after midnight was common practice for many years without regard to the exact time when surgery was to be performed. The reason why this recommendation became popular was its simplicity, practicality, and safety, and this helped provide clear instructions for patients.

From a practical perspective, in busy surgical centers, it made little sense to consider the exact time when the patient is going to undergo the procedure because there was no way of knowing it at that point in time. Moreover, it seemed safer at that time to have clear fasting rules for every patient since there was not much knowledge about stomach function at that time (Brady et al. 2003).

The adherence to this method may also be explained by institutional inertia, along with disparities in the dissemination and uptake of newer scientific evidence.

Anesthesia practices surveys have found that fasting guidelines that are no longer current still prevail in several environments owing to various obstacles, including poor communications, logistics, and medical traditions (Panjiar et al. 2019; Gebremedhn and Nagaratnam 2014).

Another factor behind prolonged fasting was medicolegal and safety issues, which have been a key driving force behind restrictive fasting guidelines. The lack of sufficient evidence in favor of fasting for shorter periods led many practitioners to adopt a safer stance in order to minimize the dangers of aspiration.

In other words, the universal acceptance and continued use of the "NPO after midnight" protocol can be attributed to various practical, structural, and historical reasons, not scientific physiological necessity.

5.3.2 Transition to Evidence-Based Guidelines

The development of perioperative medicine has led to a rethinking of fasting traditions in accordance with new physiological and clinical data. Early research into gastric emptying revealed that clear liquids leave the stomach relatively quickly, usually within 1 to 2 h in healthy subjects, without substantially expanding its capacity and acid content during this period (Brady et al. 2003; Hausel et al. 2001). This information contradicted the established idea that prolonged periods of fasting were required for the stomach to become empty before anesthesia.

At the same time, knowledge of perioperative metabolism and the principles of patient-centered care emphasized the shortcomings of existing fasting protocols. Studies indicated that a more flexible approach to the consumption of liquids might be considered without posing any threat to patients' safety, if the right conditions were met (Ljungqvist et al. 2002; Carli 2015).

However, recent developments in diagnostic methods at the patient's bedside, such as gastric ultrasonography, have shed additional light on the nature of gastric content and volume within the preoperative period. The use of point-of-care gastric ultrasound allows for a real-time non-invasive evaluation of gastric emptying and residual volume, thus providing an objective way to assess the risk of aspiration. Studies show that point-of-care gastric ultrasound has been successfully used to identify individuals with delayed gastric emptying or unusual gastric content despite following traditional fasting protocols (Bataille et al. 2014; Andrew Charlesworth and Wiles 2019).

The accumulating evidence prompted professional societies, such as the American Society of Anesthesiologists and the Enhanced Recovery After Surgery (ERAS) Society, to develop new fasting guidelines. The resulting framework suggests replacing traditional universal restrictions on fasting duration with a more rigorous scheme where the length of the fasting period depends on the kind and nature of consumption rather than applying a single threshold (Joshi et al. 2023; Ljungqvist et al. 2017).

This transition marks an important move toward making perioperative fasting consistent with current research, which will serve as the foundation for future guidelines-based perioperative care. This topic is covered extensively in the following section.

5.3.3 Current Recommendations in Practice

Current pre-operative fasting guidelines have adopted a physiology and risk stratification approach, which is based on the shift from empiric and time-based fasting protocols to physiology-based protocols that consider the nature and composition of what has been taken orally. The guidelines are recognized and developed by leading professional organizations like the ASA and ERAS Society and have strong evidence support clinically and experimentally (Joshi et al. 2023; Ljungqvist et al. 2017; Dongare et al. 2020). Table 5.1 provides the minimum fasting periods of different types of intakes as per current international guidelines.

The guidelines pertain to elective procedures involving general anesthesia, regional anesthesia, or procedural sedation. They take into account an understanding of gastric physiology, risks of aspiration, and metabolism. It is crucial to note

Table 5.1 Summary of minimum preoperative fasting durations for healthy patients undergoing elective procedures

Intake modality	Fasting duration (h)	Gastric emptying dynamics (T1/2)	Physiological rationale and ERAS perspective	Clinical and pharmacological considerations
Clear fluids (water, clear juices, carbohydrate beverages)	2	~15–20 min	Rapid transit via first-order kinetics; preserves residual volume < 1.5 mL/kg, maintaining gastric pH > 2.5. Prevents dehydration and thirst	Patients with delayed gastric emptying (e.g., severe autonomic neuropathy) may require extended durations or point-of-care ultrasound (POCUS) assessment
Breast milk	4	~25–45 min	Contains higher lipid content than clear fluids but forms softer curds than formula, facilitating faster pyloric transit	Standard for pediatric and neonatal anesthesia protocols
Non-human milk/infant formula	6	~45–75 min	High casein and fat content form dense curds in the stomach, requiring mechanical degradation and prolonged acid exposure before duodenal transit	Equivalent to a light solid meal in terms of aspiration risk profile

(Continued)

Table 5.1 (Continued)

Intake modality	Fasting duration (h)	Gastric emptying dynamics (T1/2)	Physiological rationale and ERAS perspective	Clinical and pharmacological considerations
Light meal (toast, clear tea/coffee)	6	~60–90 min	Predominantly carbohydrate-based with minimal fat content. Triggers biphasic gastric emptying	Prolongation recommended if patient is concurrently prescribed GLP-1 agonists or opioids
Heavy/fatty meal (meat, fried foods)	≥8	>120 min	Triggers cholecystokinin (CCK) release, suppressing gastric motility. Digestion requires extensive emulsification and antral grinding	Duration must be individually tailored based on total caloric load and lipid density; elevated risk of particulate aspiration

that these are minimal fasting times and not hard-and-fast guidelines that must be followed in all cases.

5.3.3.1 Clear Fluids: Gastric Physiology and Clinical Evidence

The advice for clear fluid consumption up to 2 h before anesthesia is backed up by a wealth of evidence that highlights the quick clearance rate of gastric contents. Research using scintigraphy and acetaminophen absorption methods has revealed that clear fluids leave the stomach within roughly 90–120 min in healthy individuals (Brady et al. 2003; Hausel et al. 2001).

Importantly, random clinical studies and systematic reviews have found that consuming clear fluids in this period does not result in an increase in gastric contents' volume or acidity, which are the major risk factors associated with aspiration-induced lung damage (Brady et al. 2003). This discovery contradicts the previous belief that longer periods of fasting provide extra safety.

Carbohydrate-containing clear fluids constitute a distinct category within this classification and have been adopted by ERAS guidelines for metabolic optimization to minimize insulin resistance during surgery. It is important to note that their utilization entails formulation standardization and proper patient selection, especially among those with decreased gastrointestinal motility. The topic has been extensively analyzed under the chapter on metabolic optimization (Ljungqvist et al. 2017; Ljungqvist and Jonathan 2012).

5.3.3.2 Solid Food: Composition-Dependent Gastric Emptying

In contrast to liquid diets, gastric emptying of solid food is greatly influenced by the nature of macronutrients, caloric density, and food consistency. Meals that are light and consist of easily digestible foods display gastric emptying in a predictable fashion, and therefore, 6 h can be considered as the fasting period (Joshi et al. 2023).

On the contrary, fatty and high-protein meals delay gastric emptying through hormonal control, such as cholecystokinin-induced inhibition of gastric function, requiring more fasting periods of up to 8 h. In summary, it is necessary to differentiate meals because fasting duration cannot be applied uniformly.

There have been concerns raised regarding the reliability of patients' recall of their diet history and the associated inaccuracies in defining whether meals were light or heavy. For instance, Panjiar et al. (2019) found inconsistencies among patients' descriptions of light and heavy meals (Panjiar et al. 2019).

5.3.3.3 Individualization of Fasting Practices: A Risk-Stratified Approach

Although standardized recommendations ensure safety, today's perioperative care focuses on developing personalized fasting approaches depending on individual and procedure-related factors. The process of gastric emptying depends on numerous parameters, including age, metabolic condition, autonomic nervous system regulation, medication intake, and presence of underlying diseases.

That is why personalized medicine encourages using risk stratification, combining the fasting history, physical evaluation of a patient, and additional diagnostic techniques when necessary, such as gastric ultrasonography at the point of care. This approach corresponds to the general ERAS philosophy emphasizing personalized perioperative treatment (Carli 2015; Ljungqvist et al. 2017).

5.3.3.4 Special Populations: Physiological and Clinical Considerations

Pediatric Patients

Pediatric patients have unique metabolism and physiology, which include a higher metabolic rate and reduced glycogen stores. As such, they are more prone to experiencing hypoglycemia and dehydration when fasting for a long time. Based on evidence, fasting time should be shorter with clear fluids until 2 h before anesthesia, breast milk up to 4 h before, and solids up to 6 h before anesthesia (Joshi et al. 2023). Liberal fasting practices among pediatric patients provide more comfort without posing the risk of aspiration.

Pregnant Patients

Physiological changes seen during pregnancy include the lowering of the tone of the lower esophageal sphincter and the increase in abdominal pressure that predisposes one to GERD. Nonetheless, gastric emptying is not affected in normal uncomplicated pregnancies, and therefore fasting recommendations apply. On the contrary, emergency obstetric patients have the "full stomach" principle applied to them with relevant airway precautions (Mendelson 1946; Eichelsbacher et al. 2018).

Patients with Diabetes Mellitus

Diabetic mellitus is linked with autonomic neuropathy and gastroparesis, causing erratic gastric evacuation and aspiration danger. Moreover, intraoperative glucose variations make the need for meticulous timing of fasting, insulin administration, and metabolic surveillance indispensable. The latest research has shown worries about GLP-1 receptor agonists that can cause delays in gastric evacuation (van Zuylen et al. 2024).

Obese Patients

Obesity has conventionally been viewed as one of the factors that raise the likelihood of aspirations, but research now demonstrates that obesity is not necessarily an independent risk factor that necessitates fasting for long periods. Investigations involving obese subjects have demonstrated results similar to those seen among non-obese patients under normal fasting guidelines (Harter et al. 1998). However, it is important to conduct individual assessments, especially in cases where there are other coexisting conditions like sleep apnea or reflux disorders.

Other High-Risk Conditions

Such cases include conditions like gastrointestinal obstruction, severe GERD, and delayed gastric emptying, among others. In such instances, fasting time alone is inadequate, and an in-depth assessment of the patient is required.

5.3.4 ERAS Perspective, Safety Considerations, and Individualization

Fasting is considered one of the aspects of perioperative care that is modifiable as part of the Enhanced Recovery After Surgery (ERAS) pathway and stresses the need to tailor fasting according to physiological principles. ERAS pathways encourage the development of fasting procedures not only as an aspect of restrictive management but also within the context of broader perioperative management approaches (Ljungqvist et al. 2017; Gillis et al. 2015).

One of the major concerns regarding liberalized perioperative fasting is the risk of pulmonary aspiration. It was traditionally believed that long periods of fasting lower the risk of aspiration; however, recent research showed that drinking clear fluids up until 2 h prior to surgery would not cause an increased risk of aspiration among properly chosen candidates for elective surgeries (Brady et al. 2003; Joshi et al. 2023).

It is vital that fasting advice be tailored and not provided generically to all patients. Personalized care is required since various individual and procedure-specific variables impact gastric emptying and the aspiration risk. The following situations require consideration when designing a fasting protocol for patients with poorly regulated diabetes mellitus, gastroesophageal reflux disease, pregnancy, or any condition that causes delayed gastric emptying (van Zuylen et al. 2024; Eichelsbacher et al. 2018).

When it comes to obesity, it is crucial to take a careful approach. Obesity was previously regarded as a possible risk factor for aspiration; however, there is no current scientific evidence to suggest that it warrants an extended fasting time independently. Comorbid diseases, like diabetes or gastroesophageal reflux, must be taken into account rather than BMI (Harter et al. 1998; Joshi et al. 2023).

Apart from the patient-related factors, decision-making during perioperative management must consider the nature of the surgical procedure, the anesthesia procedure, and the hospital policy. Newer technologies like bedside gastric ultrasound can also help to determine personalized risks in certain patients, especially if the status of fasting is questionable, or if the guidelines do not directly apply (Bataille et al. 2014; Charlesworth and Wiles 2019).

Generally, the ERAS approach underscores that proper fasting practices necessitate a balance between standardized evidence-based guidelines and personalized considerations in order to prioritize patient safety without any unnecessary deviation from the set guidelines.

5.3.5 Implementation Challenges and Transition to Clinical Application

However, although evidence-based fasting guidelines are available, variations in their application are still observed. Various issues, such as organizational policies, communication between perioperative care teams, and the issue of patients' safety, play an important role in implementing fasting guidelines (Panjiar et al. 2019; Gebremedhn and Nagaratnam 2014).

To enhance compliance with fasting recommendations, many organizations and institutions apply structured interventions, which involve multidisciplinary participation in the process of developing standardized fasting guidelines, training healthcare professionals, and fostering open communication within the perioperative setting. Anesthesia personnel play an important role in the process of educating and guiding patients regarding fasting protocols (Joshi et al. 2023; Lee et al. 2003).

Clinically speaking, the implementation of contemporary fasting guidelines in practice is an indication of a paradigm shift toward personalized and physiologically oriented perioperative management. Yet, the successful implementation of such recommendations entails the convergence of scientific knowledge, institutional processes, and personal patient factors. Such considerations highlight the need to transition from guidelines to implementation, which will be discussed in the following section.

5.4 Aspiration Risk and Patient Safety

Inhalation of stomach acid is a prevalent issue in anesthesia, as it can lead to complications that may prove fatal to patients. Even though the risk of the complication is relatively rare, the conditions that result from the process range from acute lung injury to respiratory failure and, in the worst-case scenarios, death (Mendelson 1946).

The reason for aspiration is that when a person undergoes general anesthesia or deep sedation, their body is unable to protect itself against inhalation of oropharyngeal and gastric content. Unlike in the past, modern research recognizes the cause of the issue as multifaceted and involving various factors such as patient-related ones, procedural factors, and perioperative management techniques (Eichelsbacher et al. 2018; Kosutova and Mikolka 2021).

The rationale behind fasting is based on the notion of minimizing the amount of contents in the stomach and their acidity in order to avoid the possibility of aspiration. Although this concept still has clinical significance, current data suggest that fasting time cannot be considered an indicator of the amount of gastric contents, as well as the likelihood of aspiration due to many factors influencing the process (Brady et al. 2003; Harter et al. 1998). Therefore, modern perioperative management implies an individualized and risk-based approach to the procedure, including the assessment of risks before the surgery, recognition of high-risk situations, and airway management.

5.4.1 Pathophysiology of Aspiration

Pulmonary aspiration refers to the introduction of gastric or oropharyngeal secretions into the lower airways and subsequent pulmonary damage that is dependent upon the composition of the aspirated material. Aspiration triggers a pathophysiological reaction, which is dependent upon the chemical nature of the aspirant, the quantity, and the burden of pathogens. It is also influenced by host defense mechanisms (Eichelsbacher et al. 2018; Kosutova and Mikolka 2021).

Aspiration pneumonitis is another type of lung injury that results from the inhalation of sterile gastric contents. Gastric juice, due to its acidity, damages the epithelium lining the bronchi and alveoli, causing an increase in capillary permeability and pulmonary edema. The condition also triggers an inflammatory response, which is driven by cytokines. The intensity of lung injury from this disease is directly related to the acidity of the aspirate and the quantity inhaled (Mendelson 1946; Kosutova and Mikolka 2021).

Aspiration pneumonia, in turn, is an infectious condition caused by the inhalation of bacteria-laden secretions from the oropharynx. The occurrence of this type of pneumonia is influenced by various parameters, such as the number of microorganisms, frequency of aspiration, and efficacy of the host defense mechanisms, including mucociliary clearance and immunity (Eichelsbacher et al. 2018).

Despite the differences in their pathogenesis, aspiration can occur concurrently with inflammation or infection, especially when discussing perioperative cases, which can start with chemical injury followed by infection. Proper differentiation is essential because of their different treatment strategies.

5.4.2 Risk Factors for Aspiration

Perioperative aspiration risk is not solely dependent on the length of fasting but rather represents an intricate balance among multiple patient-, drug-, and procedure-based variables. Under appropriate fasting and without any underlying disease conditions, patients undergoing elective surgeries have minimal risks of complications (Joshi et al. 2023; Brady et al. 2003). Certain medical conditions, however, can modify the digestive system's or airway's physiologic behavior and increase the chances of aspiration.

5.4.2.1 Patient-Related Factors

Some of the factors in patients have been shown to increase their risk for delayed gastric emptying or increased abdominal pressure, which can cause aspiration. Among these factors, the condition of diabetes mellitus has been known to increase the risk, especially when combined with conditions of autonomic neuropathy, since it can lead to a decrease in gastric emptying rate (Bataille et al. 2014).

It has been considered that obesity increases the risk of developing aspiration, although recent studies show that obesity should not be looked at on its own as a separate risk factor. Comorbid conditions like gastroesophageal reflux disease and diabetes, among others, are much more important than obesity itself (Harter et al. 1998; Joshi et al. 2023).

Other factors such as gastrointestinal obstruction, delay in gastric motility, and systemic disease may further cause an increase in residual volume and variability of gastric emptying.

5.4.2.2 Pharmacological Factors

Some drugs can affect gastric motility and can increase the chance of residual gastric content. Among those, GLP-1 agonists (such as Semaglutide, Liraglutide, Dulaglutide, Exenatide, and Tirzepatide) have been found to cause delayed gastric emptying, posing a risk of aspiration despite adherence to fasting protocols (van Zuylen et al. 2024).

5.4.2.3 Procedural Factors

Furthermore, the risk of aspiration is impacted by the procedural and perioperative factors. Emergency surgeries, where the fasting status is not always sufficient, are considered high-risk cases. In addition, other contributing factors, such as anesthesia, difficulties with managing the airway, and the depth of anesthesia, can increase the risk of aspiration (Eichelsbacher et al. 2018).

5.4.3 Preventive Strategies for Aspiration: An Integrated Approach

The prevention of pulmonary aspiration in perioperative settings is dependent on a multimodal approach that involves fasting, pharmacologic, airway management, and diagnostics. The current trends in the management of pulmonary aspiration are focused on designing risk adaptation methods tailored for each patient based on risk profiles and the procedures involved, not using one modality alone (Joshi et al. 2023; Eichelsbacher et al. 2018).

5.4.3.1 General Preventive Measures

The adherence to fasting guidelines backed up by evidence forms a critical element of aspiration management strategies. Nevertheless, fasting is not a sufficient safeguard in itself and has to be combined with proper anesthetic preparation. The pharmacological methods, such as prokinetics and antisecretory medications, may be utilized among those who have higher risks of gastric emptying delays and higher gastric acidity; however, there is no solid scientific basis to recommend using these strategies among low-risk patients (Brady et al. 2003; Joshi et al. 2023; Admass et al. 2023).

5.4.3.2 Airway Management and Mechanistic Basis of Rapid Sequence Induction

Airway management techniques play an important role in preventing aspiration, especially in cases where there is a high suspicion of a full stomach. Rapid sequence induction (RSI) is a particular technique used in anesthesia with the aim of reducing the duration from when airway reflexes are lost to establishing airway control and securing the airway.

The rationale behind the use of RSI is based on the ability of this technique to produce loss of consciousness and airway reflexes quickly followed by paralysis, leading to quick intubation of the trachea even before any regurgitation of gastric content occurs. By avoiding positive pressure ventilation before intubation, the risks of increasing intragastric pressure due to gas insufflation are reduced (Eichelsbacher et al. 2018).

RSI has traditionally been characterized by pre-oxygenation for the purpose of storing extra oxygen, administration of an induction drug rapidly, and administration of a potent neuromuscular blocking agent to allow for early laryngoscopy and tracheal intubation. The application of cricoid pressure has also been traditionally practiced to compress the esophagus to prevent passive regurgitation. Although the efficacy of cricoid pressure is controversial, there have been doubts about its consistency and possible hindrance of visualization of the airway (Eichelsbacher et al. 2018).

However, it should be noted that RSI cannot be used as a default procedure in all situations. There is ample evidence to support the need to tailor the technique to different risks, especially for patients who require emergency surgeries, have gastrointestinal obstruction, or experience obstetric complications, among other reasons (Mendelson 1946; Joshi et al. 2023). Technique selection should be personalized, considering patient-related issues, airway evaluation, and the expertise of the clinician.

5.4.3.3 Role of Point-of-Care Gastric Ultrasonography

Gastric ultrasound has become a useful complement for assessing stomach contents in perioperative care. This non-invasive bedside test allows for both qualitative and semi-quantitative analysis of gastric volume and contents, helping guide management in cases of unclear fasting status or other associated risks (Bataille et al. 2014; Charlesworth and Wiles 2019).

This method is especially applicable in situations of emergencies or abnormal stomach physiology, where routine fasting protocols do not guarantee stomach emptying. Gastric ultrasound can provide valuable real-time data that can help determine the risk of aspiration on an individual basis.

Nonetheless, it is necessary to take into account some disadvantages. This procedure is highly operator-dependent, demands sufficient training, and may not be equally accessible in all medical facilities. Furthermore, interpretation could be biased by various individual patient characteristics, including body type and positioning. Consequently, it should be considered a supplementary method, taking into account clinical knowledge.

5.4.4 Evidence and ERAS Perspective

There remain fears about allowing fluid intake nearer to the operation in fear of increasing the risk of pulmonary aspiration. Nevertheless, many clinical studies, both randomized trials and systematic reviews, have shown convincingly that drinking clear fluids up to 2 h prior to anesthesia administration neither causes gastric volume enlargement nor an elevation in acidity in properly chosen patients (Brady et al. 2003; Joshi et al. 2023).

Research on gastric emptying has revealed the rapid clearance of clear liquids in normal individuals, providing a physiologic explanation for shorter fasting times (Hausel et al. 2001). This conclusion was also backed by recommendations of guidelines, asserting the safety of liberal fasting in a perioperative context.

From the ERAS point of view, the notion of fasting cannot be understood simply as a precautionary procedure but can be seen as one of the modifiable elements of perioperative metabolism. As recommended by ERAS protocols, the need for fasting should be minimized due to a decreased amount of perioperative stress reactions without jeopardizing patient safety through proper protocol selection (Ljungqvist et al. 2017; Gillis et al. 2015). As a result, nowadays fasting is regarded as a more flexible physiological process that takes into consideration the kind of intake and particularities of both the patient and the medical procedure.

5.4.5 Medico-Legal Considerations

Medico-legal issues are significant determinants of perioperative fasting practices, especially in relation to aspiration complications. The possibility of medical malpractice claims has traditionally been one of the factors contributing to the continuation of conservative fasting guidelines, such as "nothing by mouth after midnight" practices. Nonetheless, the use of obsolete protocols in light of the available guidelines supported by evidence seems unjustified in current medical practice (Joshi et al. 2023; Brady et al. 2003).

The medico-legal environment is focused on providing medical services that meet the guidelines and policies developed by relevant organizations. In this regard, professional guidelines, including recommendations by the American Society of Anesthesiologists and ERAS Society, represent crucial standards to follow.

Effective documentation is an essential element of the medico-legal framework. The patient's fasting status, timing, and nature of food consumption before surgery, any existing risk factors that could cause delayed gastric emptying, as well as the reasons for selection of particular anesthesia and airway management approaches should be noted.

In addition, institution protocols, together with standard fasting guidelines, help minimize practice variations and increase the safety of patients and medico-legal defense. Using evidence-based fasting guidelines during the perioperative period, as well as informing patients, is crucial for improving practice.

Therefore, aspiration precautions from a medical and legal viewpoint should not be limited to fasting time alone but must involve a comprehensive approach involving guidelines, documentation, and sound clinical judgment.

5.5 Metabolic Consequences of Prolonged Fasting

After addressing the issue of aspiration risk and ways to prevent it, it is also essential to examine the physiological and clinical effects of over-fasting and prolonged fasting in the perioperative environment. Although preoperative fasting plays a crucial role in patient safety, current research suggests that the prolonged fasting period can have several physiological and clinical repercussions.

Instead of being an innocuous prolongation of physiological fasting processes, prolonged fasting before surgery has been linked to a worsening of the stress response of the surgical procedure, which triggers greater insulin resistance, increased protein breakdown, and substrate metabolism. This phenomenon affects the regulation of metabolic processes and may adversely affect perioperative patient outcomes (Ljungqvist et al. 2017; Carli 2015).

Clinically speaking, the aforementioned metabolic changes are anything but academic. Studies have shown that extended fasting has been associated with decreased intravascular volume, poor patient tolerance, and increased perioperative stress, which could negatively influence hemodynamic stability during anesthesia and impede postoperative recovery (Jacob and Chappell 2012; Gul et al. 2017). Furthermore, catabolism can result in lean tissue loss and poor recovery in patients who are at risk (Puthucheary et al. 2013).

Under ERAS guidelines, the identified effects of prolonged fasting have led to a reevaluation of current practices that promote the optimization of metabolism in the perioperative period. Today's approach involves minimizing fasting time, maintaining homeostasis, and reducing metabolic stress in the surgical context (Gillis et al. 2015).

5.5.1 Insulin Resistance and Hyperglycemia

One of the major metabolic complications associated with fasting prior to surgery is the onset of insulin resistance during the perioperative period, an effect that is exacerbated by surgical neuroendocrine stress. This involves a diminished biological action of insulin on target tissues, causing glucose uptake to be impaired and glucose production to be enhanced, especially in the liver.

From a physiological standpoint, neuroendocrine stress due to surgery causes the secretion of various counterregulatory hormones such as cortisol, catecholamines, glucagon, and growth hormone, as well as cytokines. These factors increase hepatic glucose production via gluconeogenesis and glycogenolysis, but at the same time, decrease glucose uptake mediated by insulin in muscle and fat tissues. The result of this metabolic imbalance has been called stress hyperglycemia (Khoyratty et al. 2010).

In particular, stress hyperglycemia is not exclusive to patients with diabetes. There is research indicating that the prevalence of transient hyperglycemia in the perioperative setting for non-diabetic patients undergoing surgery depends on the degree of metabolic stress but not on the presence of inherent glucose-related disorders. It has been established that the degree of insulin resistance correlates with the severity of trauma, type of anesthesia, and the metabolic status of the patient during the operation.

In terms of consequences, hyperglycemia in the perioperative setting is linked to such negative effects as an increased risk of infection at the site of the procedure, impaired wound healing, extended hospitalization time, and increased morbidity. During the surgery, it could be identified by unstable blood sugar readings.

Under the circumstances of prolonged fasting, the problem might get aggravated by the prior presence of glycogen depletion along with catabolism. Hence, in the setting of surgical operations, insulin resistance is considered a phenomenon that is mediated by multiple factors under stress conditions, where fasting is one of the contributors and not the only cause.

5.5.2 Protein Catabolism and Muscle Loss

Long fasting before the surgery is associated with the development of catabolic metabolism, where the consumption of proteins from endogenous sources becomes more intense to ensure gluconeogenesis and energetic needs. The perioperative period aggravates this process due to the additional influence of surgical stress, leading to the appearance of nitrogen deficit and the loss of body proteins.

Physiologically, muscles act as the main storage of amino acids needed for glucose production in the liver and synthesis of acute phase proteins under stressful conditions. Metabolic experiments show that surgery is characterized by a disruption of the protein balance, which is manifested by inhibition of muscle protein synthesis and accelerated protein breakdown, leading to wasting of skeletal muscles. Moreover, there are data demonstrating that fasting promotes these phenomena by increasing insulin resistance and inhibiting glucose transport into cells, accelerating the protein breakdown process (Schricker & Lattermann 2015).

Clinically, the loss of lean body mass is significant when considering patient recovery after surgery. Postoperative muscle weakness, slow mobilization, and delayed functional recovery have been attributed to even transient perioperative protein loss, especially after undergoing major surgical interventions (Gillis et al. 2015). Vulnerable patient groups, such as elderly, malnourished, or critically ill patients, may be affected by these adverse outcomes more severely, resulting in dysfunction of their respiratory muscles and making them prone to developing pulmonary issues as well as delays in the rehabilitation process.

Furthermore, it must be stressed that the perioperative protein loss should not be considered an effect of starvation alone; rather, it is one of the components of a complex metabolic phenomenon wherein starvation synergistically interacts with surgical stress, thereby increasing muscle protein degradation. This aspect of perioperative catabolism demonstrates the necessity of using catabolism-limiting approaches that are the hallmark feature of the ERAS program, with its emphasis on perioperative nutritional optimization and minimal fasting periods.

5.5.3 Dehydration and Fluid Imbalance

The combination of prolonged fasting prior to surgery with low oral fluid consumption can be related to a relative hypovolemic status in patients. While these alterations may not be clinically relevant, they have potential importance for the perioperative period and more specifically for the process of anesthetic induction.

Indeed, in physiological terms, fasting-induced hypovolemia can cause decreases in preload and inadequate cardiovascular compensation, resulting in patients being vulnerable to hemodynamic instability at the time of anesthetic induction. A variety of clinical trials and interventions have confirmed the presence of hypovolemic conditions related to prolonged fasting, thereby providing evidence of fasting-related hypovolemia (Jacob and Chappell 2012).

It should be noted that peri-induction hypotension is not only caused by fasting-induced fluid loss. Other contributory factors include vasodilation caused by drugs used for anesthesia, depression of the myocardium, the patient's cardiovascular state, and various surgical factors.

There have also been clinical studies showing that fluid optimization prior to surgery can help reduce the occurrence and severity of peri-induction hypotension, making it clear that while fluid balance is significant, it is not the only factor.

More severe cases are those where long-term fasting and low fluid intake lead to disturbances in electrolyte balance and decreased renal perfusion. Hence, one should understand that dehydration and fluid imbalance in the context of long fasts should be regarded as an intricate process involving a variety of factors, including an individual patient's volume status and anesthetic effects.

5.5.4 Enhanced Surgical Stress Response

Extended fasting prior to surgery may lead to an exaggerated perioperative stress response, especially when combined with the stress caused by surgery. Although the neuroendocrine response to fasting is reviewed above, the interplay between fasting stress and surgical stress produces an even more profound hormonal disturbance.

The insult of surgery triggers the hypothalamic-pituitary-adrenal axis and sympathetic nervous system, which causes a rise in corticosteroid and catecholamine levels and release of pro-inflammatory cytokines. These changes are necessary for ensuring cardiovascular stability and energy metabolism, but when overzealous or persistent, they could be detrimental. Findings from physiology and medicine demonstrate that chronically elevated stress hormones have a relationship with hyperglycemia, catabolism, immunomodulation, and impaired recovery (Desborough 2000).

In the setting of fasting, preexisting metabolic deficiencies and insulin resistance can make the body more sensitive to the surgical stress reaction, causing a heightened catabolic state and poor metabolism management.

In clinical practice, a more intense stress reaction might present itself through higher glucose variability, cardiovascular changes, and temporary alterations in the immune system function, thereby increasing the risk of developing postoperative complications. The impact cannot be entirely blamed on the fasting state but should rather be considered part of a comprehensive response to surgery.

When applying the principles of ERAS, one of the key goals is to reduce the surgical stress reaction. Interventions that attempt to limit fasting, improve the metabolic state, and provide multimodal perioperative care have proven their effectiveness in mitigating this response (Ljungqvist et al. 2017; Gillis et al. 2015).

5.5.5 Patient Discomfort and Psychological Effects

Extended fasting before surgery affects the patients' comfort and mental status, which are now considered crucial aspects of their perioperative management. It has been observed that patients undergoing surgery feel symptoms like thirst, hunger, tiredness, fatigue, irritability, and anxiety. These symptoms are not just a result of mere imagination by the patient. There is substantial evidence supporting these symptoms based on the findings of research work conducted on perioperative patient experience (Hausel et al. 2001; Gul et al. 2017).

Physiologically speaking, the factors of dehydration and change in metabolism caused by prolonged fasting cause fatigue and weakness, whereas preoperative anxiety and other stresses associated with surgery lead to increased irritability and anxiety. Research studies have revealed that over-fasting leads to higher levels of discomfort before surgery and low levels of satisfaction of the patient, especially when surgeries are scheduled for non-emergency situations (Francisco et al. 2015; Bopp et al. 2011).

However, in addition, they could affect patients' compliance and the experience of their perioperative care in general. In the context of ERAS programs, the improvement of patients' well-being is viewed as one of the main goals, and it has been demonstrated that the allowance of clear fluids until 2 h prior to surgery can lead to a decrease in both thirst and anxiety without any negative impact on patient safety (Hausel et al. 2001). Consequently, the psychological and comfort consequences of extended fasting should be taken into account from a medical perspective.

5.5.6 Impact on Recovery

The collective effect of perioperative metabolic alterations caused by long-term fasting, such as insulin resistance, protein breakdown, and hypovolemia, carries considerable significance when considering postoperative healing. Instead of being independent processes, each interacts with the other to weaken physiological resilience and prevent recovery to the pre-operative functional state. Recovery through contrasting paths based on conventional fasting and ERAS metabolic management is represented by the schematic model shown in Fig. 5.2.

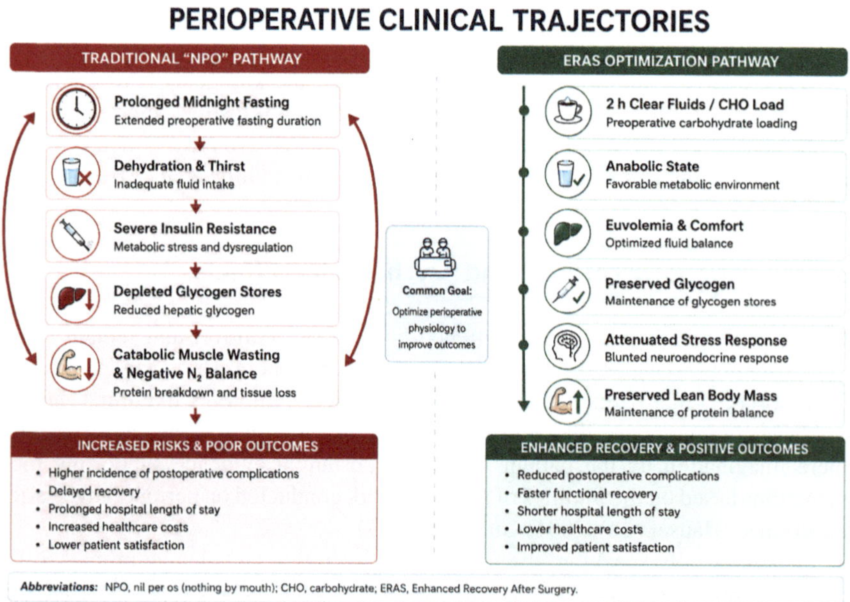

Fig. 5.2 Conceptual framework comparing the catabolic path of traditional. (Created by author using MS PowerPoint 2021)

5.5.6.1 Fasting to the Recovery-Oriented Path of ERAS Metabolic Protocols

Insulin resistance and hyperglycemia, among other findings obtained from perioperative outcome trials, are associated with an elevated risk of postoperative morbidity and complications such as surgical wound infections, delays in wound healing, and protein breakdown resulting in decreased lean body mass and functional impairment (Ljungqvist et al. 2017; Gillis et al. 2015). Furthermore, imbalances in perioperative fluid intake and volume status may also contribute to the stability of the cardiovascular system and adequate organ perfusion (Jacob and Chappell 2012).

Considering the clinical implications of this issue, the consequences of these metabolic abnormalities include an extended period of hospitalization, delayed mobilization, and an increase in morbidity, especially for patients requiring major surgery or with restricted physiological reserve capacity (Carli 2015; Puthucheary et al. 2013). However, it is also important to note that the extent of impact of each factor will be affected by individual circumstances.

Mitigation of the aforementioned metabolic disturbances is one of the key goals within the scope of the ERAS protocol, as measures are undertaken for preservation of physiological stability and accelerated recovery. It follows that long-term fasting must not be considered simply an operational preprocedure issue; rather, it is an element of the patient's condition, which needs to be modified to produce better results.

5.6 Metabolic Optimization

With the understanding that there are negative metabolic effects due to fasting prior to surgery, today's perioperative medicine practices have moved from merely restricting patients' intake to actually optimizing their metabolic function. As part of ERAS protocols, fasting has ceased being simply a means to prevent aspiration and is now considered a modifiable factor in perioperative metabolism and recovery (Ljungqvist et al. 2017).

The metabolic optimization techniques seek to reduce the effect of the stress response to surgery, maintain physiological stability, and limit metabolic disturbance during the perioperative period. The processes of metabolic optimization begin before surgery and continue even after the procedure (Gillis et al. 2015).

Notably, this paradigm underscores the need for maintaining euglycemia, hydration, and optimal substrate use, instead of the starvation induced by catabolism. This practice is in line with present-day evidence, which underscores the importance of reducing metabolic stress in order to aid the process of recovery and minimize adverse effects.

Although several techniques have been used in attempts to achieve this goal, preoperative nutrition intervention methods, including those that employ carbohydrates, have been receiving increasing focus; these will be elaborated in the following subsection. In this regard, the present section outlines the rationale behind metabolic optimization in ERAS programs.

5.6.1 Preoperative Carbohydrate Loading

Carbohydrate loading before surgery is an important nutritional intervention under ERAS principles designed to influence the metabolic response during surgery. This process entails the ingestion of a high-carbohydrate, clear solution 2–3 h before anesthesia induction in line with fasting principles (Joshi et al. 2023).

Biologically, carbohydrate loading leads to the change from fasting metabolism to fed metabolism, where there is increased insulin release, retention of liver glycogen, and decreased endogenous glucose production. These changes lead to reduced insulin resistance during surgery, a common outcome associated with surgical stress that plays a role in recovery (Ljungqvist and Jonathan 2012).

Apart from influencing carbohydrate metabolism, the intake of carbohydrates has been found to limit protein degradation and promote lean tissue maintenance, thus enhancing recovery functions after surgery (Gillis et al. 2015; Schricker & Lattermann, 2015). Nonetheless, one should consider the overall quality of perioperative care because several interacting factors determine outcomes.

A number of clinical trials have shown that consumption of carbohydrate drinks before surgery results in reduced discomfort, such as thirst, hunger, and anxiety experienced by patients undergoing surgery (Hausel et al. 2001). Additionally, some researchers argue that there can be positive changes in terms of perioperative glycemic management and other recovery functions, although their significance depends on the patient group and type of surgery (Ljungqvist et al. 2017). The comparison of the conventional fasted state and optimized metabolic state due to carbohydrate loading is provided in Table 5.2.

Although these benefits exist, the use of carbohydrate loading before surgery demands proper patient selection. The procedure is usually deemed safe among elective surgery patients who lack risk factors for delayed gastric emptying. Nonetheless, extreme caution or outright avoidance should be taken when dealing with patients suffering from:

- Uncorrected diabetes mellitus
- Gastroparesis or delayed gastric emptying
- Gastrointestinal obstruction
- States with high risk of aspiration, including some emergencies (Joshi et al. 2023; van Zuylen et al. 2024)

Also, although available scientific literature suggests that carbohydrate fluids in clear form are safe for consumption during the appropriate time before operations, the diversity of research designs and patients' sample sets requires the prudent analysis of the results.

Overall, carbohydrate loading before surgery is a scientifically supported practice within the ERAS pathway that may positively affect the metabolic and general patient experience during surgery.

Table 5.2 Comparative analysis of metabolic profiles: prolonged preoperative fasting vs. carbohydrate loading

Metabolic parameter	Prolonged fasting paradigm (>12 h)	ERAS CHO loading paradigm (up to 2 h pre-op)	Endocrine and molecular mediators	Postoperative clinical implication
Hepatic glycogen status	Rapidly depleted (~75% reduction within 12 h)	Preserved and synthesized (anabolic priming)	Glucagon ↑, Cortisol ↑	Maintained glycogen reserves prevent early reliance on gluconeogenesis
Peripheral insulin sensitivity	Pronounced resistance (~50% reduction in glucose disposal rate)	Maintained near basal levels; attenuated resistance	GLUT4 translocation ↓ (fasting); IRS-1 phosphorylation maintained (CHO)	Reduced risk of postoperative hyperglycemia; lower requirement for exogenous insulin
Protein turnover and catabolism	Accelerated proteolysis (negative nitrogen balance)	Proteolysis suppressed; nitrogen balance stabilized	Ubiquitin-proteasome pathway activation ↑; mTOR inhibition	Preservation of lean muscle mass; accelerated mobilization and functional recovery
Lipid metabolism	Enhanced lipolysis and elevated free fatty acids (FFAs)	Suppressed lipolysis; basal FFA levels	Catecholamines ↑, Hormone-Sensitive Lipase (HSL) ↑	Minimizes risk of perioperative ketoacidosis and oxidative stress
Subjective patient experience	High incidence of thirst, hunger, anxiety, and PONV	Attenuated thirst, reduced anxiety, improved comfort	Hypothalamic osmoreceptors (ADH release), Ghrelin ↑	Enhanced patient-reported outcome measures (PROMs) and compliance with early recovery milestones

5.6.2 Fluid Balance and Hemodynamic Stability

The maintenance of fluid balance in optimal condition constitutes one of the key aspects of perioperative metabolic optimization, since the occurrence of either hypovolemia or fluid overload leads to poor outcomes. However, the presence of preoperative fasting does not mean that there will be inadequate fluid status, considering that the physiological condition can be affected by various perioperative parameters (Jacob and Chappell 2012).

With regard to fluid administration during the perioperative period, there has been a shift from the application of fixed approaches to a physiology-based strategy, which involves personalized patient assessment. As a result, there has been a trend towards using goal-directed fluid therapy (GDFT), wherein dynamic indices, such as stroke volume variation, pulse pressure variation, and cardiac output measurement, determine the rate of fluid administration (Gillis et al. 2015).

The basic concept behind GDFT is ensuring optimal tissue perfusion and oxygenation without under-resuscitation and over-resuscitation. Failure to provide sufficient fluid resuscitation can affect organ perfusion, leading to hypotension, renal failure, and poor tissue oxygenation. Too much resuscitation causes edema in tissues, poor wound healing, and cardiopulmonary complications in high-risk surgical patients (Ljungqvist et al. 2017).

Several studies have demonstrated positive clinical outcomes linked to GDFT use, such as fewer complications after surgery and reduced hospitalization period, especially for major surgeries in the abdominal cavity (Gillis et al. 2015). Nevertheless, the effects of GDFT may differ according to different patient groups, types of surgery, and applied monitoring methods.

In the context of ERAS pathways, fluid management is part of the overall metabolic optimization strategy aimed at maintaining hemodynamic balance. This demonstrates the need for patient-specific approaches in fluid administration based on the patient's pre-existing conditions, surgical procedure, and hemodynamic response during surgery. The best way to achieve ideal perioperative fluid management is by adopting an individualized and evidence-based approach.

5.6.3 Attenuation of Surgical Stress Response and Role of Multimodal Analgesia

Inhibition of the surgical stress response remains one of the most important aims in the perioperative metabolic optimization process. According to ERAS guidelines, it involves using specific perioperative approaches that inhibit neuroendocrine stimulation and minimize the metabolic implications, as opposed to addressing fasting-based issues only (Patterson and Sears 2017).

Anesthetic procedures remain vital in controlling the stress response process. Measures such as maintaining an adequate level of anesthesia, using short-acting anesthetics, and employing regional anesthesia methods, including neuraxial blockage and peripheral nerve blockage, remain instrumental in inhibiting sympathetic stimulation and decreasing stress hormone production (Carli 2015; Schricker et al. 2015).

Pain control is a vital part of this treatment protocol, since uncontrolled pain further stimulates the stress response, leading to increased catabolism and metabolic instability. In this regard, the ERAS protocols emphasize the need for multimodal analgesia. It combines the usage of various types of analgesics and methods for achieving pain relief without using opioids excessively.

In addition to ensuring adequate analgesia, the application of multimodal analgesia significantly decreases the side effects associated with opioid therapy. Postoperative nausea and vomiting, sedation, and ileus are the main adverse consequences of excessive opioid consumption. Therefore, patients who received multimodal analgesia experience faster mobilization and functional recovery. These results correspond to the ERAS program objectives (Gillis et al. 2015).

One should consider that the stress response inhibition may vary depending on surgical volume, individual characteristics of patients, and perioperative period management. For this reason, analgesic and anesthetic approaches should be incorporated into a single patient treatment strategy.

5.6.4 Early Postoperative Feeding

The early onset of oral intake after surgery is one of the core elements of ERAS procedures, showing that the trend is changing from classical approaches of post-surgery fasting. Recent studies prove that it is possible to initiate early postoperative oral intake as soon as conditions allow for doing so without contraindications arising from the surgical procedure itself or the state of the patient (Ljungqvist et al. 2017).

With respect to physiology, postoperative feeding helps achieve normalization of metabolic processes, preserves the integrity of intestinal mucosa, and minimizes the level of insulin resistance. Also, the process facilitates gastrointestinal mobility, which decreases the probability of developing ileus (Gillis et al. 2015; Abela 2017).

Clinical trials and systematic reviews have shown that the early introduction of nutrition correlates positively with good recovery results, such as reduced time spent in the hospital, fewer post-surgery complications, and increased patient satisfaction. It must be stressed that these effects occur in the absence of any increase in complication rates among appropriately chosen patients (Ljungqvist et al. 2017).

Nevertheless, the time of postoperative feeding and its gradual advancement should be personalized, considering the type of surgical intervention performed, the patient's tolerance, and symptoms such as nausea or dysfunctions of the digestive tract. The usual protocol entails the initiation of clear fluid intake followed by a full-blown diet as allowed by the patient's condition.

Thus, the early feeding regimen for post-surgery patients may be considered as one of the evidence-based strategies aimed at ensuring metabolic restoration and re-establishment of functions.

5.7 Role of Anesthesiologist in Implementation of ERAS Fasting Protocols

Though the metabolic reasoning and advantages of fast optimization are detailed in the latter part of this article, the anesthesiologist's function is mainly on the application of these ERAS fasting guidelines.

5.7.1 Preoperative Verification and Risk Assessment

It is important to have a thorough preoperative assessment to apply fasting guidelines safely. This should include establishing the time and kind of the last oral intake, as well as recognizing factors that contribute to delayed gastric emptying and risk of aspiration.

Due to the possible errors of patients' recollections, cross-checking with caregivers/nursing staff may be required for accurate assessment (Joshi et al. 2023; Panjiar et al. 2019).

5.7.2 Individualized Clinical Decision-Making

However, such recommendations must be modified depending on the patient's profile. While general guidelines may suffice for the majority of elective procedures, certain patients may need tailored decisions in light of particular risk factors, including diabetes, pregnancy, gastrointestinal issues, or an unknown period of fasting.

This practice indicates a transition from risk-based preoperative management, where safety will always come first, but unnecessary fasting will not be extended unnecessarily.

5.7.3 Intraoperative Planning and Management

The anesthesia provider can significantly influence the decision-making process during anesthesia according to fasting status and other clinical factors. The strategy used for the induction procedure, airway management, and monitoring procedures depends on the assessed risks of aspiration and the general patient condition.

It is essential to note that the peri-induction hemodynamic changes occur due to several reasons, so the treatment strategy should be based on clinical assessments of the situation and not on fasting times (Jacob and Chappell 2012).

5.7.4 Airway Strategy and Safety

Airway management is intimately related to the evaluation of the risk of aspiration. Conventional induction methods are suitable for low-risk patients who have been appropriately fasted, while those with an unclear fasting status or other risk factors might benefit from airway modification.

The selection of the procedure should be patient-centered and grounded in sound science without resorting to overly invasive techniques unless indicated.

5.7.5 Communication and Multidisciplinary Coordination

For the successful application of the fasting protocol, effective communication between anesthesia, surgery, and nursing teams is necessary. Disagreement in instructions may result in inappropriate fasting times, while misunderstanding will cause problems in performing a procedure. It is common practice for anesthesiologists to ensure that the perioperative team follows protocols according to the latest evidence base.

5.7.6 Documentation and Medico-Legal Responsibility

It is important to document patients' fast status, risk factors, and anesthesia technique to ensure consistency in patient care and prevent medical legal problems (Lee et al. 2003; Baril and Portman 2007).

In general, the anesthesiologist plays an important role in implementing the ERAS fasting regimen by making sure that the evidence-based recommendations are implemented safely and consistently.

5.8 Implementation, Clinical Impact, and Future Directions

Even with robust scientific evidence and recommended guidelines, adherence to contemporary fasting protocols is inconsistent among various organizations. There are multiple reasons why there is a difference between evidence and practice regarding this issue.

5.8.1 Barriers to Implementation

One of the biggest challenges is the continued practice of conventional preoperative fasting guidelines like "nil per oral after midnight." These guidelines remain relevant because they are easy to understand and remember, although there is no scientific evidence behind them. Furthermore, insufficient knowledge and misunderstanding about preoperative fasting guidelines by medical professionals, including nurses and young doctors, often cause them to err on the side of caution (Panjiar et al. 2019).

Poor communication among operating room personnel also plays a significant role in this issue. Failure to follow through and communicate effectively among surgeons, anesthetists, and nurses can sometimes lead to unnecessary fasting.

Operational issues also hold considerable importance in the matter. Operating room delays, changes in surgery sequence, and emergency interventions often mean that fasting times become much higher than they should be under recommended guidelines. Patients who have been advised to fast in the morning but end up undergoing procedures later in the day can find themselves having fasted for much longer than is required.

Medico-legal issues provide yet another factor in the situation. Fear of aspirative consequences and legal liability might make medical personnel more cautious about fasting times. Cultural beliefs among patients also contribute to unnecessary fasting times.

5.8.2 Strategies for Effective Implementation

Dealing with such challenges would call for a well-planned approach based on systems thinking.

Key strategies include:

- Standardizing institutional protocols in accordance with up-to-date recommendations
- Training healthcare professionals to raise awareness
- Concise, patient-oriented communication, such as written fasting orders
- Enhancing cooperation among various healthcare professionals to avoid contradictory instructions
- Regularly documenting and auditing protocol compliance

The anesthesiologist has a leading role in this process by implementing protocols, following evidence-based practice guidelines, and coordinating perioperative pathways.

5.8.3 Clinical Impact of Evidence-Based Fasting Practices

The implementation of ERAS-based fasting guidelines has been associated with a number of positive perioperative outcomes. The clinical research evidence shows that patients who followed the contemporary fasting guidelines during their operations had a more successful perioperative period when compared to their counterparts, who underwent the classic prolonged fasting regime (Ljungqvist et al. 2017).

From the standpoint of the intra-operative period, the implementation of the optimal fasting approach will allow for stabilization of the patient's hemodynamics, which is associated with the improved initial volume state and lower level of stress (Jacob and Chappell 2012). Postoperatively, these patients will demonstrate early mobility and faster restoration of gut motility (Gillis et al. 2015).

The list of benefits provided by the new approach does not end here; from the standpoint of patient-oriented care, one should mention the reduction of the feeling of thirst and preoperative anxiety due to permission to have clear fluid intake within a certain timeframe (Hausel et al. 2001).

5.8.4 Future Directions

With further advances in perioperative care, it is anticipated that advancements will emphasize more personalized and precise management of fasting and metabolism. Future research may include:

- Individualized fasting guidelines tailored to the patient's risk profile and associated diseases

- Leveraging of point-of-care gastric ultrasonography for objective evaluation of stomach content in ambiguous situations
- Application of biomarkers and metabolic assessment techniques to customize perioperative nutrition and metabolism plans
- Utilization of digital solutions and guided care pathway strategies to improve adherence and minimize variability
- Capitalizing on continuous quality improvement programs and audit processes for ensuring ongoing compliance with ERAS standards

Such changes represent the general movement towards precision perioperative medicine, whereby the fasting and nutrition techniques have been designed with consideration to enhancing safety and recovery.

In summary, although there have been remarkable achievements concerning the definition of fasting approaches based on scientific evidence, putting these approaches into use becomes the most critical issue. In this case, it is important to make certain efforts that will involve the institution, clinicians, and patients in order to be able to utilize the benefits.

5.9 Conclusion

The management of fasting in patients undergoing surgery has significantly evolved from being strict in terms of timing to becoming evidence-based and flexible. Although the prevention of pulmonary aspiration is still considered as an important objective, current research has shown that excessive fasting confers no extra advantage for the patients and can even negatively impact their metabolic status.

The introduction of the ERAS approach to fasting in surgical patients has revolutionized the process by advocating for faster times to achieve a more balanced physiologic state. Even though there is sufficient supportive evidence, variations in clinical practice continue to exist, stressing the importance of more work being done on education, protocols, and implementation.

In conclusion, adequate fasting in surgery involves balancing both patient safety and metabolic issues, and proper adherence to the principles of ERAS is important in this regard.

References

Abela G. The potential benefits and harms of early feeding post-surgery: a literature review. Int Wound J. 2017;14(5):870–3. https://doi.org/10.1111/iwj.12750.

Admass BA, Abebe MM, Aretayne NR, Temesgen MM. Assessment of preoperative preventive measures for pulmonary aspiration in surgical patients: a cross-sectional study. Heliyon. 2023;9(6):e17109. https://doi.org/10.1016/j.heliyon.2023.e17109.

Baril P, Portman H. Preoperative fasting: knowledge and perceptions. AORN J. 2007;86(4):609–17. https://doi.org/10.1016/j.aorn.2007.09.003.

Bataille A, Rousset J, Marret E, Bonnet F. Ultrasonographic evaluation of gastric content during labour under epidural analgesia: a prospective cohort study. Br J Anaesth. 2014;112(4):703–7. https://doi.org/10.1093/bja/aet435.

Bopp C, Höper S, Klein A, Weigand MA, Martin E, Gust R. A liberal preoperative fasting regimen improves patient comfort and satisfaction with anesthesia care in day-stay minor surgery. Minerva Anestesiol. 2011;77:680–6. PMID: 19190563

Brady M, Kinn S, Stuart P, Ness V. Preoperative fasting for adults to prevent perioperative complications. Cochrane Database Syst Rev. 2003;4:CD004423. https://doi.org/10.1002/14651858.CD004423.

Carli F. Physiologic considerations of enhanced recovery after surgery (ERAS) programs: implications of the stress response. Can J Anesth. 2015;62(2):110–9. https://doi.org/10.1007/s12630-014-0264-0.

Charlesworth M, Wiles MD. Pre-operative gastric ultrasound—should we look inside Schroedinger's gut? Anaesthesia. 2019;74:109–12. https://doi.org/10.1111/anae.14516.

Desborough JP. The stress response to trauma and surgery. Br J Anaesth. 2000;85(1):109–17. https://doi.org/10.1093/bja/85.1.109.

Dongare PA, Bhaskar SB, Harsoor SS, Garg R, Kannan S, Goneppanavar U, et al. Preoperative fasting and feeding in adults, obstetric, paediatric and bariatric population: practice guidelines from the Indian Society of Anaesthesiologists. Indian J Anaesth. 2020;64:556–84. https://doi.org/10.4103/ija.IJA_923_20.

Eichelsbacher C, Ilper H, Noppens R, Hinkelbein J, Loop T. Rapid sequence induction and intubation in patients with risk of aspiration: recommendations for action for practical management of anesthesia. Anaesthesist. 2018;67(8):568–83. https://doi.org/10.1007/s00101-018-0460-3.

Francisco F, Batista ST, Pena GDG. Fasting in elective surgical patients: comparison among the time prescribed, performed and recommended on perioperative care protocols. Arq Bras Cir Dig. 2015;28(4):250–4. https://doi.org/10.1590/S0102-6720201500040008.

Gebremedhn EG, Nagaratnam VB. Audit on preoperative fasting of elective surgical patients in an African academic medical center. World J Surg. 2014;38:2200–4. https://doi.org/10.1007/s00268-014-2582-3.

Gillis C, et al. Promoting perioperative metabolic and nutritional care. Anesthesiology. 2015;123(6):1455–72. https://doi.org/10.1097/ALN.0000000000000795.

Gul A, Andsoy I, Ozkaya B. Preoperative fasting and patients' discomfort. Indian J Surg. 2017;80:549–53. https://doi.org/10.1007/s12262-017-1657-4.

Hamid S. Pre-operative fasting: a patient centered approach. BMJ Qual Improv Rep. 2014;3(1):1–4. https://doi.org/10.1136/bmjquality.u605.w1252.

Harter RL, Kelly WB, Kramer MG, Perez CE, Dzwonczyk RR. A comparison of the volume and pH of gastric contents of obese and lean surgical patients. Anesth Analg. 1998;86(1):147–52. https://doi.org/10.1097/00000539-199801000-00030.

Hausel J, Nygren J, Lagerkranser M, Hellström PM, Hammarqvist F, Almström C, Jeppsson B. A carbohydrate-rich drink reduces preoperative discomfort in elective surgery patients. Anesth Analg. 2001;93:1344–50. https://doi.org/10.1097/00000539-200111000-00063.

Jacob M, Chappell D. Effects of perioperative fasting on haemodynamics and intravascular volumes. Best Pract Res Clin Anaesthesiol. 2012;26(4):421–30. https://doi.org/10.1016/j.bpa.2012.10.002.

Joshi GP, Abdelmalak BB, Weigel WA, Harbell MW, Kuo CI, Soriano SG, Stricker PA, Tipton T, Grant MD, Marbella AM, Agarkar M, Blanck JF, Domino KB. 2023 American Society of Anesthesiologists practice guidelines for preoperative fasting: carbohydrate-containing clear liquids with or without protein, chewing gum, and pediatric fasting duration—a modular update of the 2017 American Society of Anesthesiologists Practice Guidelines for Preoperative Fasting. Anesthesiology. 2023;138(2):132–51. https://doi.org/10.1097/ALN.0000000000004381.

Khoyratty S, Modi BN, Ravichandran D. Preoperative starvation in elective general surgery. J Perioper Pract. 2010;20:100–2. https://doi.org/10.1177/175045891002000302.

Kosutova P, Mikolka P. Aspiration syndromes and associated lung injury: incidence, pathophysiology and management. Physiol Res. 2021;70(Suppl 4):S567–83. https://doi.org/10.33549/physiolres.934767.

Lee A, Chui PT, Gin T. Educating patients about anesthesia: a systematic review of randomized controlled trials of media-based interventions. Anesth Analg. 2003;96:1424–31. https://doi.org/10.1213/01.ANE.0000055806.93400.93.

Ljungqvist O, Jonathan E. Rhoads lecture 2011: insulin resistance and enhanced recovery after surgery. JPEN J Parenter Enteral Nutr. 2012;36(4):389–98. https://doi.org/10.1177/0148607112445580.

Ljungqvist O, Nygren J, Thorell A. Modulation of post-operative insulin resistance by pre-operative carbohydrate loading. Proc Nutr Soc. 2002;61(3):329–36. https://doi.org/10.1079/PNS2002168.

Ljungqvist O, Scott M, Fearon KC. Enhanced recovery after surgery: a review. JAMA Surg. 2017;152(3):292–8. https://doi.org/10.1001/jamasurg.2016.4952.

Mendelson CL. The aspiration of stomach contents into the lungs during obstetric anesthesia. Am J Obstet Gynecol. 1946;52:191–205. https://doi.org/10.1016/s0002-9378(16)39829-5.

Panjiar P, Kochhar A, Vajifdar H, Bhat K. A prospective survey on knowledge, attitude and current practices of pre-operative fasting amongst anaesthesiologists. Indian J Anaesth. 2019;63:350–5. https://doi.org/10.4103/ija.IJA_50_19.

Patterson RE, Sears DD. Metabolic effects of intermittent fasting. Annu Rev Nutr. 2017;37:371–93. https://doi.org/10.1146/annurev-nutr-071816-064634.

Puthucheary ZA, Rawal J, McPhail M, Connolly B, et al. Acute skeletal muscle wasting in critical illness. JAMA. 2013;310(15):1591–600. https://doi.org/10.1001/jama.2013.278481.

Schricker T, & Lattermann R. Perioperative catabolism. Canadian Journal of Anesthesia/Journal canadien d anesthésie, 2015;62(2):182-193. https://doi.org/10.1007/s12630-014-0274-y

van Zuylen ML, Siegelaar SE, Plummer MP, Deane AM, Hermanides J, Hulst AH. Perioperative management of long-acting glucagon-like peptide-1 (GLP-1) receptor agonists. Br J Anaesth. 2024;132(4):64-8. https://doi.org/10.1016/j.bja.2024.01.001.

Carbohydrate Loading and Early Postoperative Feeding

6

Luxita Sharma, Mansi Joon, Shristi Gupta, and Dhananjay Sharma

Abstract

In modern perioperative nutritional management, the postoperative feeding practices and carbohydrate loads are the key components. While in traditional surgical practices, often need to extend fasting before and after the surgery, which could involve metabolic stress, insulin resistance, and delayed recovery. Whereas, the current researches support the balancing of controlled carbohydrate intake in preoperative surgery, and early reintroduction of nutrition just after the surgery for better outcome of the patient health. This chapter explores the clinical outcome and physiological basis of carbohydrate drinks in preoperative patients, which helps in energy preservation and reduces the metabolic imbalance linked with surgical stress. By restoring the muscle mass and improving the insulin sensitivity, the carbohydrate load can improve the postoperative recovery and the patient's outcome. The chapter also focuses on the significance of introducing nutritional feeding in postoperative feeding, especially the enteral feeding, to sustain the gastrointestinal functioning, tissue building, and immune responses. The practical guidelines for the introduction of carbohydrate liquids before the surgery, and its execution would be the safe feeding strategies after the surgeries are planned. Additionally, patient selection and possible challenges are considered to safeguard the proper application of these applications. Focusing on the integration of sugar load and early feeding enhanced the recovery pathways. Overall, this chapter focuses on how to introduce and integrate the proper nutri-

L. Sharma · M. Joon · S. Gupta · D. Sharma (✉)
Department of Dietetics and Applied Nutrition, Amity Medical School, Amity University Haryana, Manesar (Gurugram), Haryana, India
e-mail: lshrama@ggn.amity.edu

P. K. Bhattacharyya et al. (eds.), *Integrated Anesthesia and Nutrition Approaches to Enhanced Recovery after Surgery*,
https://doi.org/10.1007/978-981-92-3294-9_6

tional management in perioperative access that can reduce patient complications and improve outcomes, also minimize muscle loss, reduce hospital stays, and improve surgical recovery.

Keywords

Carbohydrate loading · Postoperative feeding · Insulin resistance · Metabolic stress · Insulin sensitivity

6.1 Introduction to Perioperative Carbohydrate Management

The carbohydrate loading and perioperative feeding interventions are some of the important elements of the current nutritional care of surgical patients. The conventional practice of perioperative care entailed long periods of preoperative fasting and delayed postoperative feeding, which was supposed to reduce the risk of aspiration. Nonetheless, there has been a lot of clinical data that proved that these fasting methods can be harmful to metabolic balance and slow down the recuperation instead of enhancing security (Weimann et al. 2017). Surgery causes a physiological stress response (hormonal and metabolic changes). This involves augmented release of cortisol, catecholamines, and glucagon, which altogether provoke gluconeogenesis, lipolysis, and protein degradation. The processes result in a catabolic condition, a negative nitrogen balance, and lean body mass loss (Thorell et al. 2016). Postoperative insulin resistance is one of the most clinically significant effects of this stress response that leads to poor glucose metabolism and functional recovery (Ljungqvist et al. 2017).

Insulin resistance has been linked to several negative effects such as hyperglycemia, risk of infections, delayed wound healing, and extended hospitalization. Such metabolic imbalances underscore the importance of interventions to minimize surgical stress and maintain metabolic homeostasis (Gustafsson et al. 2013). In this background, the use of carbohydrates during perioperation and the feeding of the patient early after the operation has received good scientific support. These procedures are meant to sustain energy, enhance insulin sensitivity, and gastrointestinal recovery, which leads to better functioning after surgery.

6.1.1 Metabolic Changes During Surgical Stress

The surgical trauma leads to a well-coordinated neuroendocrine and inflammatory response that cannot sustain normal metabolic homeostasis, which is mainly caused by the activation of the hypothalamic-pituitary-adrenal (HPA) axis and sympathetic nervous system, which causes an increase in cortisol, catecholamines, and glucagon (Thorell et al. 2016; Desborough 2000). This hormonal burst is enhanced by the activation of pro-inflammatory cytokines like interleukin-6 and tumor necrosis factor-a that all cause the metabolism to shift toward a catabolic state (Weimann et al. 2017; Thorell et al. 2016).

One significant metabolic effect of this reaction is higher levels of hepatic glucose production due to increased glycogenolysis and gluconeogenesis, which causes perioperative hyperglycemia (Ljungqvist et al. 2017; Thorell et al. 2016). Meanwhile, skeletal muscle peripheral glucose uptake is decreased by a combination of disrupted insulin receptor signaling and diminished GLUT-4 translocation, resulting in systemic insulin resistance (Ljungqvist et al. 2017; Thorell et al. 2016). Figure 6.1 illustrates the metabolic response to surgical stress, where hormones and inflammation lead to insulin resistance, increased glucose production, and stress hyperglycemia. It also highlights how perioperative nutrition (e.g., carbohydrate intake vs fasting) influences blood glucose and insulin levels.

The insulin resistance that is postoperative usually occurs hours following surgical trauma and can be continued over several days based on the extent of tissue injury and the prior metabolic condition (Ljungqvist et al. 2017; Thorell et al. 2016). This condition is associated with a decreased use of glucose even when the glucose levels in the body are high, and the body has to use other energy sources. Compensation for the damaged carbohydrate use is provided by a greater release of free fatty acids out of the adipose tissue through greater lipolysis (Weimann et al. 2017; Desborough 2000). But in cases where the energy needs surpass the lipid oxidation potential, skeletal muscle protein catabolism turns into a significant source of gluconeogenic substances, resulting in the loss of lean body mass and negative nitrogen balance (Weimann et al. 2017; Deutz et al. 2014).

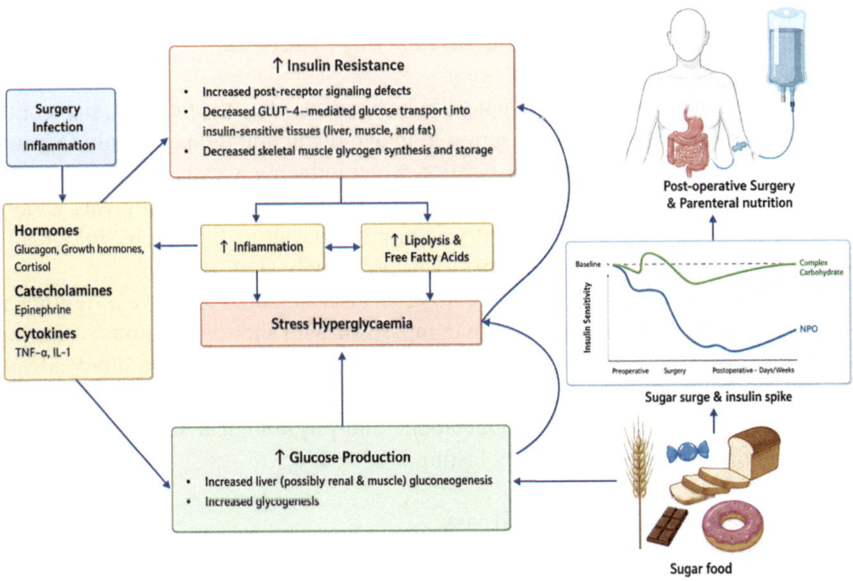

Fig. 6.1 Carbohydrate metabolic and hormonal changes during surgical stress. (Created by the author using PowerPoint 2021)

The clinical importance of muscle proteolysis as a stress response to surgery is evident as it is directly related to postoperative weakness, slow mobilization, and a long recovery time (Deutz et al. 2014). The reduction of skeletal muscle mass in patients with existing malnutrition or sarcopenia, in which the baseline protein reserves are already impaired, worsens the situation (Cruz-Jentoft et al. 2019). The insulin-related hyperglycemia also has some negative impacts on immune performance, due to its inability to chemoattract neutrophils, decrease phagocytic activity, and increase oxidative stress (Calder 2020; Weimann et al. 2017). Such immune changes lead to increased risk of postsurgical infectious complications and delayed wound repair (Calder 2020; Ljungqvist et al. 2017).

Moreover, metabolism changes under the influence of stress are linked to the elevated energy expenditure at rest and a shift in the use of the substrate, but the degree of change depends on the severity of surgery and the nutritional condition of an individual (Thorell et al. 2016; Desborough 2000). Patients already inflamed or having a chronic illness tend to have exaggerated metabolic responses, which further augment catabolic load (Weimann et al. 2017; Cederholm et al. 2019). In general, the metabolic responses before, during, and after surgery are insulin-resistant, hyperglycemic, characterized by an augmented protein catabolism and expedited muscle wasting, all of which have adverse impacts on the progression of recovery (Ljungqvist et al. 2017; Weimann et al. 2017). The knowledge of these processes gives the physiological foundation to perioperative nutritional plans to maintain lean body mass and enhance metabolic stability (Deutz et al. 2014; Ljungqvist et al. 2017).

6.1.2 Limitations of Traditional Fasting Practices

Historical preoperative fasting practices have been based on the fact that, since midnight before surgery, patients are required to avoid any oral intake (mainly to minimize the chances of pulmonary aspiration when inducing anesthesia) (Brady et al. 2003; Weimann et al. 2017). Such a nil per os after midnight policy was widely adopted in surgical care, although it was more of a routine than a physiologically sound decision in the current perioperative care (Brady et al. 2003).

Nevertheless, recent data show that long-term fasting does not have a significant effect on gastric volume or acidity in comparison with shorter durations of fasting on clear fluids, which is why long-term restriction may not offer extra safety advantages in well-chosen patients (Weimann et al. 2017; Brady et al. 2003). Rather, patients are prone to unnecessary metabolic and physiological stress prior to surgery brought about by unnecessary fasting.

6.1.2.1 Increased Metabolic Stress

Long-term fasting causes the depletion of the hepatic glycogen stores and premature activation of gluconeogenesis, which switches the body to the catabolic metabolic state before surgical injury can take place (Thorell et al. 2016; Ljungqvist et al. 2017). This preoperative catabolic priming has the potential to enhance the ensuing stress response to surgery by elevating the need to use protein breakdown as a source of energy substances (Weimann et al. 2017). Consequently, patients can go to surgery in a metabolically impaired condition, and this can adversely affect the postoperative recovery patterns (Thorell et al. 2016).

6.1.2.2 Dehydration and Patient Discomfort

Frequently, prolonged fasting (both of solid and fluid forms) leads to dehydration, especially in geriatric patients and those with underlying comorbidities (Søreide et al. 2005; Weimann et al. 2017). Thirst, dry mouth, headache, dizziness, and fatigue are common clinical symptoms that manifest the restriction of fluids as well as the lack of energy (Søreide et al. 2005). These symptoms may also lead to hemodynamic instability during the induction of anesthesia in predisposed people.

6.1.2.3 Worsening Insulin Resistance

Preoperative fasting is a factor that worsens perioperative insulin resistance as it involves becoming more dependent on endogenous glucose production and decreasing insulin sensitivity before surgical insult (Ljungqvist et al. 2017; Thorell et al. 2016). Without exogenous carbohydrate consumption, hepatic glucose production rises, and peripheral glucose uptake falls, and stress-induced hyperglycemia in the postoperative period is magnified (Weimann et al. 2017). This disruption in metabolism is linked to a poor immune system and susceptibility to postoperative complications (Calder 2020; Ljungqvist et al. 2017).

6.1.2.4 Reduced Patient Comfort and Psychological Burden

Long-term starvation can also be linked with more discomfort and anxiety in patients and less satisfaction with the perioperative process (Søreide et al. 2005; Weimann et al. 2017). Preoperative hunger and thirst are also some of the factors that cause psychological stress and can further activate neuroendocrine stress pathways and exacerbate metabolic responses to surgery (Thorell et al. 2016). Comfort and satisfaction are key elements of the quality of care in perioperative care that have been noted in patient-centered outcomes research (Søreide et al. 2005).

6.1.2.5 Clinical Implications and Guideline Evolution

Modern perioperative fasting practices have added to the mounting evidence base by greatly decreasing the duration of fasting and allowing clear fluids up to 2 h and light meals up to 6 h prior to anesthesia, in suitably-selected patients (Brady et al. 2003; Gustafsson et al. 2013). The new protocols are designed to reduce metabolic stress and ensure patient safety by reducing the risk of aspiration in comparison with physiological stability (Weimann et al. 2017).

In general, these restrictions of the conventional fasting methods demonstrate that long-term preoperative starvation is not clinically healthy and can be a cause of metabolic abnormalities, discomfort, and poor postoperative outcomes of surgery. This has contributed to the change towards more individualized and evidence-based perioperative nutritional management solutions (Ljungqvist et al. 2017; Gustafsson et al. 2013).

6.2 Preoperative Carbohydrate Loading

Preoperative carbohydrate loading is a strategic nutrition therapy used to reduce metabolic stress before surgery. It mainly helps in maintaining insulin sensitivity to ensure better glucose control and reduce postoperative insulin resistance. Liver glycogen stores are preserved to maintain a readily available source of glucose, thereby providing energy and minimizing excessive fat and protein catabolism. This will reduce muscle loss and promote metabolic stability. In addition, it also aids in patient comfort by decreasing hunger, thirst, and anxiety. Overall, carbohydrate loading helps in faster recovery, early return of gastrointestinal function, reduced complications, and shorter hospital stay, making it an essential component of modern perioperative care practices.

6.2.1 Purpose and Physiological Benefits of Preoperative Carbohydrate Loading

Nutritional approach to preoperative carbohydrate loading is aimed at mitigating the negative metabolic impact of preoperative fasting and stress in the course of surgery. It has the main goal to ensure the optimal metabolic homeostasis of perioperative patients through the endogenous availability of energy and the enhancement of insulin sensitivity before surgical insult (Ljungqvist et al. 2017; Weimann et al. 2017). Figure 6.2 shows how preoperative carbohydrate loading improves insulin release and sensitivity, leading to better glucose utilization in the liver and muscles.

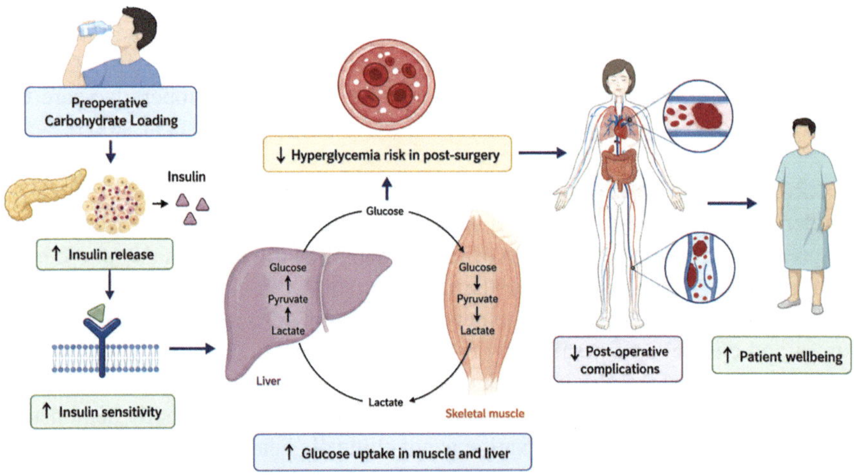

Fig. 6.2 Preoperative and postoperative carbohydrate loading. (Created by author using PowerPoint 2021)

As a result, it reduces postoperative hyperglycemia, complications, and enhances overall patient recovery and well-being.

6.2.1.1 Reduction in Insulin Resistance

Preoperative carbohydrate intake has been well-established as a beneficial factor in the reduction of insulin resistance postoperatively. The preoperative carbohydrate intake preserves insulin receptor sensitivity and decreases excessive endogenous glucose production caused by hormonal alterations in response to fasting (Ljungqvist et al. 2017). Carbohydrate loading prevents the excessive metabolic switch and use of gluconeogenesis instead of glycolysis, and enhances perioperative glycemic control (Thorell et al. 2016). Clinical significance of this stabilization of glucose metabolism is due to the fact that there is a strong association between insulin resistance and postoperative morbidity.

6.2.1.2 Preservation of Energy Reserves

Preoperative carbohydrate beverages can also be used to maintain the glycogen levels in the liver and act as a ready source of energy during the perioperative period (Thorell et al. 2016; Weimann et al. 2017). During the fasting condition, glycogen reserves are quickly burned off, and the body is compelled to utilize other energy sources, such as lipolysis and proteolysis. Carbohydrate loading keeps the body in reserve glycogen and therefore enables the body to maintain metabolic stability during surgical stress because of maintaining metabolic balance that shifts to catabolism (Thorell et al. 2016).

6.2.1.3 Reduction of Protein Catabolism

The other important physiological advantage is the decreased skeletal muscle protein breakdown. When in a fasting and/or stress state, muscle tissue amino acids are utilized in the process of hepatic gluconeogenesis, which leads to lean body mass loss (Deutz et al. 2014; Weimann et al. 2017). Carbohydrate intake prior to the operation blocks this response by offering an easily accessible energy source and thus decreasing the necessity to break down endogenous proteins (Thorell et al. 2016). This muscle maintenance is crucial, especially in surgical patients who are at risk of malnutrition or sarcopenia (Cruz-Jentoft et al. 2019).

6.2.1.4 Improved Patient Well-Being

Carbohydrate loading has also been implicated as a cause of better subjective patient comfort during the preoperative period. Research has indicated a decrease in hunger, thirst, irritability, and anxiety among patients who consume carbohydrate-rich beverages as opposed to patients who undergo a long period of starvation (Søreide et al. 2005; Weimann et al. 2017). Such patient-reported outcome improvements also have the potential to indirectly decrease neuroendocrine responses to stress, thus leading to more favorable metabolic stability in the preoperative period (Thorell et al. 2016).

6.2.1.5 Improved Postoperative Recovery Outcomes

A better metabolic control during perioperative using carbohydrate loading has been linked to better postoperative recovery parameters. These consist of the earlier restoration of the gastrointestinal activity, the enhanced mobilization, and shorter stay in the hospital among surgical patients (Gustafsson et al. 2013; Ljungqvist et al. 2017). Carbohydrate loading helps to facilitate a quicker physiological recovery and lessen postoperative complications associated with metabolic stress through attenuation of insulin resistance and metabolic homeostasis.

6.2.1.6 Overall Clinical Significance

All these physiological advantages prove the point that preoperative carbohydrate loading is not a supportive procedure but a specific metabolic policy that is focused on decreasing the severity of stress response during surgery. Carbohydrate loading is essential in improving the metabolic state of the perioperative period and improving the recovery processes through preservation of energy stores, decreased protein breakdown, and increased insulin sensitivity (Weimann et al. 2017; Ljungqvist et al. 2017).

6.2.2 Recommended Protocols and Timing for Preoperative Carbohydrate Loading

Carbohydrate loading protocols (preoperative) are designed nutritional interventions, which are formulated in order to maximize the perioperative metabolism status without compromising patient safety. These guidelines are mainly based on perioperative nutrition guidelines and the controlled clinical trials of gastric emptying, insulin sensitivity, and postoperative recovery rates (Weimann et al. 2017; Gustafsson et al. 2013).

6.2.2.1 Standard Carbohydrate Loading Regimen

The most popular carbohydrate loading method is a two-dosage regimen aimed at euglycemic conditions and minimizing the metabolic stress during fasting. In the majority of cases, a carbohydrate-rich liquid with about 12.5% of maltodextrin solution is given to the patients the evening before the surgery, and a repeat dose is administered 2–3 h before the induction of anesthesia (Weimann et al. 2017; Gustafsson et al. 2013).

The evening dose (which is usually approximately 800 mL) aims to restore the insulin levels of hepatic glycogen stores and decrease catabolism overnight, whereas the preoperative one (usually about 400 mL) is expected to bring the insulin sensitivity levels nearer to those at the time of surgical stress exposure (Thorell et al. 2016; Ljungqvist et al. 2017). This two-stage method will reduce the metabolic effects of long-term starvation and surgery (Fig. 6.2).

6.2.2.2 Physiological Rationale of Timing

The time of carbohydrate intake is essential to the attainment of an ideal effect on metabolism without affecting gastric safety. Gastric emptying tests indicate that clear carbohydrate solutions are normally emptied out of the stomach in the span of 90–120 min in healthy people and can be safely administered 2–3 h prior to administration of anesthesia (Søreide et al. 2005; Gustafsson et al. 2013). This is also a quick clearance method that reduces the risk of aspiration and maintains metabolic advantages.

Preoperative intake of carbohydrates will decrease the activation of hormones in response to fasting, which limits the insulin resistance mediated by cortisol and catecholamine (Thorell et al. 2016). Also, keeping carbohydrate levels near the perioperative surgery enhances the efficiency of glucose use and minimizes the intraoperative hyperglycemia (Ljungqvist et al. 2017).

6.2.2.3 Composition of Carbohydrate Solutions

Maltodextrin is the main underlying carbohydrate loading formula in most of the cases because of its high molecular weight, low osmolality, and quick gastric emptying properties (Weimann et al. 2017; Gustafsson et al. 2013). In comparison to hyperosmolar glucose solutions, maltodextrin-based drinks are well tolerated and cause little gastrointestinal discomfort.

These are the formulations that are set to provide quickly absorbable carbohydrates and do not stimulate excessive insulin secretion and evoke gastrointestinal intolerance. The low protein, low-fat content will guarantee that there is less delay in the gastric clearance and quick metabolic availability (Thorell et al. 2016).

6.2.2.4 Safety Profile and Clinical Considerations

The clinical experience has always proved that gastric residual volume and the risk of aspiration do not increase with preoperative carbohydrate loading that is performed within the recommended guidelines (Gustafsson et al. 2013; Søreide et al. 2005). Comparison of carbohydrate drinks and more conventional fasting regimens has indicated equal or quicker emptying of the stomach with clear carbohydrate solutions, which contributes to their safety in elective surgical patients.

Nevertheless, there are some groups of patients who need special evaluation prior to carbohydrate intake. These are patients with known delayed gastric emptying, severe gastroesophageal reflux disease, and those who are subjected to emergency surgery, and the gastric emptying status is not known (Weimann et al. 2017). Carbohydrate loading is cautiously recommended and should be accompanied by proper glycemic surveillance in patients with poorly controlled diabetes mellitus, though it is not contradictory in all patients (Ljungqvist et al. 2017; Gustafsson et al. 2013).

6.2.2.5 Clinical Outcomes and Evidence Base

Randomized clinical trials and systematic reviews have shown that preoperative carbohydrate loading enhances insulin sensitivity, postoperative insulin resistance, and patient comfort without augmenting the complications of the perioperative period (Awad et al. 2013; Gustafsson et al. 2013). Other positive effects are decreased preoperative thirst, hunger, and anxiety that result in a better patient experience and psychological health (Søreide et al. 2005).

Metabolically, carbohydrate loading decreases the dependence on and the catabolic response to endogenous glucose synthesis and counteracts the catabolic response of muscle protein in the perioperative period (Thorell et al. 2016; Deutz et al. 2014). All of these effects lead to better recovery outcomes, such as an earlier mobilization process and a shorter time in hospital among elective surgical patients (Ljungqvist et al. 2017). The carbohydrate loading and early postoperative feeding are explained in Table 6.1.

Table 6.1 Carbohydrate loading vs early postoperative feeding

Aspect	Carbohydrate loading (preoperative)	Early postoperative feeding	References
Definition	Intake of carbohydrate-rich clear fluid before surgery	Initiation of oral/enteral feeding soon after surgery	Bilku et al. (2014)
Standard Dose	50–100 g carbohydrate drink (usually 12.5% solution, ~400 mL night before +200 mL 2–3 h before surgery)	Start with liquids → advance to solids within 24–48 h	Lopez-Betancourt and Afonso (2021)
Timing	Up to 2 h before anesthesia (as per ERAS guidelines)	Within 6–24 h post-surgery	Kumar et al. (2025) and Robinson et al. (2021)
Effect on insulin resistance	Reduces postoperative insulin resistance by ~30–50%	Helps restore insulin sensitivity faster	Bilku et al. (2014) and Robinson et al. (2021)
Glycogen stores	Maintains liver glycogen (~70–90% preserved vs fasting depletion)	Prevents further depletion post-surgery	Lopez-Betancourt and Afonso (2021)
Nitrogen loss/ muscle breakdown	Reduces nitrogen loss by ~10–15%	Decreases muscle protein catabolism significantly	Robinson et al. (2021)
Patient comfort	Reduces thirst, hunger, and anxiety by ~40–60%	Improves overall well-being and satisfaction	Bilku et al. (2014)
Gastric emptying time	Clear fluids empty within 90–120 min	Feeding resumed once GI motility returned	Kumar et al. (2025)

(Continued)

Table 6.1 (Continued)

Aspect	Carbohydrate loading (preoperative)	Early postoperative feeding	References
Length of hospital stay	Reduced by ~0.5–1.5 days	Reduced by ~1–2 days	Şanlı et al. (2025) and Robinson et al. (2021)
Complication rate	No increase in aspiration risk (if guidelines followed)	↓ infections by ~20–30%, ↓ ileus	Robinson et al. (2021) and Şanlı et al. (2025)
GI function	Safe if gastric emptying normal	Stimulates gut motility, reduces ileus duration	Lopez-Betancourt and Afonso (2021)
Blood glucose effect	Mild increase (controlled in diabetics with monitoring)	Requires glucose monitoring, especially in the ICU	Kumar et al. (2025)
Mortality/morbidity	↓ overall complications (trend ~10–20%)	↓ postoperative morbidity significantly	Robinson et al. (2021)
ERAS recommendation	Strongly recommended (Grade A evidence)	Core ERAS component (Grade A evidence)	Kumar et al. (2025)
Contraindications	Gastroparesis, bowel obstruction, high aspiration risk	Severe ileus, hemodynamic instability	Lopez-Betancourt and Afonso (2021)
Recent research trends	Safe in well-controlled type 2 diabetes	Feeding even within 6 hrs in some surgeries	Şanlı et al. (2025)

6.3 Early Postoperative Feeding

Catabolism of protein is additionally caused due to pre-operative, peri-operative, and postoperative fasting, thereby resulting in associated morbidities and mortality. Postoperatively, the most common management of patients undergone elective abdominal surgery is to hold back the food till the reinstatement of bowel function. Moreover, in some of the patients, prolonged postoperative fasting for 3–4 days is suggested. This management is contemplated to be harmless for reducing complications like malabsorption and disruption of the anastomosis of intestines due to physical stress. Although prolonged fasting might cause depletion of significant nutrients, thus resulting in complications such as delay in wound healing and higher rate of infections, which further leads to longer period of stay in hospitals (Abela 2017).

By tradition, oral feeding among patients is put on hold till the restoration of bowel function in their postoperative stage. The reason is supposed to be that it can cause severe emesis, paralytic ileus, consequent aspiration pneumonia, anastomotic leakage, and wound dehiscence. During the postoperative period, the initiation of gastric emptying and minor absorption through intestines takes place on the first day. Additionally, reactivation of the colon takes place only after 48 hours of operation, and only 1–2 l of liquid, which is absorbed in the intestine, is secreted by the stomach and pancreas. Thus, it can be concluded that the gastrointestinal tract does not work properly in the initial days of the postoperative stage. However, the psychological aspect is also the point of consideration, as early feeding leads to improvement in the patient's well-being and thus has a significant role in the process of recovery followed by surgery. An additional point of consideration is cost-reduction, as patients who start eating earlier are likely to have reduced time of hospitalization (Ludwig et al. 2013).

Enhanced recovery after surgery (ERAS) protocols have developed as a standard for the management of patients in the postoperative stage for optimizing the postoperative outcomes. Internationally, nutrition is the core component of ERAS. The fundamental aspect of this nutritional component of ERAS protocols includes avoiding prolonged fasting periods and following the recent guidelines which recommend the initiation of oral intake on the first postoperative day. Conversely, though stronger evidence of introducing early oral intake in ERAS protocols has been reported in the case of colorectal surgery, the evidence for upper gastrointestinal surgery is yet to be established (Carmichael et al. 2022). Figure 6.3 outlines the progressive nutritional support strategy across different phases of critical illness and recovery. In the acute phase, feeding is gradually initiated while avoiding overfeeding, followed by full nutritional support and early mobilization in the ICU phase. As the patient recovers, calorie and protein requirements increase to support exercise and rehabilitation. Post-discharge, higher nutritional intake is emphasized to promote convalescence, muscle recovery, and overall functional improvement.

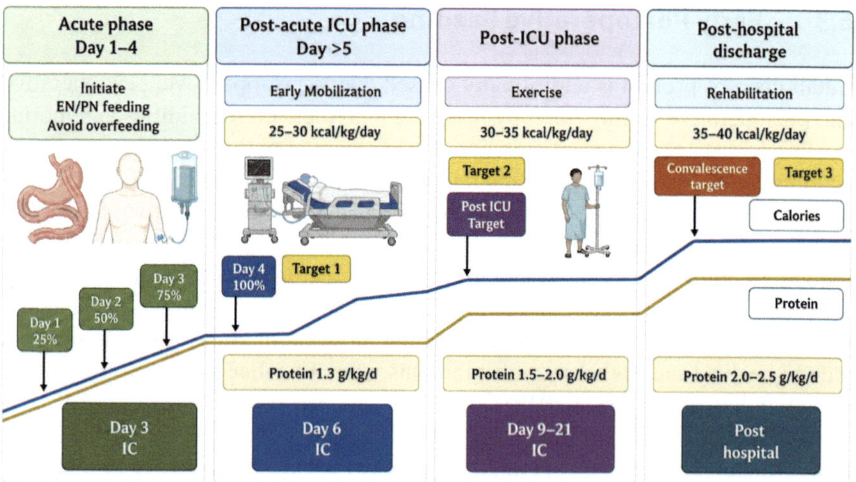

Fig. 6.3 Early postoperative feeding. (Created by author using PowerPoint 2021)

6.3.1 Benefits of Early Nutritional Intake

Early feeding supports gut function, improves energy balance, and promotes faster recovery. The expenditure of energy and loss of protein is increased by the surgical stress, thus necessitating the early nutritional support (Dervenis et al. 2003). ERAS is a multimodal care pathway intended toward the attainment of early recovery among patients going through major surgical procedures (Parks et al. 2018). The implementation process of ERAS comprises a team that consists of surgeons, anesthetists, an ERAS coordinator (usually a nurse or a physician assistant), and staff from units that take care of the surgical patients (Ljungqvist et al. 2017).

ERAS has been introduced to accelerate the time of recovery subsequent to surgery. Nutritional preparation with carbohydrate loading prior to surgery and early feeding with carbohydrates during the initial 24 h after surgery is recommended by the ERAS protocols (Abela 2017). The ERAS Society is an international non-profit professional society working to promote, develop, and implement ERAS programs. It publishes updated guidelines for several operations including evidence-based modern care changes where overnight fasting has been changed to serving carbohydrate drinks 2 h prior to surgery, minimal invasive approaches in place of large incisions, management of fluids for seeking balance instead of providing larger volumes of intravenous fluids, avoiding drains and tubes or removing them early, timely mobilization, and serving the food and drinks on the day of the operation.

ERAS protocols have led to a reduced time span of stay in the hospital by 30–50% and likewise a decrease in the complications, along with reductions in readmissions and costs. The components of the ERAS protocol result in reducing the operation-associated stress for retaining the anabolic homeostasis (Ljungqvist et al. 2017). The ERAS items being the sturdiest predictors for the reduced stay at hospital, along with decreased morbidities included the absenteeism of a nasogastric tube, timely mobilization, early oral nutrition, removal of the epidural and urinary catheter as early as possible, and use of non-opioid analgesics (Parks et al. 2018). Early oral nutrition (EON) has been reported of improving the recovery of gastrointestinal (GI) function, reducing the duration of hospital stay, and reducing associated mortalities subsequent to abdominal surgery. Although EON is also reported to frequently fail during the first week subsequent to surgery (Sun et al. 2017).

Early feeding is not only beneficial in stimulating GI peristalsis and promoting GI function, but also beneficial in nourishing the intestine, maintaining the integrity of the structure and function of intestinal mucosa, reducing the intestinal flora balance, and therefore reducing the incidence of wound infection as well as additional complications. Early feeding by means of laparoscopy-assisted colectomy leads to reduced time of stay in hospital and decreased postoperative morbidities among the elderly (DiFronzo et al. 2003). During the intervention by ERAS mode, drug analgesics are not utilized, and thus the inhibition of GI peristalsis is less, being beneficial in decreasing the time duration of intestinal peristalsis and anal exhaust. Additionally, early enteral nutrition support can result in promoting the repair of intestinal immunity and the biological barrier, blood circulation, and additionally accelerating the recovery of GI function, reducing complications like infections, and shortening the time duration of stay at the hospital (Kennedy et al. 2020) (Fig. 6.3).

6.3.2 Enteral Nutrition in the Immediate Postoperative Period

Enteral feeding is preferred because it maintains intestinal integrity and supports immune function. Conventional treatment followed by bowel resection necessitates starvation by administering intravenous fluids till the flatulence occurs. Postoperative gastric stasis results in nausea and vomiting, thereby obstructing the oral intake; however, continuation of small bowel function is still observed. Early enteral feeding results in improved outcomes among patients suffering from burns and trauma. Improvement in wound healing among a patient fed through enteral feeding subsequent to bowel resection was reported; however, the dietary requirements were met only upon introducing the normal diet (Carr et al. 1996).

Malnutrition is associated with suppression of humoral and cellular immune function, changes in the inflammatory responses, and delay or failure of the process of wound healing. Consequently, such patients showed higher incidences of severe complications during the immediate postoperative period. Supplementation of enteral formulas with arginine, RNA, and omega-3 fatty acids is specifically gaining attention as they combine such components that are beneficial in improving wound healing, the immune response, and the inflammatory reaction. Such immune-enhanced formulas introduced during the early postoperative period consistently showed significant improvement in the immunological status and inflammatory response among the patients (Farreras et al. 2005).

The very early postoperative enteral nutrition intervention provided on the basis of ERAS theory to patients undergoing gastrointestinal surgery is able to lessen the stress response. It is caused as the perioperative stress response among the patients is decreased and the rehabilitation process is reduced by the integration of nutritional support, anesthesia, and other nursing measures provided during the very early postoperative enteral nutrition intervention on the basis of ERAS theory. The major reason behind it is the ERAS concept, which, by means of improvement in the perioperative nursing measures like pain and injury control, results in combining the epidural block technology with general anesthesia for reducing the perioperative stress response of patients, effectively reducing the myocardial oxygen consumption of patients, and therefore promoting the postoperative recovery (Shao et al. 2023).

Enteral nutrition follows the normal physiological characteristics and possess the characteristic of greater utilization of nitrogen, that can be beneficial in maintaining the nitrogen balance during the postoperative stage, maintaining the metabolism of tissue and organ, maintaining the integrity of intestinal mucosal barrier function, promoting recovery of GI function, reducing the abdominal distension, and contributing in the prevention and treatment of anastomotic oedema and postoperative delayed gastric functional emptying syndrome (Lowen et al. 2022). Patients suffering from GI tumors are nutritionally vulnerable; thus, early enteral nutrition support programs can be beneficial in improving the nutritional status of such patients along with speedy postoperative recovery. Early enteral nutrition is not only beneficial in improving the immune function and protecting the intestinal function among patients, but is also helpful in improving the patient's quality of life (Chen et al. 2023).

Early enteral nutrition not only possesses the potential of providing nutrients to the body as per its requirements but also aids in the recovery of GI peristalsis function, boosts the protective function of the GI mucosal barrier, and reduces the incidence of bacterial flora disorders (Lin et al. 2025). Enteral nutrition is also advantageous in avoiding stomach mucosa atrophy and speeding up the recovery of GI function.

6.4 Impact on Recovery and Muscle Preservation

Early postoperative feeding is associated with a decrease in infection-associated complications, improvement in healing, and reduction in the duration of stay at the hospital. Therefore, resuming oral feeding as early as possible after the surgery, along with the aim of introducing solid foods within 24 h, is recommended. During the initial hours after surgery, the appetite of the patient is usually repressed, which leads to difficulty in consuming solid foods. Encouraging the intake of free-form EAAs is recommended to be valuable at this time. Free-form EAAs have negligible influence on the appetite (Paddon-Jones et al. 2005). Though the effects of EAA are yet not analyzed during the post-surgical period, the early intake of free-form EAA after surgery could be extremely beneficial as it provides the amino acids required for supporting healing and recovery, devoid of concern related to a large gastric load. The consumption of amino acids during the immediate postoperative period could also be beneficial in supporting the immune response (Muyskens et al. 2019).

6.4.1 Reduction of Muscle Loss and Fatigue

Adequate carbohydrate and nutrient intake helps reduce protein breakdown after surgery. Surgical trauma results in an induced state of stress in the patient, thus resulting in imbalanced homeostasis. Stress response possesses a nature of a survival mechanism for providing energy and maintaining the cardiovascular equilibrium. However, an excessive or continuing response, as observed in the case of surgery, results in adverse outcomes such as catabolism of protein, hypertension, hyperglycemia, immunosuppression, and tachycardia.

The major objectives of the multidisciplinary, multimodal, and comprehensive ERAS pathways include blunting the surgical stress response by optimizing the nutritional and functional status, limiting the preoperative fasting, promoting individualized fluid management, encouraging opioid-sparing analgesia, utilizing minimally invasive surgery, and promoting early post-operative ambulation as well as feeding (Brown et al. 2018). Providing carbohydrate or carbohydrate with peptide drinks orally during the preoperative phase as an alternative to fasting could be beneficial in improving the strength of voluntary muscles, ambulation, and consumption of nutrients during the post-operative stage, along with decreasing the anxiety, exhaustion, and distress observed postoperatively and reducing the endocrine response toward surgery (Henriksen et al. 2003).

The consumption of nutrients around the operative phase aims to support the enhanced nutritional needs in the hypermetabolic and inflammatory state, manage the post-surgical resistance to insulin, and reduce muscle atrophy. The strategies opted initially have emphasized carbohydrate/glucose intake, in efforts to reduce post-surgical insulin resistance and the rise in gluconeogenesis (Ackerman et al. 2020). Compared to fasting conditions, pre-operative glucose intake (8–10 oz. containing 50 g, 2 h before surgery) has been shown to reduce post-operative insulin resistance by up to 50%. In addition, pre-operative glucose intake has been shown to positively impact lean body mass maintenance and muscle function. Ingesting 125 mg/mL carbohydrate orally during the night before and until 3 h prior to surgery effectively sustained the protein balance of the whole body after 24 h of surgery (Hirsch et al. 2021). The supplementation of amino acids after surgery effectually reduced the catabolism of muscles and the whole body, increasing the protein synthesis in the whole body by 40%, and reducing the protein breakdown in the whole body by 20% (Rittig et al. 2016).

6.4.2 Improved Patient Comfort and Functional Recovery

Early nutrition can decrease weakness and support quicker return to normal activity.

Carbohydrates rapidly increase the levels of glucose in the blood, thus resulting in hyperglycemia. A biphasic rise in insulin is caused, which further leads to increased oxidation of glucose and synthesis of glycogen, along with inhibiting the oxidation of fatty acids. However, alterations in such a biphasic response are observed in the conditions of insulin resistance, like post-surgical insulin resistance or type 2 diabetes. In contrast, the intake of protein results in increased concentration of amino acids in the blood, thereby stimulating insulin and the synthesis of muscle protein. Insulin resistance does not negatively impact the insulin response observed after the consumption of protein. In essence, combined consumption of amino acid and glucose could lessen the loss of muscle loss and its strength, specifically when consumed before surgery (Hirsch et al. 2021).

Intake levels of protein are usually recommended to be not less than 1.6 g/kg/day and up to 2.0–3.0 g/kg/day at the time of rehabilitation (Tipton 2015). A decreased appetite is usually observed after surgery, thereby causing difficulty in meeting the dietary protein needs. Intake of EAAs and/or protein supplements between meals can be beneficial in attaining greater levels of protein consumption and optimizing the consumption of nutrients throughout the day, at the time of repressed appetite (Smith-Ryan et al. 2020).

In case of surgeries necessitating physical rehabilitation, like the joint replacement, the timings related to nutrient consumption during the rehabilitation sessions also need to be measured. Consumption of nutrients during the exercise/rehabilitation session could be beneficial in increasing the strength, lean mass, and functionality, eventually resulting in quickly returning to day-to-day activities of livelihood (Hirsch et al. 2021). Prior to 3–4 h of a therapy session, a small meal comprising complex carbohydrates (50–100 g) and high biological value protein (30–40 g) should be consumed by the patients. Thereafter, a beverage that consists of protein and carbohydrate needs to be consumed before 15–45 min of therapy.

Additionally, a protein beverage should be consumed subsequent to the therapy session (Smith-Ryan et al. 2020). In addition to protein, supplements like β-hydroxy-β-methylbutyrate (HMB), omega-3 fatty acids, creatine monohydrate, and probiotics have shown effectiveness in supporting the strength and functionality of muscles (Burgess et al. 2018), and thus might be worthy of being considered. Adequate intake of nutrients is necessary to address the surgical stress response and mitigate the loss of mass, strength, and functionality of muscles. Consumption of carbohydrate is valuable in meeting the increased needs of energy related to the altered metabolism and wound healing observed after surgery. On the other hand, consumption of protein is favorable in providing the amino acids needed for supporting wound healing, immune function, and preservation of muscles.

Consumption of protein during the whole surgical process, specifically at the time of the post-surgical time period, should be emphasized, as it results in reduced catabolism of muscles and reduced functionality associated with loss. Though maintaining the good quality whole food sources of protein and carbohydrate is important, inclusion of supplemental sources allows continuous consumption of nutrients immediately before and after hours of surgery. Intake of free-form EAAs, solely or additionally with protein sources, is specifically advantageous in controlling anabolic resistance, demanding their usage both prior to and post-surgery for attenuating muscle atrophy among older adults (Hirsch et al. 2021).

6.5 Clinical Considerations and Implementation

Two recent perioperative nutritional methods gaining increasing acceptance as essential parts of the modern surgical treatment are carbohydrate loading and early postoperative feeding. Their successful deployment, however, heavily depends on the careful choice of the patients, the safety, and the incorporation into structured therapeutic approaches such as the Enhancement Recovery After Surgery (ERAS) (Şanlı et al. 2025). Although these treatment methods possess a number of benefits, such as; reduced insulin resistance, reduced recovery time, and reduced hospital stay, recent studies point out that the modalities are only effective when administered in a patient-based, protocol-focused and multidisciplinary manner (Wolosowicz et al. 2022).

6.5.1 Patient Selection and Safety Considerations

6.5.1.1 Importance of Patient Selection in Perioperative Nutrition

Patient selection is significant in ensuring a safe and effective use of carbohydrate load and early postoperative nutrition. Variables that need to be considered in clinical decisions may include the type of operation, metabolic status, comorbidities, and intestinal status, since not every surgical client will be the best candidate. Considering the heterogeneity of the patients in surgery departments, the modern perioperative guidelines emphasize the individual approach to dietary planning and do not focus on the universal approach (Bilku et al. 2014).

6.5.1.2 Preoperative Carbohydrate Loading: Indications and Benefits

Patients undergoing elective surgery with a functioning gastrointestinal system who do not pose a considerable risk of aspiration are often advised to undergo preoperative carbohydrate loading (PCL). Surgical outcomes, prolonged insulin resistance, and an amplification of metabolic stress due to long-term fasting have been demonstrated not just as detrimental to the current surgical practice. Carbohydrate loading, in turn, helps conserve glycogen stores, decrease catabolic responses, and become more sensitive to insulin. They are commonly administered as a transparent, carbs-rich beverage two to three hours prior to anesthesia (Kumar et al. 2025).

6.5.1.3 Evidence from Clinical Studies and Surgical Outcomes

Recent meta-analyses and randomized controlled studies indicate that carbohydrate loading can dramatically reduce patient hospitalization and add to patient comfort in comparison with fasting (2024–2025). The importance of proper patient selection is stressed by the fact that the degree of said benefits varies depending on the surgical setting and patient groups. As an example, larger abdominal and colorectal surgeries, where metabolic load is predominant, tend to demonstrate more benefits (Sebestyén et al. 2025).

6.5.1.4 Special Considerations in Diabetic Patients

Carbohydrate loading of patients with metabolic diseases, with diabetes mellitus being a particular concern, is the subject of recent studies and the treatment debate. Its use in diabetic patients has been somewhat limited since the worries were hyperglycemia and delayed gastric emptying, as well as risk of aspiration. Nevertheless, when using glycemic monitoring and individualized insulin therapy, most recent systematic reviews show that carbohydrate loading can be used safely in individuals with controlled type 2 diabetes. Also, studies refute past limited solutions by presenting more patient comfort and presumably no evident increase in issues in this group (Robinson et al. 2021).

6.5.1.5 Gastrointestinal Factors and Contraindications

One such SAF area is gastrointestinal, which transcends metabolic state. Early feeding could be inappropriate in patients with issues such as gastroparesis, intestinal blockage, severe reflux disease, or high risk of aspiration. In some cases, alternative ways of diet such as parenteral assistance or delaying feeding may be required. Moreover, given that a low quality of administration can increase perioperative risks, guidelines on such issues as the time and combination of carbohydrate drinks should be followed to the letter (Miao et al. 2023).

6.5.1.6 Early Postoperative Feeding: Safety and Clinical Benefits

The other critical area of perioperative nutrition is early postoperative feeding that requires selective nursing. Patients may previously be kept nil per os (NPO) until they are digesting again, but the current studies recommend that they receive oral or enteral food within 24–48 h after surgery. Early feeding has been proven to enhance recovery, reduce infectious issues, and enhance gastrointestinal motility. However, not all patients can react to early nutrition. The factors that should be considered include individual gastrointestinal tolerance, aesthetic effects, and surgical intricacy (Abunnaja et al. 2013).

6.5.1.7 Feeding Intolerance and Management Strategies

One of the issues that must be carefully observed is feeding intolerance, which may manifest itself as nausea, vomiting, distension of the stomach or ileus. Sometimes in these cases, it may be necessary to switch to alternative dietary practices, prokinetic medications, or make a progressive change in feeding. Importantly, new studies indicate that, in the right amount, early feeding does not increase the chances of anastomotic leakage or other severe issues, another fact that proves its safety in certain individuals (Ortigoza 2022).

6.5.1.8 Aspiration Risk and Fasting Guidelines

Another significant safety aspect is the risk of aspiration under the induction of anesthesia. Recent studies report that carbohydrate clear drinks to a maximum of 2 times in the pre-surgery time help to improve metabolic state and avoid injuries as they empty the stomach rapidly and do not increase the gastrointestinal volume. Consequently, explicit liquids, such as beverage that includes carbohydrates, can now be taken nearer to the working time with new fasting guidelines (Zhang et al. 2020).

6.5.1.9 Emerging Trends: Biomarkers and Personalized Nutrition

Risk assessment methods and use of biomarkers to guide dietary therapy are a new development in patient selection. Such indicators as metabolic and insulin resistance index and inflammatory markers are also in use increasingly in place of clinical examination to understand which patients will benefit most by carbohydrate loading and early feeding. Moreover, personalized medicine techniques include patient genomics, metabolic, and real-time, which are emerging as possible options of the future in perioperative nutrition (Kosmas et al. 2024).

6.5.1.10 Safety Considerations

In this context, patient selection and safety concerns are imperative in the establishment of successful implementation of carbohydrate loading and early postoperative feeding. Although the benefits of these methods are evident, they should be tailored on the health of the patient, surgery, and risk profile. The individualization and evidence-based procedure of perioperative nutritional therapy have reached a new level, and the recent research is concerned with the use of safety policies, and the implementation of prequalification standards. The patient selection and safety considerations have been explained in Table 6.2.

Table 6.2 Patient selection and safety considerations

Aspect	Carbohydrate loading	Early postoperative feeding	References
Definition	Intake of carbohydrate-rich drinks before surgery (2–3 h prior)	Initiation of oral/enteral feeding within 24–48 h after surgery	Awad et al. (2013) and Ludwig et al. (2013)
Ideal candidates	Elective surgery patients with functional GI tract	Patients with stable condition and functional GI tract	Lopez-Betancourt and Afonso (2021) and Osland et al. (2011)
Not suitable for	Gastroparesis, bowel obstruction, high aspiration risk	Severe ileus, bowel obstruction, hemodynamic instability	Awad et al. (2013) and Lopez-Betancourt and Afonso (2021)
Metabolic benefit	Reduces insulin resistance, preserves glycogen	Reduces catabolism, improves recovery	Lopez-Betancourt and Afonso (2021) and Yi et al. (2020)
Safety concerns	Risk of hyperglycemia (especially in diabetes)	Feeding intolerance (nausea, vomiting, distension)	Ludwig et al. (2013) and Osland et al. (2011)
Aspiration risk	Low if given within guidelines (clear fluids ≤2 h)	Minimal if patient monitored properly	Lopez-Betancourt and Afonso (2021) and Yi et al. (2020)
Diabetic consideration	Safe in controlled diabetes with monitoring	Requires glucose monitoring and gradual feeding	Awad et al. (2013) and Osland et al. (2011)
Monitoring needed	Blood glucose, gastric emptying	GI tolerance, bowel function	Ludwig et al. (2013) Yi et al. (2020)
Recent trends	Personalized carbohydrate dosing, use in diabetics	Early oral feeding protocols, tolerance-based advancement	Awad et al. (2013) and Lopez-Betancourt and Afonso (2021)
Evidence-based outcome	Reduced hospital stay, improved comfort	Reduced complications, faster recovery	Lopez-Betancourt and Afonso (2021), Ludwig et al. (2013) and Yi et al. (2020)

6.5.2 Integration with Enhanced Recovery Programs

6.5.2.1 Introduction to ERAS and Nutritional Integration

The introduction of early postoperative nutrition and carbohydrate loading into the Enhanced recovery after surgery (ERAS) is one of the considerable changes that have occurred on the field of perioperative care. ERAS is a multimodal, evidence-based approach which is normally aimed at speeding up the recovering process, sustaining physiological processes and minimizing surgical stress. An early eating and carbohydrate loading are important factors in these pathways, known as nutritional optimization (Jain et al. 2023).

6.5.2.2 Avoidance of Prolonged Fasting and Role of Carbohydrate Loading

One of the principal tenets of ERAS is the prevention of the prolonged fasting, an experiment that has traditionally been one of the preoperative practices. Instead, the ERAS guidelines recommend preoperative carbohydrate loading to metabolically prepare a patient to surgery. Evidence to support this change includes decreasing rates of insulin resistance in the presence of carbohydrate loading, maintaining muscle mass, and postoperative outcome improvements. Surgery stresses patients and makes their recovery slow when they are maintained in a well-nourished metabolism (Steenhagen 2016).

6.5.2.3 Synergistic Effect of ERAS Components

These current research findings have demonstrated the advantages of including carbohydrate loading with other elements of the ERAS that comprise: goal-oriented hydration therapy, less-invasive surgery and early mobility. Research shows that the benefits of including carbohydrate loading into a complete ERAS protocol are greater than when it as a stand-alone intervention. This brings out the importance of a holistic approach, where a number of evidence-based approaches are used to complement each other to enhance the recovery (Tong et al. 2022).

6.5.2.4 Early Postoperative Feeding in ERAS Protocols

Early postoperative nutrition is another critical element of ERAS processes. ERAS recommends initiating oral nutrition within the first few hours after surgery, but does not wait until there is a restoration of bowel movements or the presence of flatus. This plan has been observed to enhance gastrointestinal health, reduce complications, and decreased hospitalization. Moreover, early feeding is beneficial in terms of nutritional integrity during critical postoperative period, and enhancement of immunological activity (Canzan et al. 2022).

6.5.2.5 Continuity of Nutritional Care Across Perioperative Phases

The combination of early feeding with carbohydrate loading leads to a continuous nutritional plan in the future, during the perioperative phase. Although preoperative carbohydrate intake reduces catabolic processes and prepares the body to begin a surgical procedure, early postoperative nutrition will foster the process and inhibit it. One of the main characteristics of ERAS routes is continuity, which enhances therapeutic results (Tong et al. 2022).

6.5.2.6 Clinical Outcomes and Benefits of ERAS Integration

Recent trials (2024–2025) suggested that early feeding and carbohydrate loading regimens using ERAS protocols are crucial in decreasing the duration of stay, surgery-related and medical cost problems by a large margin. This has also been linked with more satisfaction in the patients and lower ratings of pain and an earlier time to resume normal activity (Yi et al. 2020).

The other important development is the adjustment of ERAS protocols to specific fields of surgery and patient demographics. Special ERAS routes (examples include carbohydrate loading with early feeding) have been created to meet the needs of the corresponding groups, e.g. gynecologic oncology, orthopedic surgery, and colorectal surgery. Such specialty-friendly processes have also demonstrated the efficacy of the ERAS procedure and have proceeded to improve the results (Melnyk et al. 2011).

6.5.2.7 Technological Advancements in ERAS Implementation

The use of ERAS feeding techniques is also being improved by technological developments. Digital health technologies and the processes of guiding patients on preoperative planning and postoperative recovery are being implemented through the use of digital health technologies in both remote monitoring systems and as mobile applications. The technologies help to improve compliance with the ERAS processes by monitoring the recovery state, tracking of nutritional intake, and offering personalized nutritional advice (Abosheisha et al. 2025).

6.5.2.8 Challenges in Implementation of ERAS Programs

ERAS program implementation is fraught with challenges, in spite of its benefits. They consist of diversity to clinical practice, a lack of knowledge of healthcare professionals, and an inability to abandon traditional practices. Successful integration requires a team of professionals, who comprise surgeons, anesthesiologists, nutritionists, nurses, and physiotherapists. To overcome these barriers, education, standardization of procedures, and continuous quality improvement are needed (Özçelik 2024).

6.5.2.9 Emerging Trends: Immunonutrition and Personalized Nutrition

There is another recent trend of integrating the use of functional foods and immunonutrition into the ERAS pathways. Besides carbohydrate loading, nutritional supplements supplemented with nucleotides, omega-3 fatty acids, and arginine are being used to boost the immune responses and recovery. What is more, research is carried out on the role of personalized diet according to genetic and metabolic profile, which in the future can enhance ERAS procedures.

6.5.2.10 Role of Patient Education and Engagement

Importantly, patient education and involvement are key components of ERAS programs. Through well-defined information on preoperative intake of carbohydrates, postoperative diet, and exercises to recover, patients are involved in the treatment procedures. By applying this patient-centered approach, adherence will be enhanced and favor deeper outcomes (Martínez-Ortega et al. 2022).

Table 6.3 Integration with ERAS programs

Component	Role in ERAS	Clinical benefit	References
Preoperative fasting avoidance	Allows clear fluids + carbohydrate drinks	Reduces stress response	Kennedy et al. (2020) and Özçelik (2024)
Carbohydrate loading	Maintains metabolic state before surgery	Reduces insulin resistance	Özçelik (2024)
Early postoperative feeding	Starts feeding within 24 h	Improves gut motility and healing	Melnyk et al. (2011)
Multimodal approach	Combined with early mobilization, minimal invasive surgery	Faster recovery	Kennedy et al. (2020) and Melnyk et al. (2011)
Nutritional continuity	Pre-operational + Post-operational nutrition integration	Prevents catabolism	Özçelik (2024) and Thorell et al. (2016)
Hospital stay	Reduced duration	Cost-effective care	Melnyk et al. (2011)
Complication rate	Lower infections and morbidity	Better outcomes	Özçelik (2024) and Thorell et al. (2016)
Patient comfort	Less thirst, hunger, anxiety	Improved satisfaction	Kennedy et al. (2020)
Specialized protocols	Tailored for colorectal, orthopedic, oncology surgeries	Better targeted outcomes	Melnyk et al. (2011) and Özçelik (2024)
Recent innovations	Digital monitoring, AI-based nutrition plans	Personalized care	Kennedy et al. (2020) and Thorell et al. (2016)

6.5.2.11 ERAS as a Paradigm Shift in Perioperative Care

Lastly, there is the paradigm shift of carbohydrate loading and the early feeding, postoperative care in the ERAS programs of perioperative care. ERAS guidelines improve the stability of metabolisms, reduce the occurrence of complications, and increase recovery through the replacement of outdated practices of fasting and late feeding with evidence-based nutrition measures. Further research and innovation are still improving these techniques and the future of a personal, efficient, and patient-centered surgery (Lopez-Betancourt and Afonso 2021) (Table 6.3).

6.6 Conclusion

Metabolic stress, delayed recovery, and insulin resistance fluctuate the carbohydrate loading and show the impact on the pre-post-operative condition. The scrupulous carbohydrate intake helps in preoperative surgery and early reintroduction of nutrition just after surgery, for better outcomes in the patient's health. Based on the clinical evidence and physiological basis, carbohydrate intake helps in energy preservation and mitigates the metabolic imbalance in preoperative surgical conditions. Restoring the carbohydrates, it also helps in improving the muscle mass and insulin sensitivity in the postoperative patients' outcome. The enteral feeding helps in sustaining the gastrointestinal functioning, immune response boost, and tissue building. The supplementation of personalized nutritional management improves the patient's complications and outcomes in perioperative cases.

References

Abela G. The potential benefits and harms of early feeding post-surgery: a literature review. Int Wound J. 2017;14(5):870–3. https://doi.org/10.1111/iwj.12750.

Abosheisha M, Nasr E, Abdellatif M, Swealem A, Ammar A, Hasan MAS, et al. The future of enhanced recovery after surgery in general surgery: integrating artificial intelligence, personalized care, and technological advances. Cureus. 2025;17(9). https://doi.org/10.7759/cureus.91528.

Abunnaja S, Cuviello A, Sanchez JA. Enteral and parenteral nutrition in the perioperative period: state of the art. Nutrients. 2013;5(2):608–23. https://doi.org/10.3390/nu5020608.

Ackerman RS, Tufts CW, DePinto DG, Chen J, Altshuler JR, Serdiuk A, Cohen JB, Patel SY. How sweet is this? A review and evaluation of preoperative carbohydrate loading in the enhanced recovery after surgery model. Nutr Clin Pract. 2020;35(2):246–53. https://doi.org/10.1002/ncp.10427.

Awad S, Varadhan KK, Ljungqvist O, Lobo DN. A meta-analysis of randomised controlled trials on preoperative oral carbohydrate treatment in elective surgery. Clin Nutr. 2013;32(1):34–44. https://doi.org/10.1016/j.clnu.2012.10.011.

Bilku DK, Dennison AR, Hall TC, Metcalfe MS, Garcea G. Role of preoperative carbohydrate loading: a systematic review. Ann R Coll Surg Engl. 2014;96(1):15–22. https://doi.org/10.1308/003588414x13824511650614.

Brady M, Kinn S, Stuart P. Preoperative fasting for adults to prevent perioperative complications. Cochrane Database Syst Rev. 2003;(4):CD004423. https://doi.org/10.1002/14651858.CD004423.

Brown JK, Singh K, Dumitru R, Chan E, Kim MP. The benefits of enhanced recovery after surgery programs and their application in cardiothoracic surgery. Methodist Debakey Cardiovasc J. 2018;14(2):77. https://doi.org/10.14797/mdcj-14-2-77.

Burgess LC, Phillips SM, Wainwright TW. What is the role of nutritional supplements in support of total hip replacement and total knee replacement surgeries? A systematic review. Nutrients. 2018;10(7):820. https://doi.org/10.3390/nu10070820.

Calder PC. Nutrition, immunity and inflammation. Nutrients. 2020;12(1):118. https://doi.org/10.3390/nu12010118.

Canzan F, Caliaro A, Cavada ML, Mezzalira E, Paiella S, Ambrosi E. The effect of early oral postoperative feeding on the recovery of intestinal motility after gastrointestinal surgery: protocol for a systematic review and meta-analysis. PLoS One. 2022;17(8):e0273085. https://doi.org/10.1371/journal.pone.0273085.

Carmichael L, Rocca R, Laing E, Ashford P, Collins J, Jackson L, et al. Early postoperative feeding following surgery for upper gastrointestinal cancer: a systematic review. J Hum Nutr Diet. 2022;35(1):33–48. https://doi.org/10.1111/jhn.12930.

Carr CS, Ling KE, Boulos P, Singer M. Randomised trial of safety and efficacy of immediate postoperative enteral feeding in patients undergoing gastrointestinal resection. BMJ. 1996;312(7035):869–71. https://doi.org/10.1136/bmj.312.7035.869.

Cederholm T, Jensen GL, Correia MITD, Gonzalez MC, Fukushima R, Higashiguchi T, et al. GLIM criteria for the diagnosis of malnutrition: A consensus report. Clin Nutr. 2019;38(1):1–9. https://doi.org/10.1016/j.clnu.2018.08.002.

Chen Z, Hong B, He JJ, Ye QQ, Hu QY. Examining the impact of early enteral nutritional support on postoperative recovery in patients undergoing surgical treatment for gastrointestinal neoplasms. World J Gastrointest Surg. 2023;15(10):2222–33. https://doi.org/10.4240/wjgs.v15.i10.2222.

Cruz-Jentoft AJ, Bahat G, Bauer J, Boirie Y, Bruyère O, Cederholm T, et al. Sarcopenia: Revised European consensus on definition and diagnosis. Age Ageing. 2019;48(1):16–31. https://doi.org/10.1093/ageing/afy169.

Dervenis, C., Avgerinos, C., Lytras, D., & Delis, S. (2003). Benefits and limitations of enteral nutrition in the early postoperative period. Langenbeck's Arch Surg, 387(11), 441–449. https://doi.org/10.1007/s00423-003-0350-1.

Desborough JP. The stress response to trauma and surgery. Br J Anaesth. 2000;85(1):109–17. https://doi.org/10.1093/bja/85.1.109.

Deutz NEP, Bauer JM, Barazzoni R, Biolo G, Boirie Y, Bosy-Westphal A, et al. Protein intake and exercise for optimal muscle function with aging: recommendations from the ESPEN Expert Group. Clin Nutr. 2014;33(6):929–36. https://doi.org/10.1016/j.clnu.2014.04.007.

DiFronzo AL, Yamin N, Patel K, O'Connell TX. Benefits of early feeding and early hospital discharge in elderly patients undergoing open colon resection. J Am Coll Surg. 2003;197(5):747–52. https://doi.org/10.1016/s1072-7515(03)00794-4.

Farreras N, Artigas V, Cardona D, Rius X, Trias M, González JA. Effect of early postoperative enteral immunonutrition on wound healing in patients undergoing surgery for gastric cancer. Clin Nutr. 2005;24(1):55–65. https://doi.org/10.1016/j.clnu.2004.07.002.

Gustafsson UO, Scott MJ, Schwenk W, Demartines N, Roulin D, Francis N, et al. Guidelines for perioperative care in elective colonic surgery: Enhanced Recovery After Surgery (ERAS®) Society recommendations. World J Surg. 2013;37(2):259–84. https://doi.org/10.1016/j.clnu.2012.08.013.

Henriksen MG, Hessov I, Dela F, Vind Hansen H, Haraldsted V, Rodt SÅ. Effects of preoperative oral carbohydrates and peptides on postoperative endocrine response, mobilization, nutrition and muscle function in abdominal surgery. Acta Anaesthesiol Scand. 2003;47(2):191–9. https://doi.org/10.1034/j.1399-6576.2003.00047.x.

Hirsch KR, Wolfe RR, Ferrando AA. Pre-and post-surgical nutrition for preservation of muscle mass, strength, and functionality following orthopedic surgery. Nutrients. 2021;13(5):1675. https://doi.org/10.3390/nu13051675.

Jain SN, Lamture Y, Krishna M. Enhanced recovery after surgery: exploring the advances and strategies. Cureus. 2023;15(10). https://doi.org/10.7759/cureus.47237.

Kennedy GT, Hill CM, Huang Y, So A, Fosnot J, Wu L, Farrar J t, Tchou J. Enhanced recovery after surgery (ERAS) protocol reduces perioperative narcotic requirement and length of stay in patients undergoing mastectomy with implant-based reconstruction. Am J Surg. 2020;220(1):147–52. https://doi.org/10.1016/j.amjsurg.2019.10.007.

Kosmas CE, Sourlas A, Oikonomakis K, Zoumi EA, Papadimitriou A, Kostara CE. Biomarkers of insulin sensitivity/resistance. J Int Med Res. 2024;52(10):03000605241285550. https://doi.org/10.1177/03000605241285550.

Kumar M, Patil NS, Mohapatra N, Yadav A, Sindwani G, Dhingra U, et al. Preoperative carbohydrate loading reduces perioperative insulin resistance and hastens functional recovery of remnant liver after living donor hepatectomy: an open-label randomized controlled trial. Hepatol Int. 2025;19(5):1151–61. https://doi.org/10.1007/s12072-025-10831-5.

Lin XJ, Xu JZ, Hu Q, Chen J. Effects of enhanced recovery after surgery on postoperative intestinal function and intestinal flora during laparoscopic gastric cancer surgery. World J Gastrointest Surg. 2025;17(9):106286. https://doi.org/10.4240/wjgs.v17.i9.106286.

Ljungqvist O, Scott M, Fearon KC. Enhanced recovery after surgery: a review. JAMA Surg. 2017;152(3):292–8. https://doi.org/10.1001/jamasurg.2016.4952.

Lopez-Betancourt R, Afonso AM. Carbohydrate loading and fluid management within enhanced recovery. Semin Colon Rectal Surg. 2021;32(3):100828). WB Saunders. https://doi.org/10.1016/j.scrs.2021.100828.

Lowen DJ, Hodgson R, Tacey M, Barclay KL. Does deep neuromuscular blockade provide improved outcomes in low pressure laparoscopic colorectal surgery? A single blinded randomized pilot study. ANZ J Surg. 2022;92(6):1447–53. https://doi.org/10.1111/ans.17458.

Ludwig RB, Paludo J, Fernandes D, Scherer F. Lesser time of preoperative fasting and early postoperative feeding are safe? ABCD Arquivos Brasileiros de Cirurgia Digestiva (São Paulo). 2013;26:54–8. https://doi.org/10.1590/s0102-67202013000100012.

Martínez-Ortega AJ, Piñar-Gutiérrez A, Serrano-Aguayo P, González-Navarro I, Remón-Ruíz PJ, Pereira-Cunill JL, García-Luna PP. Perioperative nutritional support: a review of current literature. Nutrients. 2022;14(8):1601. https://doi.org/10.3390/nu14081601.

Melnyk M, Casey RG, Black P, Koupparis AJ. Enhanced recovery after surgery (ERAS) protocols: time to change practice? Can Urol Assoc J. 2011;5(5):342. https://doi.org/10.5489/cuaj.11002.

Miao P, Zhang Y, Zhong A. Risk factors of aspiration occurrence with different feeding patterns in elderly intensive care unit patients: a cross-sectional study. J Thorac Dis. 2023;15(5):2585. https://doi.org/10.21037/jtd-23-430.

Muyskens JB, Foote DM, Bigot NJ, Strycker LA, Smolkowski K, Kirkpatrick TK, Lantz BA, Shah SN, Mohler CG, Jewett BA, Dreyer HC. Cellular and morphological changes with EAA supplementation before and after total knee arthroplasty. J Appl Physiol. 2019;127(2):531–45. https://doi.org/10.1152/japplphysiol.00869.2018.

Ortigoza EB. Feeding intolerance. Early human development. 2022;171:105601. https://doi.org/10.1016/j.earlhumdev.2022.105601.

Osland E, Yunus RM, Khan S, Memon MA. Early versus traditional postoperative feeding in patients undergoing resectional gastrointestinal surgery: a meta-analysis. J Parenter Enter Nutr. 2011;35(4):473–87. https://doi.org/10.1177/0148607110385698.

Özçelik M. Implementation of ERAS protocols: in theory and practice. Turkish J Anaesthesiol Reanim. 2024;52(5):163. https://doi.org/10.4274/tjar.2024.241723.

Paddon-Jones D, Sheffield-Moore M, Aarsland A, Wolfe RR, Ferrando AA. Exogenous amino acids stimulate human muscle anabolism without interfering with the response to mixed meal ingestion. Am J Physiol-Endocrinol Metab. 2005;288(4):E761–7. https://doi.org/10.1152/ajpendo.00291.2004.

Parks L, Routt M, De Villiers A. Enhanced recovery after surgery. J Adv Pract Oncol. 2018;9(5):511. https://pmc.ncbi.nlm.nih.gov/articles/PMC6505539/.

Rittig N, Bach E, Thomsen HH, Johannsen M, Jørgensen JO, Richelsen B, Jessen N, Møller N. Amino acid supplementation is anabolic during the acute phase of endotoxin-induced inflammation: a human randomized crossover trial. Clin Nutr. 2016;35(2):322–30. https://doi.org/10.1016/j.clnu.2015.03.021.

Robinson KN, Cassady BA, Hegazi RA, Wischmeyer PE. Preoperative carbohydrate loading in surgical patients with type 2 diabetes: are concerns supported by data? Clin Nutr ESPEN. 2021;45:1–8. https://doi.org/10.1016/j.clnesp.2021.08.023.

Şanlı D, Kundakçı GA, Katırcıoğlu K, Yurt A, Akçay E. The effects of preoperative carbohydrate loading on postoperative outcomes in neurosurgery: a systematic review and meta-analysis. BMC Anesthesiol. 2025;25(1):575. https://doi.org/10.1186/s12871-025-03468-2.

Sebestyén AR, Turan C, Szemere A, Virág M, Ocskay K, Dembrovszky F, et al. Preoperative carbohydrate loading reduces length of stay after major elective, non-cardiac surgery when compared to fasting: a systematic review and meta-analysis. Sci Rep. 2025;15(1):19119. https://doi.org/10.1038/s41598-025-00767-z.

Shao YR, Ke X, Luo LH, Xu JD, Xu LQ. Application of early enteral nutrition nursing based on enhanced recovery after surgery theory in patients with digestive surgery. World J Gastrointest Surg. 2023;15(9):1910. https://doi.org/10.4240/wjgs.v15.i9.1910.

Smith-Ryan AE, Hirsch KR, Saylor HE, Gould LM, Blue MN. Nutritional considerations and strategies to facilitate injury recovery and rehabilitation. J Athl Train. 2020;55(9):918–30. https://doi.org/10.4085/1062-6050-550-19.

Søreide E, Eriksson LI, Hirlekar G, et al. Pre-operative fasting guidelines. Acta Anaesthesiol Scand. 2005;49(8):1041–7. https://doi.org/10.1111/j.1399-6576.2005.00781.x.

Steenhagen E. Enhanced recovery after surgery: it's time to change practice! Nutr Clin Pract. 2016;31(1):18–29. https://doi.org/10.1177/0884533615622640.

Sun DL, Li WM, Li SM, Cen YY, Xu QW, Li YJ, Lu QP, Xu PY. Comparison of multi-modal early oral nutrition for the tolerance of oral nutrition with conventional care after major abdominal surgery: a prospective, randomized, single-blind trial. Nutr J. 2017;16(1):11. https://doi.org/10.1186/s12937-017-0228-7.

Thorell A, MacCormick AD, Awad S, et al. Guidelines for perioperative care in ERAS. World J Surg. 2016;40(9):2065–83. https://doi.org/10.1007/s00268-016-3492-3.

Tipton KD. Nutritional support for exercise-induced injuries. Sports Med. 2015;45(Suppl 1):93–104. https://doi.org/10.1007/s40279-015-0398-4.

Tong E, Chen Y, Ren Y, Zhou Y, Di C, Zhou Y, et al. Effects of preoperative carbohydrate loading on recovery after elective surgery: a systematic review and Bayesian network meta-analysis of randomized controlled trials. Front Nutr. 2022;9:951676. https://doi.org/10.3389/fnut.2022.951676.

Weimann A, Braga M, Carli F, et al. ESPEN guideline: clinical nutrition in surgery. Clin Nutr. 2017;36(3):623–50. https://doi.org/10.1016/j.clnu.2017.02.013.

Wolosowicz M, Prokopiuk S, Kaminski TW. Recent advances in the treatment of insulin resistance targeting molecular and metabolic pathways: fighting a losing battle? Medicina. 2022;58(4):472. https://doi.org/10.3390/medicina58040472.

Yi HC, Ibrahim Z, Abu Zaid Z, Mat Daud ZA, Md. Yusop NB, Omar J, et al. Impact of enhanced recovery after surgery with preoperative whey protein-infused carbohydrate loading and postoperative early oral feeding among surgical gynecologic cancer patients: an open-labelled randomized controlled trial. Nutrients. 2020;12(1):264. https://doi.org/10.3390/nu12010264.

Zhang Z, Wang RK, Duan B, Cheng ZG, Wang E, Guo QL, Luo H. Effects of a preoperative carbohydrate-rich drink before ambulatory surgery: a randomized controlled, double-blinded study. In: Med Sci Monit, vol. 26; 2020. p. e922837–1. https://doi.org/10.12659/MSM.922837.

Multimodal Analgesia Protocols Optimising Metabolism

7

Hemani Sarbadhikary and Debasrita Banerjee

Abstract

Over the past 30 years, one of the most important developments in perioperative medicine has been Enhanced Recovery After Surgery (ERAS), which has revolutionised the care of surgical patients before, during, and after surgery in almost all surgical disciplines. ERAS is premised on the concept of minimising surgical stress via a bundled approach to care, and pain management has a distinctive place in this bundle because pain is not just a symptom to treat but a powerful trigger for the neuroendocrine response that drives postoperative catabolism, immunosuppression, and metabolic dysfunction.

Conventional pain management protocols that are centred on high doses of opioid analgesics, though effective in reducing pain, are associated with a constellation of adverse effects that oppose the ERAS strategy. Postoperative nausea and vomiting, delayed return of bowel function, oversedation, respiratory depression, and urinary retention all delay the return of oral feeding, hinder mobilisation, and contribute to insulin resistance, producing a metabolically hostile milieu. By contrast, multimodal analgesia (deliberate integration of multiple analgesic agents and techniques that target different mechanisms of pain to improve pain relief while minimising opioid use) has become a central tenet of ERAS and a metabolically savvy approach to surgical recovery.

The objective of this chapter is to offer a detailed exploration of multimodal analgesia protocols that can be developed and applied not just to treat pain but

H. Sarbadhikary
Department of Clinical Nutrition, Yathra Hospital, New Delhi, India

D. Banerjee (✉)
Department of Nutrition and Dietetics, Medhavi Skills University, Singtam, Sikkim, India

P. K. Bhattacharyya et al. (eds.), *Integrated Anesthesia and Nutrition Approaches to Enhanced Recovery after Surgery*,
https://doi.org/10.1007/978-981-92-3294-9_7

proactively to improve metabolic recovery. It examines the physiological basis of the relationship between pain, stress, and metabolism; reviews the key pharmacologic and regional analgesic techniques used during ERAS; describes their impact on insulin resistance, gut motility, inflammation, protein catabolism, and functional recovery; and explains the link between multimodal analgesia and perioperative nutrition. The chapter also discusses protocol design, multidisciplinary stewardship, challenges, and the future of multimodal analgesia, including precision analgesia and digital data collection and monitoring. Multimodal analgesia, well understood, is not an analgesic approach. It is a critical pathway for successful integration of anaesthesia and nutrition strategies in ERAS, resulting in better metabolic outcomes, fewer complications, and more rapid and complete recovery.

Keywords

Multimodal analgesia · Enhanced recovery after surgery · Opioid-sparing strategies · Metabolic recovery · Insulin resistance · Perioperative nutrition · Postoperative ileus · Regional anaesthesia

7.1 Introduction

Enhanced Recovery After Surgery (ERAS) pathways have revolutionised perioperative care since their inception in colorectal surgery in the 1990s, and are now slowly being applied in orthopaedic, thoracic, gynaecological, urologic, hepatopancreatobiliary, bariatric and cardiac surgery (Kehlet and Wilmore 2002; Ljungqvist et al. 2017). Such pathways bundle a series of evidence-based interventions aimed at minimising the stress of surgery and maintaining physiological status, along with promoting early recovery. ERAS interventions include preoperative optimisation and education, short fasting times with carbohydrate loading, standardised anaesthesia and pain management, goal-directed fluid management, minimally invasive surgery where feasible, prevention of nausea and vomiting, early mobilisation, and early feeding (Gustafsson et al. 2018; Lassen et al. 2009). In hundreds of randomised controlled trials and meta-analyses, implementation of ERAS has been shown to reduce the length of stay by 30–50%, major and minor complications, hospital costs, and improve quality of life without increasing readmissions or death (Sarin et al. 2016; Nelson et al. 2016; Thiele et al. 2015).

In this multidisciplinary system, pain management is one of the most important areas as it influences more than just patient comfort. Poorly managed postoperative pain maintains activation of the hypothalamic-pituitary-adrenal axis and sympathetic nervous system, leading to peaks of cortisol, catecholamines, glucagon, and pro-inflammatory cytokines that trigger and sustain the traditional catabolic stress response to surgery (Tan et al. 2015; Nimmo et al. 2017). This catabolic stress response is a metabolic nightmare: it induces peripheral insulin resistance and hyperglycaemia, exacerbates skeletal muscle and fat catabolism, depresses the immune system, alters gastrointestinal blood flow and motility, and provides a biochemical milieu hostile to wound healing and repair (Kehlet and Wilmore 2002; Lassen et al. 2009). Ineffective pain relief also makes patients less capable and motivated to engage in early mobilisation and rehabilitation, exacerbating the physical and functional consequences of catabolism (Tan et al. 2015; Popping et al. 2014).

Traditional approaches to postoperative pain management, particularly the use of escalating opioid doses, effectively relieve pain but often introduce additional barriers to recovery. Opioids induce dose-dependent nausea and vomiting, ileus, constipation, sedation, respiratory depression, urinary retention, and pruritus, which delay discharge and compromise nutritional recovery (Oderda et al. 2007; Koo et al. 2014). The issue with opioid-based pain management from the viewpoints of ERAS and integrated anaesthesia-nutrition care is that it substitutes one impediment to recovery, pain, for a number of others that are similarly or more problematic for metabolic and functional recovery (Cheung et al. 2022; Weimann et al. 2017).

Multimodal analgesia overcomes this conundrum by using agents and approaches with different mechanisms of action to deliver effective, even superior analgesia with greatly reduced opioid use and its side effects (Kehlet 1997; Beverly et al. 2017). Multimodal opioid-sparing analgesia is advocated as best practice for pain management in the ERAS guidelines for colorectal, gynaecological, orthopaedic, thoracic, bariatric, and other surgeries (Gustafsson et al. 2018; Carmichael et al. 2017; Batchelor et al. 2019; Thorell et al. 2016). But the justification for multimodal analgesia in ERAS goes beyond opioid-sparing. Multimodal analgesia, with its impact on stress, inflammation, bowel motility, blood glucose control, and physical function, is appropriately recognised as an intervention for metabolic recovery (Nimmo et al. 2017; Cusack et al. 2020).

This chapter explores multimodal analgesia within the context of integrated anaesthesia and nutrition strategies in ERAS. It suggests that analgesic interventions should be considered not just for their effects on pain, but also for their downstream consequences on the metabolic milieu, nutritional recovery, and overall recovery of the individual patient. By recognising the metabolic effects of multimodal analgesia, anaesthesia and nutrition practitioners can develop ERAS pathways that leverage the complementary effects of anaesthesia and nutrition for outcomes that are not possible with either discipline acting alone.

7.2 Pain, Surgical Stress, and Metabolic Dysregulation

7.2.1 The Surgical Stress Response

Surgical trauma activates a consistent, predictable neuroendocrine and immune response that starts at the time of the skin incision and can last for days to weeks (depending upon the extent of the surgical procedure, quality of perioperative care, and the individual's homeostatic capacity) (Kehlet and Wilmore 2002; Scott et al. 2015). The response is initiated at the periphery by nociceptors and is relayed via spinal afferent pathways to the hypothalamus to activate the hypothalamic-pituitary-adrenal (HPA) axis and sympathoadrenal (SA) system (Nimmo et al. 2017). At the same time, the tissue trauma of surgery results in the release of local inflammatory mediators, such as prostaglandins, bradykinin, histamine, substance P, and cytokines, which sensitise peripheral and central nociceptors, facilitate the amplification of the pain signal, and activate the systemic inflammatory response (Tan et al. 2015; Scott et al. 2015) (Fig. 7.1).

The efferent responses to this neuroendocrine activation are dramatic. Plasma cortisol and catecholamines increase markedly, leading to hepatic glycogenolysis and gluconeogenesis, and peripheral insulin resistance due to post-receptor signalling defects, resulting in intraoperative insulin resistance and hyperglycaemia (Thiele et al. 2015; Lassen et al. 2009). Muscle protein degradation is increased, providing amino acids for gluconeogenesis and negative nitrogen balance. Inflammatory cytokines (including interleukin-1β, interleukin-6, and tumour necrosis factor-α) also adversely affect insulin signalling, decrease food intake, disrupt the gut barrier, and stimulate the acute-phase response, redirecting hepatic protein synthesis away from functional proteins such as albumin and towards acute-phase proteins such as C-reactive protein (Scott et al. 2015; Weimann et al. 2017).

7.2.2 Pain as a Stress Response

Pain is a symptom of surgical trauma. It is a major way by which the stress response is perpetuated and intensified following surgery. Pain impulses transmitted through spinal afferents continually activate the hypothalamus and adrenal glands; poorly

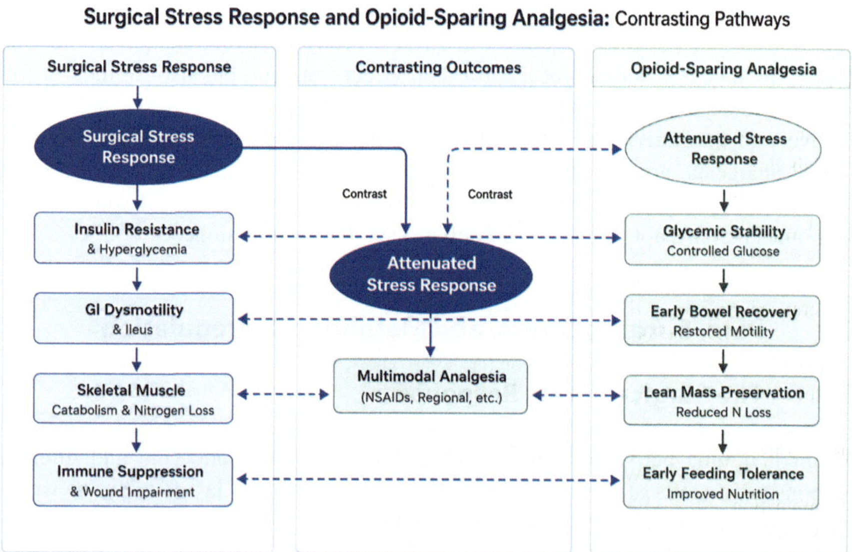

Fig. 7.1 The pain stress metabolism nutrition axis in perioperative ERAS care. (Created by author using MS PowerPoint)

managed pain keeps the cortisol and catecholamine levels high, and results in persistent insulin resistance, gut dysmotility, and reduced perfusion (Tan et al. 2015; Nimmo et al. 2017). Unrelieved pain also prevents patients from participating in early ambulation and deep breathing exercises, and from taking early oral nutrition, eliminating the benefits of early mobilisation to insulin sensitisation and of early feeding to anabolic substrate delivery (Weimann et al. 2017; Gillis et al. 2014).

So, good pain relief can directly improve metabolic outcomes not just through the pain-relieving effect but by establishing the physiological milieu that allows recovery-enhancing activities (Kehlet and Wilmore 2002; Popping et al. 2014). In ERAS, the aim is not just to achieve a numerical rating scale below a certain threshold but to have an awake patient, comfortable at rest and with movement, who can eat and walk, and is metabolically stable (Nimmo et al. 2017).

7.2.3 The Metabolic Costs of Opioid-Dominant Analgesia

Opioids activate μ-opioid receptors throughout the gastrointestinal tract, inhibiting propulsive peristalsis, reducing lower oesophageal sphincter tone, delaying gastric emptying, impairing small bowel and colonic motility, and promoting constipation (Koo et al. 2014; Carroll et al. 2004). These effects collectively produce postoperative ileus, nausea, vomiting, abdominal distension, and bloating, which in turn delay oral intake, necessitate prolonged intravenous fluid administration, reduce the feasibility of early enteral nutrition, and impair the delivery of protein and energy substrates at a time when the patient's anabolic needs are greatest (Oderda et al. 2007; Weimann et al. 2017).

Sedation and respiratory depression associated with opioids impair mobilisation and respiratory mechanics, increasing the risk of atelectasis, pneumonia, deep vein thrombosis, and prolonged decubitus with its attendant muscle deconditioning and pressure injury risks (Tan et al. 2015; Brindle et al. 2020). Together, these effects mean that opioid-dominant pain management, while superficially addressing the symptom of pain, may paradoxically worsen the metabolic environment, impair the delivery of nutritional therapy, and prolong the very recovery that ERAS is designed to accelerate (Cheung et al. 2022; Nimmo et al. 2017).

7.3 Principles and Pharmacology of Multimodal Analgesia

7.3.1 Definition and Rationale

Multimodal analgesia is the simultaneous administration of two or more pharmacologically dissimilar analgesic drugs or techniques that interact to produce additive or synergistic analgesia with reduced dose and side effects from each component (Kehlet 1997; Beverly et al. 2017). There are many pharmacologically targetable sites along the pain pathway, including the peripheral nociceptors, spinal dorsal horn, and supraspinal processing (Zhang et al. 2021). Multimodal analgesia can achieve pain relief equivalent to or better than high-dose opioid analgesia with a dramatic reduction in opioid use and its metabolic and functional side effects (Joshi et al. 2010; Tan et al. 2015) (Table 7.1).

Table 7.1 Core components of multimodal analgesia and their metabolic relevance in ERAS

Component	Mechanism	Primary ERAS role	Metabolic/ nutritional benefit	Key precautions
Acetaminophen	Central and peripheral inhibition of prostaglandin synthesis	Baseline non-opioid analgesia; opioid-sparing	Reduces opioid-related nausea and sedation; supports mobilisation and appetite (Tan et al. 2015)	Adjust the dose in hepatic dysfunction
NSAIDs/ COX-2 inhibitors	Cyclooxygenase-mediated prostaglandin inhibition	Opioid-sparing anti-inflammatory analgesia	Reduces inflammatory catabolism; improves bowel function (Nimmo et al. 2017)	Renal impairment, GI bleeding risk
Thoracic epidural analgesia	Blockade of afferent nociception and sympathetic efferents	Major abdominal/ thoracic analgesia	Attenuates stress response and insulin resistance; improves ileus and enables early feeding (Popping et al. 2014; Cusack et al. 2020)	Hypotension; anticoagulation contraindication
TAP/fascial plane blocks	Peripheral local anaesthetic nerve blockade	Procedure-specific opioid-sparing analgesia	Reduces systemic opioid burden; supports early mobilisation (Cheung et al. 2022)	Technique and expertise dependent
IV lidocaine infusion	Systemic anti-inflammatory and analgesic Na^+ channel blockade	Analgesic adjunct with prokinetic properties	Reduces opioid consumption; accelerates bowel recovery and early feeding (Imani et al. 2022)	Requires continuous cardiac monitoring
Low-dose IV ketamine	NMDA receptor antagonism; prevents central sensitisation	Reduces opioid consumption in high-pain procedures	Supports functional recovery and early mobilisation (Imani et al. 2022)	Dysphoric effects in susceptible patients

(Continued)

Table 7.1 (Continued)

Component	Mechanism	Primary ERAS role	Metabolic/ nutritional benefit	Key precautions
Alpha-2 agonists	Supraspinal and spinal sympatholysis	Stress attenuation; adjunct opioid-sparing	Hemodynamic stability; reduced catabolic hormone response (Cheung et al. 2022)	Bradycardia; hypotension risk

7.3.2 Acetaminophen and NSAIDs

Acetaminophen (paracetamol) is a well-established non-opioid background medication in nearly all ERAS protocols due to its safety, reliable opioid-sparing effect (20–30%), and improvement in dynamic pain (typically during mobilisation) (Tan et al. 2015; Cheung et al. 2022). Acetaminophen administered around-the-clock is generally more effective than on-demand and is part of ERAS guidelines across a range of surgical subspecialities (Gustafsson et al. 2018; Carmichael et al. 2017).

NSAIDs and selective COX-2 inhibitors have effective analgesic and anti-inflammatory properties due to inhibition of peripheral and central prostaglandin synthesis. They are opioid-sparing (30–50% in many scenarios), improve dynamic pain, and may have a positive effect on inflammation-induced catabolism and insulin resistance (Tan et al. 2015; Nimmo et al. 2017). But they must be used with caution due to the risk of renal dysfunction, gastrointestinal bleeding, and platelet dysfunction in at-risk populations.

7.3.3 Regional and Neuraxial Anaesthesia

Regional and neuraxial anaesthesia are the most significant components of multimodal ERAS analgesia as they can provide intense anaesthesia for the surgical site and block or reduce afferent nociceptive input to the hypothalamus, thus reducing the neuroendocrine stress response at its source (Kehlet 1997; Popping et al. 2014). Thoracic epidural analgesia for major open abdominal surgery offers superior dynamic pain relief, reduces intraoperative and postoperative opioid use to near zero in the area blocked, blunts the rise in cortisol and catecholamines, shortens the period of postoperative ileus, and may prevent major pulmonary and cardiovascular complications (Popping et al. 2014; Melloul et al. 2016). Thoracic epidural analgesia is confirmed by meta-analysis to reduce postoperative mortality, major morbidity, and hospital stay following major abdominal surgery (Popping et al. 2014).

Transversus abdominis plane (TAP) blocks, erector spinae plane blocks, and other fascial plane blocks can be used when epidurals are contraindicated, technically difficult, or not justified by the nature of the procedure (Cheung et al. 2022; Batchelor et al. 2019). These blocks offer targeted analgesic effects, systemic opioid-sparing, and are becoming staples of ERAS for colorectal, thoracic, gynaecologic, and hepatobiliary surgery.

7.3.4 Intravenous Ketamine and Lidocaine

Intravenous ketamine is an NMDA receptor antagonist that denies central sensitisation and opioid-induced hyperalgesia, and provides analgesia and opioid sparing in major surgery (Imani et al. 2022). Perioperative sub-anaesthetic infusions of ketamine decrease postoperative pain intensity, opioid consumption, and opioid requirements, especially in those with high preoperative opioid tolerance, or those having surgery that is associated with a high degree of postoperative pain (Imani et al. 2022; Carli et al. 2011).

The analgesic, anti-inflammatory, and pro-kinetic effect of intravenous lidocaine infusion has a systemic effect. It has been shown in clinical trials and meta-analyses that perioperative intravenous lidocaine infusion leads to decreased pain scores and opioid consumption, and faster return of flatus and bowel motility, and may shorten hospital stay in patients undergoing open abdominal surgery and colorectal surgery in particular (Imani et al. 2022; Scott et al. 2015). The prokinetic effect is important in ERAS nutrition, as it allows earlier return of bowel function and earlier commencement of oral nutrition and/or enteral nutrition.

7.3.5 Alpha-2 Agonists and Adjuncts

Alpha-2 adrenoceptor agonists (e.g. dexmedetomidine) have sedative, anxiolytic, and mild analgesic effects via supraspinal and spinal pathways, as well as sympatholytic effects that blunt the hemodynamic stress response (Cheung et al. 2022). Gabapentinoids are opioid-sparing but need to be titrated cautiously in the elderly or frail, as sedative effects may be problematic (Cheung et al. 2022; Batchelor et al. 2019).

7.3.6 Opioid Stewardship, Discharge Planning, and Prevention of Persistent Opioid Exposure

Multimodal analgesia aims to decrease the amount of opioids used for pain control in perioperative settings; nevertheless, it is also necessary to practise opioid stewardship in line with ERAS principles throughout the complete pathway of recovery. This involves minimising post-discharge opioid exposure using non-opioid medication prescribed regularly, limiting opioid prescription to rescue usage only, and educating the patient in relation to dosage, duration of usage, titration, and proper disposal of leftover pills (Cheung et al. 2022; Wick et al. 2017). This is especially crucial in patients with pre-operative opioid use, chronic pain conditions, frailty, and anxiety disorders, where excessive postoperative opioid dependency may lead to limited mobility, appetite, and involvement in rehab activities (Tan et al. 2015; Cheung et al. 2022).

Opioid stewardship in the setting of ERAS should be perceived as an element of the recovery process itself, and not simply an individual's drug choice. The best scenario includes the presence of adequate pain relief when moving around and being at rest, with opioid exposure being minimal, time-limited, and directly associated with achievement of functional endpoints such as walking, eating, and sleeping (Wick et al. 2017; Tan et al. 2015). Moreover, another reason for the application of multimodal analgesia in ERAS is the possibility that it may help minimise the likelihood of converting acute post-surgical pain into chronic post-operative pain. Minimising nociceptive inputs, limiting central sensitisation, and diminishing the need for increased use of opioids can be consistent with a recovery process that strives to not only provide immediate relief, but one that focuses on sustained functional improvement (Kehlet 1997; Imani et al. 2022).

The benefits of providing better pain management through multimodal analgesia in the early stages of recovery without the need for high doses of opioids may help facilitate better recovery outcomes.

7.4 Metabolic Effects of Multimodal Analgesia

7.4.1 Insulin Resistance and Glycaemic Control

Insulin resistance is a well-described and clinically relevant perioperative metabolic dysfunction of major surgery, and can be influenced by analgesic approach (Kehlet and Wilmore 2002; Thiele et al. 2015). Neuraxial multimodal analgesia has been shown to result in lower levels of postoperative cortisol and interleukin-6, insulin resistance indices, and improved glycaemic control when compared with systemic opioid-based approaches in colorectal and other major abdominal surgeries (Cusack et al. 2020; McEvoy et al. 2016). This is achieved by the blockade of nociceptive and sympathetic efferent by the neuraxial blockade, avoiding the stress-induced impairment of insulin signalling (Table 7.2).

Better glycaemic management in ERAS leads to improved rates of infection, wound healing, and immune function, and tolerability of nutritional strategies, such as carbohydrate loading and early enteral nutrition (Weimann et al. 2017; Thiele et al. 2015). In patients with diabetes and other metabolically at-risk patients, where the risk of adverse effects of perioperative hyperglycaemia is high, the role of multimodal analgesia on glucose homeostasis may be particularly important.

Table 7.2 How multimodal analgesia influences perioperative nutrition and recovery milestones in ERAS

Recovery domain	Effect of opioid-dominant analgesia	Effect of multimodal opioid-sparing analgesia	Clinical significance
Gastrointestinal function	Ileus, delayed gastric emptying, constipation, and feeding intolerance (Koo et al. 2014)	Earlier return of peristalsis, flatus, and bowel movement (Carroll et al. 2004)	Enables earlier oral/enteral feeding and nutrition delivery
Postoperative nausea and vomiting	High incidence; impairs oral intake and hydration (Oderda et al. 2007)	Substantially reduced incidence with opioid sparing	Facilitates progressive diet advancement per ERAS nutrition targets
Insulin resistance	Sustained stress response; persistent hyperglycaemia (Thiele et al. 2015)	Attenuated cortisol/catecholamine surge; improved glucose handling (Li et al. 2020)	Better tolerance of carbohydrate loading and early nutrition therapy
Protein catabolism	Amplified nitrogen loss through sustained cortisol elevation	Reduced catabolic stress; better protein substrate utilisation (Kehlet and Wilmore 2002)	Supports lean mass preservation and wound healing
Mobilisation capacity	Sedation, orthostatic effects, and motor impairment limit mobility (Tan et al. 2015)	Adequate dynamic analgesia enables early ambulation (Sarin et al. 2016)	Improves insulin sensitivity, appetite, and recovery pace
Oral intake timeline	Delayed first intake; slower diet advancement (Oderda et al. 2007)	Earlier first oral intake; faster diet advancement (Teoh et al. 2007; Weimann et al. 2017)	Reduces IV fluid dependence; shortens length of stay

7.4.2 Early Nutrition and Gut Motility

A key metabolic impact of opioid-sparing multimodal analgesia in ERAS is the maintenance of gastrointestinal function. Multimodal pain regimens that avoid or minimise the influence of opioids on μ-receptors in the gut by relying primarily on regional anaesthesia, non-steroidal anti-inflammatory drugs (NSAIDs), acetaminophen, and intravenous adjuncts enable early return of gastrointestinal motility (Koo et al. 2014; Carroll et al. 2004). An earlier return of bowel function equates to earlier tolerance of oral diet, which in turn minimises the duration of fasting-induced catabolism, and allows the ERAS nutrition team to progress diet more quickly to clear fluids, free fluids and solid diet (Weimann et al. 2017; Steenhagen 2016).

Published results from randomised controlled trials (RCTs) in colorectal and gynaecologic surgery show that patients following opioid-sparing ERAS protocols pass flatus and stool sooner, tolerate foods and fluids sooner, require less antiemetics, and are less reliant on fluid support (Sarin et al. 2016; Teoh et al. 2007). All of these are key steps towards improved ability to deliver the nutritional support the patient needs for metabolic recovery.

7.4.3 Reduction of Catabolism and Maintenance of Lean Mass

The stress response to surgery is the major driver of catabolism and multimodal analgesia, by reducing the stress response via reduced pain and reduction in the levels of cortisol and catecholamines, as well as inflammatory signalling, can help minimise the magnitude of catabolism and nitrogen loss in the immediate postoperative period (Kehlet and Wilmore 2002; Cusack et al. 2020). This is significant because just a few days of severe catabolism can lead to substantial losses of muscle and function, especially in older or sarcopenic patients who have a reduced physiological reserve (Weimann et al. 2017; Gillis et al. 2014).

Multimodal analgesia, in combination with ERAS nutrition support, helps maintain lean mass, suppress catabolic hormone levels, and allow earlier enteral protein intake, thus providing the conditions for the patient to initiate anabolic recovery sooner. This translates into more rapid recovery of physical activity, quicker recovery of function, and improved quality of life in the postoperative period (Gillis et al. 2014; Sarin et al. 2016).

7.4.4 Mobilisation, Respiratory Function, and Metabolic Recovery

Postoperative physical activity is an integral part of the ERAS protocol because such activities increase insulin sensitivity of the skeletal muscle, stimulate intestinal motility, minimise the risks of venous thromboembolism, maintain mechanical functions of breathing, and prevent deconditioning from prolonged bed rest (Memtsoudis et al. 2019; Sarin et al. 2016). Early mobilisation can be achieved through multimodal pain management protocols that provide sufficient pain relief during active movements, avoiding sedation, orthostatic hypotension, and extreme drowsiness caused by an opioid-based regimen (Tan et al. 2015; Cheung et al. 2022). Walking, sitting, and deep breathing on the same or the next day after the operation have some metabolic implications, such as increased glucose metabolism, muscle fibre performance, and improved lung elasticity (Memtsoudis et al. 2019).

7.4.5 Patient-Reported Recovery, Functional Status, and Quality of Recovery

An analysis in ERAS must go further than just looking at clinical parameters such as time of hospitalisation, development of ileus, and incidence of complications. Instead, one needs to consider patient-recovery outcomes, which demonstrate the extent to which a given analgesic strategy actually helped in recovery, especially when it came to pain interfering with walking and movement, eating comfortably, sleeping, dealing with fatigue, and general satisfaction with recovery (Sarin et al. 2016; Cheung et al. 2022).

Such issues as the use of multimodal analgesia are pertinent to patient recovery because, through multimodal analgesia, the patient can walk sooner, take deep breaths sooner, and start eating without suffering from sedation and other side effects common to the use of opioids (Tan et al. 2015; Oderda et al. 2007). Hence, it is important to measure not just the levels of pain through pain scores, but functional recovery in a sense as well (Memtsoudis et al. 2019; Sarin et al. 2016).

7.4.6 Sleep, Sedation Burden, and Recovery Quality

ERAS recovery is also dependent on the proper balance between adequate pain control and oversedation. If there is a strategy that will alleviate pain but leads to oversedation, daytime sleepiness, or an inability to participate in physiotherapy, then the core aim of ERAS in restoring functions is not achieved (Tan et al. 2015; Cheung et al. 2022). Hence, multimodal analgesia must be formulated such that it does not induce oversedation and maintains consciousness and participation in eating and mobilisation within the initial 24–72 h post-operatively.

Here, minimising the use of opioids is effective not only to minimise nausea or ileus but also to maintain consciousness and behaviours needed for eating, mobilising, and participating in recovery activities (Oderda et al. 2007; Wick et al. 2017).

7.5 Multimodal Analgesia Across the Perioperative ERAS Timeline

7.5.1 Preoperative Phase

During the screening phase, the opportunity exists to identify individuals who may have complex analgesic needs, such as chronic pain, current opioid prescription, high levels of anxiety, metabolic syndrome, diabetes, frailty, or malnutrition (Weimann et al. 2017; Tan et al. 2015). Multimodal prehabilitation strategies that include exercise, nutrition, and psychological interventions have been shown to enhance postoperative recovery and decrease complications (Gillis et al. 2014). Pre-emptive analgesia techniques, such as preoperative acetaminophen and (where appropriate) NSAIDs, prepare the system for better response to analgesics (Carmichael et al. 2017). Here, the nutrition team is coordinated to ensure compatibility between analgesic strategies and carbohydrate loading and fasting schedules (Weimann et al. 2017).

7.5.2 Intraoperative Phase

During surgery, the anaesthesia and analgesic choices determine the physiological response to surgery. Neuraxial or regional techniques should be initiated prior to incision for pre-emptive analgesia and early blockage of "stress" signals (Nimmo et al. 2017; Popping et al. 2014). Intravenous adjuncts (ketamine, lidocaine) can be started intraoperatively and continued into the early postoperative period. Normothermia, normovolemia, and hemodynamic stability provided by goal-directed fluid management support the analgesic management in maintaining gastrointestinal function and motility (McEvoy et al. 2016; Mythen et al. 2012).

7.5.3 Early Postoperative Phase

Early after surgery is the time when the success of multimodal analgesia has a direct impact on nutrition and metabolism. Regular doses of non-opioid analgesics should be administered. Infusions should be continued for large abdominal and thoracic surgery. PONV treatment should be given alongside analgesics as nausea is a major factor preventing early oral intake (Gustafsson et al. 2018; Carmichael et al. 2017). Opioids should be used only for "rescue" pain control, for the shortest time possible, and with the lowest dose. The nursing and nutrition teams should integrate the assessment of pain, nausea, bowel sounds, flatus, and oral intake and adjust analgesic and nutritional interventions accordingly, as the patient's condition develops (Weimann et al. 2017; Sarin et al. 2016).

7.5.4 Discharge and Beyond

Discharge from the hospital is a critical time for analgesia and nutrition for ambulatory and short-stay ERAS programs. Analgesic prescriptions at discharge should prioritise non-opioids; if opioids are prescribed, they should be in minimal amounts with education provided to the patient (Wick et al. 2017). Dietitian support and symptom monitoring apps can help ensure appropriate nutritional progress is being made, and that pain doesn't impact eating, mobility, or sleep in the home environment (Cheung et al. 2022; Macones et al. 2019) (Fig. 7.2).

7.5.5 Procedure-Specific Examples of Multimodal Analgesia within ERAS

An ideal multimodal approach must take into account the type of surgery, pain intensity, and risk of complications involving the gastrointestinal and respiratory systems. For instance, surgeries involving the colon, rectum, liver, pancreas, and bile ducts will gain most by incorporating regional techniques in addition to acetaminophen, NSAIDs, and other intravenous drugs to enhance early bowel function

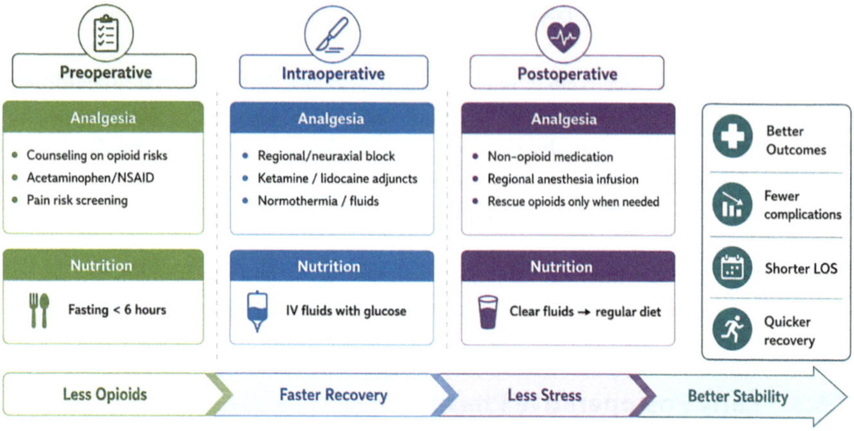

Fig. 7.2 Integrated multimodal analgesia and perioperative nutrition pathway within ERAS. (Created by the author using MS PowerPoint)

and feeding, while thoracic surgery protocols must focus more on neuraxial or paravertebral techniques to maintain normal respiratory dynamics and allow for early ambulation (Gustafsson et al. 2018; Melloul et al. 2016; Batchelor et al. 2019).

Likewise, bariatric, gynaecologic, and obstetric ERAS protocols may need adjustments in their anaesthesia strategies through prioritising opioid-sparing techniques, early enteral nutrition, and prompt ambulation while maintaining hemodynamic stability and reducing nausea and drowsiness (Thorell et al. 2016; Nelson et al. 2016; Macones et al. 2019).

7.6 The Analgesia–Nutrition Interface in ERAS

7.6.1 Early Feeding as an ERAS Priority

Early oral and enteral nutrition is a key nutrition intervention in the ESPEN guidelines for clinical nutrition in surgery and the ERAS Society guidelines for several surgical specialties and should be initiated as soon as possible after surgery, preferably within 24 h (Weimann et al. 2017; Gustafsson et al. 2018). Early nutrition prevents loss of nitrogen via catabolic hormones, provides fuel for immune responses and wound healing, maintains gut mucosal integrity and barrier, alters the microbiome, and reduces length of stay (Weimann et al. 2017; Steenhagen 2016). But the success of early feeding is dependent on effective pain relief, and patients with excessive nausea, vomiting, abdominal bloating, or those who are oversedated with an opioid-based pain relief plan are unlikely to be able to tolerate early feeding (Nimmo et al. 2017; Oderda et al. 2007).

7.6.2 Carbohydrate Loading and Metabolic Preparation

Oral carbohydrate loading in the hours before surgery decreases preoperative insulin resistance, increases patient comfort during fasting hours, decreases postoperative nausea and vomiting, and may improve surgical outcomes (Weimann et al. 2017; Thorell et al. 2016). The metabolic advantages of carbohydrate loading require the postoperative period to also be managed in a way that reduces insulin resistance, which is affected by the quality of analgesia. Multimodal analgesia that reduces the stress response and facilitates early feeding is therefore complementary to preoperative carbohydrate loading and helps to improve the perioperative metabolic trajectory (Weimann et al. 2017; Cusack et al. 2020).

7.6.3 Protein Feeding and Lean Mass Loss

Catabolism and lean mass degradation are more pronounced in malnourished or nutritionally vulnerable patients who undergo major surgery. The ESPEN surgical nutritional guidelines recommend pre-operative nutritional support (including protein-enriched oral supplements) for at-risk patients and as soon as possible after surgery (Weimann et al. 2017). Immunonutrition formulas with arginine, omega-3 fatty acids, and glutamine have been shown to be beneficial in terms of infection rates and recovery in malnourished patients undergoing cancer surgery (Weimann et al. 2017; Feldheiser et al. 2016). To benefit from these nutritional interventions, the gut must be able to absorb the delivered substrates, which is more likely to be true following early recovery of bowel function following opioid-sparing multimodal analgesia (Steenhagen 2016; Carroll et al. 2004).

7.7 Implementation: Building Metabolically Informed ERAS Protocols

7.7.1 Procedure-Specific Protocol Development

Effective implementation of metabolically oriented multimodal analgesia requires procedure-specific, patient-centred protocol development integrated within the broader ERAS pathway (Gustafsson et al. 2018; Carmichael et al. 2017). A thoracic surgery ERAS protocol requires different regional techniques and respiratory-focused analgesic considerations than a colorectal or gynaecologic surgery protocol (Batchelor et al. 2019; Melloul et al. 2016). Frail, elderly, or renal-impaired patients will require NSAID cautious protocols with heavier reliance on neuraxial or wound infiltration techniques. Protocol development should involve anaesthesiologists, surgeons, nurses, pharmacists, and dietitians, and should explicitly map analgesic interventions to nutrition milestones.

7.7.2 Multidisciplinary Governance and Education

Institutional implementation of ERAS-aligned multimodal analgesia requires multidisciplinary governance structures that include regular audit, protocol review, and education programs (Scott et al. 2015; Wick et al. 2017). ERAS coordinators play a critical role in monitoring adherence, identifying patients who are failing to progress on the expected analgesic-nutrition recovery trajectory, and facilitating prompt escalation or adjustment of care. Clinical decision support tools embedded in the electronic health record can provide real-time guidance on analgesic choices, dose adjustments, and nutrition advancement cues (Cheung et al. 2022).

7.7.3 Audit and Quality Improvement

Meaningful audit of multimodal analgesia within ERAS should extend beyond pain scores and opioid consumption to include outcomes that directly reflect metabolic recovery: time to first oral intake, time to solid diet, daily caloric and protein intake, time to first ambulation, PONV incidence, ileus rates, glycaemic control metrics, length of stay, and complication rates (Sarin et al. 2016; Thiele et al. 2015). These audit metrics create accountability for the metabolic as well as analgesic consequences of clinical practice and support continuous improvement toward the goal of fully integrated anaesthesia-nutrition ERAS care. Performance dashboards that display both analgesic and nutritional compliance metrics simultaneously reinforce the interdependency of these two domains to the entire clinical team.

7.7.4 ERAS Compliance, Bundle Fidelity, and Recovery Dashboards

In practice, ERAS success does not merely depend on the prescription of ERAS elements but also depends on how strictly the pathway has been adhered to. Hence, audit of ERAS protocols can encompass indicators for consistency, such as percentage usage of non-opioid analgesics, regional blocks, no unnecessary opioids, and timely resumption of oral intake and activity, alongside conventional audit indicators like pain score and LOS (Sarin et al. 2016; Thiele et al. 2015).

The ideal ERAS dashboard will also incorporate both compliance with analgesics and nutrition, as these two variables interact with one another in the process of recovery. This will make it easy to detect failures that might occur within the process and correct the problems, such as continuous nausea, poor oral consumption, or opioid overdoses (Cheung et al. 2022; Weimann et al. 2017; Wick et al. 2017).

7.8 Future Directions

As ERAS continues to evolve, the future of multimodal analgesia lies in increasing precision and individualisation of protocols based on patient-specific metabolic, genetic, and physiological phenotypes. Pharmacogenomic profiling holds promise for identifying patients who are poor metabolisers of certain opioids or who carry genetic variants associated with heightened postoperative pain or opioid-related adverse effects, enabling pre-emptive selection of the most appropriate analgesic combination before surgery (Cheung et al. 2022). Integration of continuous glucose monitoring, wearable activity trackers, and digital symptom-reporting platforms into ERAS pathways will allow analgesic and nutritional interventions to be adjusted in real time based on objective physiological data rather than scheduled review intervals (Macones et al. 2019).

Machine learning algorithms trained on large perioperative datasets may identify patient phenotypes and procedure combinations where specific multimodal regimens produce the greatest metabolic benefit, moving ERAS analgesia from evidence-based population-level guidelines toward precision-based individual-level care (Cheung et al. 2022). At the intersection of anaesthesia and nutrition, predictive models may ultimately be able to specify not only which analgesic technique is optimal for a given patient but when that patient's gut function will be restored, what nutritional formulation they are most likely to tolerate, and how rapidly their diet can be advanced, creating a fully integrated, data-driven perioperative recovery plan. Digital twin technology, computational models of individual patient physiology, may further allow preoperative simulation of different analgesic and nutritional scenarios to identify the most metabolically favourable ERAS pathway for each patient before they enter the operating room.

Future approaches to analgesia in ERAS should therefore progress from one-size-fits-all strategies based on population-based protocols toward approaches that utilise biomarkers or phenotypes. The metabolic effect of any chosen strategy could be objectively monitored through glucose levels during the perioperative period, insulin resistance indices, inflammatory markers, and signs of functional recovery, thus enabling assessment of whether any given strategy is only analgesic but also metabolically protective (Thiele et al. 2015; B., Cusack et al. 2020; Zhang et al. 2021).

The importance of this concept becomes especially evident in diabetics, patients with metabolic syndrome, frail elderly patients, and those suffering from sarcopenia, because small differences in their levels of physiological stress, time required for bowel recovery, and the ability to maintain oral nutrition will result in significantly divergent results regarding their functional recovery (Weimann et al. 2017; Tan et al. 2015). From a long-term perspective, precision analgesia may become a key tool in the determination of the best combination of analgesic drugs for every patient undergoing a particular procedure.

7.9 Conclusion

Multimodal analgesia is a foundational strategy within ERAS whose importance extends far beyond the relief of postoperative pain. By minimising opioid exposure, attenuating the neuroendocrine stress response, preserving gastrointestinal function, improving glycaemic control, supporting early mobilisation, and facilitating earlier and more effective nutritional rehabilitation, well-designed multimodal analgesic protocols actively optimise the metabolic trajectory of surgical patients. The evidence across surgical specialties consistently demonstrates that opioid-sparing, multimodal approaches are associated with superior recovery outcomes: shorter length of stay, fewer complications, earlier oral intake, and better patient-reported functional recovery.

In the context of integrated aesthesia and nutrition approaches to ERAS, multimodal analgesia is the critical bridge between perioperative anaesthetic care and nutritional rehabilitation. It creates the physiological conditions, reduced pain, reduced nausea, functional gut motility, metabolic stability, and physical capacity, without which perioperative nutrition strategies cannot achieve their full potential. Understanding and harnessing this relationship is essential for any perioperative team committed to delivering the full benefits of ERAS to their surgical patients and to the vision of this book: a fully integrated, evidence-based approach to anaesthesia and nutrition in surgical recovery.

References

Batchelor TJP, Rasburn NJ, Abdelnour-Berchtold E, Brunelli A, Cerfolio RJ, Gonzalez M, Ljungqvist O, Petersen RH, Popescu WM, Slinger PD, Naidu B. Guidelines for enhanced recovery after lung surgery: recommendations of the Enhanced Recovery After Surgery (ERAS®) Society and the European Society of Thoracic Surgeons (ESTS). Eur J Cardiothorac Surg. 2019;55(1):91–115. https://doi.org/10.1093/ejcts/ezy301.

Beverly A, Kaye AD, Ljungqvist O, Urman RD. Essential elements of multimodal analgesia in enhanced recovery after surgery (ERAS) guidelines. Anesthesiol Clin. 2017;35(2):115–43. https://doi.org/10.1016/j.anclin.2017.01.018.

Brindle ME, McDiarmid C, Short K, Miller K, MacRobie A, Lam JYK, Brockel M, Raval MV, Howlett A, Lee KS, Offringa M, Wong K, de Beer D, Wester T, Skarsgard ED, Wales PW, Fecteau A, Haliburton B, Goobie SM, Nelson G. Consensus guidelines for perioperative care in neonatal intestinal surgery: Enhanced Recovery After Surgery (ERAS®) society recommendations. World J Surg. 2020;44(8):2482–92. https://doi.org/10.1007/s00268-020-05530-1.

Carli F, Kehlet H, Baldini G, Steel A, McRae K, Slinger P, Hemmerling T, Salinas F, Neal JM. Evidence basis for regional anesthesia in multidisciplinary fast-track surgical care pathways. Reg Anesth Pain Med. 2011;36(1):63–72. https://doi.org/10.1097/AAP.0b013e31820307f7.

Carmichael JC, Keller DS, Baldini G, Bordeianou L, Weiss E, Lee L, Wick E, Augustine M, Feingold D, Steele SR. Clinical practice guidelines for enhanced recovery after colon and rectal surgery. Dis Colon Rectum. 2017;60(8):761–84. https://doi.org/10.1097/DCR.0000000000000883.

Carroll IR, Angst MS, Clark JD. Management of perioperative pain in patients chronically consuming opioids. Reg Anesth Pain Med. 2004;29(6):576–91. https://doi.org/10.1016/j.rapm.2004.06.009.

Cheung CK, Adeola JO, Beutler SS, Urman RD. Postoperative pain management in enhanced recovery pathways. J Pain Res. 2022;15:123–35. https://doi.org/10.2147/JPR.S231774.

Cusack B, Buggy DJ. Anaesthesia analgesia and the surgical stress response BJA Education 2020;20(9):321-328 10.1016/j.bjae.2020.04.006

Feldheiser A, Aziz O, Baldini G, Cox BPBW, Fearon KCH, Feldman LS, Gan TJ, Kennedy RH, Ljungqvist O, Lobo DN, Miller T, Radtke FF, Ruiz Garces T, Schricker T, Scott MJ, Thacker JK, Ytrebø LM, Carli F. Enhanced Recovery After Surgery (ERAS) for gastrointestinal surgery, part 2: consensus statement for anaesthesia practice. Acta Anaesthesiol Scand. 2016;60(3):289–334. https://doi.org/10.1111/aas.12651.

Gillis C, Li C, Lee L, Awasthi R, Augustin B, Gamsa A, Liberman AS, Stein B, Charlebois P, Feldman LS, Carli F. Prehabilitation versus rehabilitation: a randomized control trial in patients undergoing colorectal resection for cancer. Anesthesiology. 2014;121(5):937–47. https://doi.org/10.1097/ALN.0000000000000393.

Gustafsson UO, Scott MJ, Hubner M, Nygren J, Demartines N, Francis N, Rockall TA, Young-Fadok TM, Hill AG, Soop M, de Boer HD, Urman RD, Chang GJ, Fichera A, Kessler H, Grass F, Whang EE, Fawcett WJ, Carli F, et al. Guidelines for perioperative care in elective colorectal surgery: Enhanced Recovery After Surgery (ERAS®) Society recommendations: 2018. World J Surg. 2018;43(3):659–95. https://doi.org/10.1007/s00268-018-4844-y.

Imani F, Bagheri AR, Arvin E, Gatt SP, Sarveazad A. Effects of ketamine and lidocaine infusion on acute pain after elective open abdominal surgery, a randomised, double-blinded study. Med J Islam Repub Iran. 2022;36:60. https://doi.org/10.47176/mjiri.36.60.

Joshi GP, Chung F, Vann MA, Ahmad S, Gan TJ, Goulson DT, Merrill DG, Twersky R, Society for Ambulatory Anesthesia. Society for Ambulatory Anesthesia consensus statement on perioperative blood glucose management in diabetic patients undergoing ambulatory surgery. Anesth Analg. 2010;111(6):1378–87. https://doi.org/10.1213/ANE.0b013e3181f9c288.

Kehlet H. Multimodal approach to control postoperative pathophysiology and rehabilitation. Br J Anaesth. 1997;78(5):606–17. https://doi.org/10.1093/bja/78.5.606.

Kehlet H, Wilmore DW. Multimodal strategies to improve surgical outcome. Am J Surg. 2002;183(6):630–41. https://doi.org/10.1016/S0002-9610(02)00866-8.

Koo KC, Rha KH, Kim SM, Choi YD, Hong SJ, Cho KS. Analgesic opioid dose is an important indicator of postoperative ileus following radical cystectomy with ileal conduit. Yonsei Med J. 2014;55(5):1359–65. https://doi.org/10.3349/ymj.2014.55.5.1359.

Lassen K, Soop M, Nygren J, Cox PBW, Hendry PO, Spies C, von Meyenfeldt MF, Fearon KCH, Revhaug A, Norderval S, Ljungqvist O, Lobo DN, Dejong CHC. Consensus review of optimal perioperative care in colorectal surgery: Enhanced Recovery After Surgery (ERAS) Group recommendations. Arch Surg. 2009;144(10):961–9. https://doi.org/10.1001/archsurg.2009.170.

Ljungqvist O, Scott M, Fearon KC. Enhanced recovery after surgery: a review. JAMA Surg. 2017;152(3):292–8. https://doi.org/10.1001/jamasurg.2016.4952.

Macones GA, Caughey AB, Wood SL, Wrench IJ, Huang J, Norman M, Petrou S, Dande A, Wilson J, Collis R, Habiba M, Brocklehurst P, Plaat F, Cheyne H, Pasupathy D, Sultan A. Guidelines for postoperative care in cesarean delivery: Enhanced Recovery After Surgery (ERAS) Society recommendations (part 3). Am J Obstet Gynecol. 2019;221(3):247–58. https://doi.org/10.1016/j.ajog.2019.04.012.

McEvoy MD, Wanderer JP, King AB, Geiger TM, Tiwari V, Terekhov M, Ehrenfeld JM, Furman WR, Lee LA, Sandberg WS. A perioperative consult service results in reduction in cost and length of stay for colorectal surgical patients: evidence from a healthcare redesign project. Perioperative medicine (London, England). 2016;5:3. https://doi.org/10.1186/s13741-016-0028-1.

Melloul E, Hübner M, Scott M, Snowden C, Prentis J, Dejong CHC, Garden OJ, Farges O, Kokudo N, Vauthey J-N, Clavien P A, Demartines N. Guidelines for perioperative care for liver surgery: Enhanced Recovery After Surgery (ERAS) Society recommendations. World J Surg. 2016;40(10):2425–40. https://doi.org/10.1007/s00268-016-3700-1.

Memtsoudis SG, Poeran J, Zubizarreta N, Cozowicz C, Mörwald EE, Mariano ER, Mazumdar M. Association of multimodal pain management strategies with perioperative outcomes and resource utilization. Anesthesiology. 2019;128(5):891–902. https://doi.org/10.1097/ALN.0000000000002132.

Mythen MG, Swart M, Acheson N, Crawford R, Jones K, Kuper M, McGrath JS, Horgan A. Perioperative fluid management: consensus statement from the enhanced recovery partnership. Perioperative Medicine. 2012;1(1):2. https://doi.org/10.1186/2047-0525-1-2.

Nelson G, Altman AD, Nick A, Meyer LA, Ramirez PT, Achtari C, Antrobus J, Huang J, Scott M, Wijk L, Acheson N, Ljungqvist O, Dowdy SC. Guidelines for pre- and intra-operative care in gynecologic/oncology surgery: Enhanced Recovery After Surgery (ERAS®) Society recommendations—Part I. Gynecol Oncol. 2016;140(2):313–22. https://doi.org/10.1016/j.ygyno.2015.11.015.

Nimmo SM, Foo ITH, Paterson HM. Enhanced recovery after surgery: pain management. J Surg Oncol. 2017;116(5):583–91. https://doi.org/10.1002/jso.24814.

Oderda GM, Said Q, Evans RS, Stoddard GJ, Lloyd J, Jackson K, Rublee D, Samore MH. Opioid-related adverse drug events in surgical hospitalizations: impact on costs and length of stay. Ann Pharmacother. 2007;41(3):400–6. https://doi.org/10.1345/aph.1H386.

Popping DM, Elia N, Van Aken HK, Marret E, Schug SA, Kranke P, Wenk M, Tramèr MR. Impact of epidural analgesia on mortality and morbidity after surgery: systematic review and meta-analysis of randomized controlled trials. Ann Surg. 2014;259(6):1056–67. https://doi.org/10.1097/SLA.0000000000000237.

Sarin A, Litonius ES, Naidu R, Yost CS, Varma MG, Chen L-L. Successful implementation of an enhanced recovery after surgery program shortens length of stay and improves post-operative pain, and bowel and bladder function after colorectal surgery. BMC Anesthesiol. 2016;16(1):55. https://doi.org/10.1186/s12871-016-0223-0.

Scott MJ, Baldini G, Fearon KCH, Feldheiser A, Feldman LS, Gan TJ, Ljungqvist O, Lobo DN, Rockall TA, Schricker T, Carli F. Enhanced Recovery After Surgery (ERAS) for gastrointestinal surgery, part 1: pathophysiological considerations. Acta Anaesthesiol Scand. 2015;59(10):1212–31. https://doi.org/10.1111/aas.12601.

Steenhagen E. Enhanced Recovery After Surgery: It's Time to Change Practice! Nutrition in clinical practice: official publication of the American Society for Parenteral and Enteral Nutrition. 2016;31(1):18–29. https://doi.org/10.1177/0884533615622640.

Tan M, Law LS-C, Gan TJ. Optimizing pain management to facilitate enhanced recovery after surgery pathways. Can J Anesth. 2015;62(2):203–18. https://doi.org/10.1007/s12630-014-0275-x.

Teoh WHL, Shah MK, Mah CL. A randomised controlled trial on beneficial effects of early feeding post-Caesarean delivery under regional anaesthesia. Singapore Med J. 2007;48(2):152–7. https://pubmed.ncbi.nlm.nih.gov/17304396/

Thiele RH, Rea KM, Turrentine FE, Friel CM, Hassinger TE, Goudreau BJ, Umapathi BA, Sawyer RG, Stukenborg GJ, Hedrick TL, Evans HL. Standardization of care: impact of an enhanced recovery protocol on length of stay, complications, and direct costs after colorectal surgery. J Am Coll Surg. 2015;220(4):430–43. https://doi.org/10.1016/j.jamcollsurg.2014.12.042.

Thorell A, MacCormick AD, Awad S, Reynolds N, Roulin D, Ljungqvist O, Fearon KCH. Guidelines for perioperative care in bariatric surgery: Enhanced Recovery After Surgery (ERAS) Society recommendations. World J Surg. 2016;40(9):2065–83. https://doi.org/10.1007/s00268-016-3492-3.

Weimann A, Braga M, Carli F, Higashiguchi T, Hübner M, Klek S, Laviano A, Ljungqvist O, Lobo DN, Martindale R, Waitzberg DL, Bischoff SC, Singer P. ESPEN guideline: clinical nutrition in surgery. Clin Nutr. 2017;36(3):623–50. https://doi.org/10.1016/j.clnu.2017.02.013.

Wick EC, Grant MC, Wu CL. Postoperative multimodal analgesia pain management with non-opioid analgesics and techniques. JAMA Surg. 2017;152(7):691–7. https://doi.org/10.1001/jamasurg.2017.0898.

Zhang Y, Su T, Li R, Yan Q, Zhang W, Xu G. Effect of multimodal analgesia on perioperative insulin resistance in patients with colon cancer. Indian J Cancer. 2021;58(3):349–54. https://doi.org/10.4103/ijc.IJC_197_19.

Insulin Resistance Management and Glycemic Control

8

Prachi Bansal, Hema Deupa, Priyanka Shankar, and A. C. Kar

Abstract

Insulin resistance is a major metabolic condition leading to reduced sensitivity of insulin-targeted tissues, impairing glucose uptake and raising BGLs. The metabolic response to insulin resistance contributes to hyperglycemia, inflammation, vascular pathology, hypertension, dyslipidemia, hyperuricemia, and endothelial dysfunction. Insulin resistance in surgical patients is common and is associated with increased mortality and morbidity. To prevent perioperative complications, patients with diabetes and insulin resistance undergoing surgery need optimal perioperative care, including appropriate preoperative glucose-lowering therapies such as oral carbohydrate administration and frequent glucose monitoring on the day of surgery. Guidelines recommend maintaining intraoperative glucose levels typically between 140–180 mg/dL, though optimal targets vary by patient population and surgical context. Effective management of glycemic control level and insulin resistance requires multimodal perioperative strategies, perioperative strategies, and approaches to prevent complications. Therefore, this chapter provides a comprehensive overview of the pathophysiology of perioperative insulin resistance and its impact on clinical outcomes, immediate preoperative prepara-

P. Bansal · A. C. Kar
Department of Vikriti Vigyan, Faculty of Ayurveda, Institute of Medical Sciences, Banaras Hindu University, Varanasi, Uttar Pradesh, India

H. Deupa (✉)
Department of Food and Nutrition, Babasaheb Bhimrao Ambedkar University, Lucknow, Uttar Pradesh, India

P. Shankar
Department of Human Development and Family Studies, Babasaheb Bhimrao Ambedkar University, Lucknow, Uttar Pradesh, India
e-mail: Priyanka.fn@bbau.ac.in

P. K. Bhattacharyya et al. (eds.), *Integrated Anesthesia and Nutrition Approaches to Enhanced Recovery after Surgery*,
https://doi.org/10.1007/978-981-92-3294-9_8

tion, intraoperative glucose monitoring, postoperative and nutrition strategies, including enhanced recovery after surgery protocols (ERAS) to improve insulin resistance and glucose management.

Keywords

Insulin resistance · Glycemic control · Diabetes Mellitus · Perioperative strategies · Nutritional strategies

8.1 Introduction

Diabetes mellitus (DM) is a metabolic disorder characterized by persistent hyperglycemia caused by defects in insulin secretion, insulin action, or both. The vast majority of cases are classified into type 1 DM and type 2 DM. In former cases, there is an autoimmune destruction of β-cells resulting in a deficiency of insulin, while in the latter, 90–95% of cases are characterized by the progressive secretory dysfunction within the setting of insulin resistance (American Diabetes Association, 2014). Additionally, perioperative hyperglycemia or hypoglycemia has emerged as a crucial determining factor in surgical outcomes in parallel with the increasing global burden of metabolic disease. According to the World Health Organisation (WHO), global diabetes prevalence rose from approximately 200 million in the 1990s to over 830 million adults by 2022. Almost half of the population was not taking medicine for treatment. Low- and middle-income nations had the lowest rates of diabetes treatment (World Health Organization 2024). Furthermore, 589 million adults (20–79 years old) were living with diabetes mellitus in 2024. Over the following ten years, this number is predicted to rise significantly, reaching 853 million in 2050 (International Diabetes Federation 2025). This epidemiological shift has major implications in surgical practice and anesthesia, as increasing numbers of patients presented for surgery have pre-existing diabetes or undiscovered problems related to glucose metabolism. Furthermore, the incidence of stress-induced hyperglycemia in non-diabetic patients having surgery ranges from 20% to 80%, depending on the kind and severity of postoperative stress (Umpierrez and Pasquel 2021). These trends suggest the growing relevance of perioperative glycemic response.

Insulin resistance is a pathophysiological condition of type 2 diabetes mellitus, where insulin action is mostly impaired in target tissues, especially affecting carbohydrate metabolism. It repeatedly leads to hyperinsulinemia, which contributes to multisystem effects and underlies conditions grouped as metabolic syndrome. During severe insulin resistance, there is impaired glucose response to endogenous and exogenous insulin, and substantial hyperinsulinemia. Further, a large amount of exogenous insulin is required to maintain euglycemia (a normal concentration of glucose in the blood, indicating good glycemic control) during abnormal glucose homeostasis (Angelidi et al. 2021). Chronic hyperglycemia is strongly associated with other comorbidities such as cardiovascular disease, neuropathy, nephropathy, and retinopathy, making effective glycemic control a cornerstone of diabetes management. In symptomatic individuals, the standard diagnostic criteria include elevated glycated hemoglobin (HbA1c > 6.5%), random plasma glucose >200 mg/dL, fasting plasma glucose ≥126 mg/dL, and an oral glucose tolerance test (Finney et al. 2003). Although maintaining optimal glycemic control is important for not only preventing chronic complications but also reducing medical expenses and improving survival rates (Van den Berghe et al. 2001, 2006).

Perioperative surgical conditions commonly induce insulin resistance in both diabetic and non-diabetic individuals, characterized by hepatic gluconeogenesis, glycogenolysis, lower peripheral glucose uptake, and resultant hyperglycemia (Lipshutz et al. 2009). Anesthesia, surgical factors, and baseline metabolic factors all affect the response to a certain extent. Perioperative hyperglycemic complications are majorly associated with increased morbidity rates, including infections, acute renal injury, myocardial infarction, and neurological dysfunction (Finney et al. 2003; McGirt et al. 2006). The best glycemic objective to regulate the perioperative phase is conflicting. In some evidence-based study of Van den Berge et al.. (2001, 2006) demonstrated that normalizing glucose with intense insulin administration considerably reduces the risks of mortality and morbidity in ICU patients. Later studies showed normoglycemia has beneficial effects rather than insulin dose administration (Van den Berghe et al. 2003). However, many studies were unable to prove these results, and the issue was heavily debatable (Gandhi et al. 2007; Finfer et al. 2009).

It is unclear whether there is an effect of perioperative glucose levels on postoperative outcomes. Previous literature mostly focused on cardiac surgery with diabetes. Consequently, glycemic control is increasingly recognized as an important preliminary step for achieving positive postoperative outcomes in surgical and critically ill patients. It is crucial to understand the mechanism and therapeutic implication of disturbed glucose homeostasis because of the interaction between insulin resistance and perioperative hyperglycemia. Thus, this chapter provides a detailed description of the pathophysiology of perioperative glucose regulation and its impact on clinical outcomes and management of perioperative care via immediate preoperative preparation, intraoperative glucose monitoring, nutrition strategies, including enhanced recovery after surgery (ERAS).

8.2 Pathophysiology of Perioperative Glucose Regulation

There are several factors influencing perioperative glucose management, such as degree of glucose control prior to hospital admission, glucose dysfunction related to type 1 and type 2 diabetes, nutritional status, and the type of anesthesia administered during surgery (Fig. 8.1). An integrated neuroendocrine and inflammatory reaction to surgical stress causes perioperative glucose dysregulation, which leads to a change toward hyperglycemia and insulin resistance. Surgical stress increases counter-regulatory hormones, including cortisol, catecholamines, glucagon, and growth hormone, because the hypothalamic-pituitary-adrenal axis and sympathetic nervous system are activated during surgical injury (Desborough 2000; Umpierrez

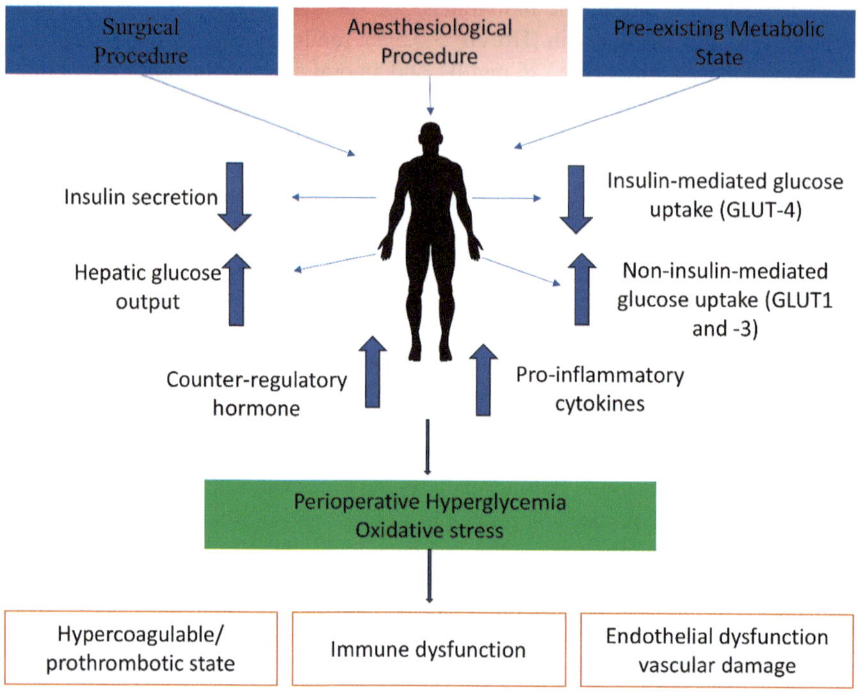

Fig. 8.1 Pathophysiology of perioperative glucose regulation. (Created using MS PowerPoint Presentation)

and Pasquel 2021). Depending on the anesthetic depth and modality, these reactions may be controlled by anesthetic procedures, which can reduce or alter the intensity of the stress response (Duggan et al. 2017). Collectively, these mechanisms create a catabolic state that disrupts normal glucose homeostasis and increases substrate availability for metabolic demands.

Increased hepatic glucose production is a key mechanism. Cortisol increases the transcription of gluconeogenic enzymes, while elevated glucagon and catecholamines promote glycogenolysis and gluconeogenesis (Petersen and Shulman 2018). Concurrently, hepatic glucose production is further increased, and insulin signaling pathways are compromised by proinflammatory cytokines like interleukin-6 and tumor necrosis factor-α, which are generated in reaction to surgical trauma (Ceriello et al. 2020). Hepatic glucose production consequently becomes comparatively resistant to insulin suppression. Concurrently, tissue-specific insulin resistance impairs peripheral glucose absorption. Surgical stress and inflammatory mediators interfere with insulin receptor substrate-1 (IRS-1) signaling and downstream pathways such as phosphoinositide 3-kinase and Akt in skeletal muscle, which reduces glucose uptake and the translocation of glucose transporter type 4 (GLUT4) to the cell membrane (Petersen and Shulman 2018). In adipose tissue, catecholamine-driven lipolysis raises circulating free fatty acids, which worsen insulin resistance by having lipotoxic effects on the liver and muscles (Thorell et al. 1999; Ceriello et al. 2020).

The combination of increased hepatic glucose output and decreased peripheral glucose consumption causes acute hyperglycemia in those people without a history of diabetes. This metabolic disruption frequently lasts into the postoperative phase, where continued inflammation, immobility, and dietary variables all contribute to persistent insulin resistance (Umpierrez and Pasquel 2021). The magnitude and duration of this response correlate with the severity of surgical trauma and influence recovery trajectories.

This integrated pathophysiological response has important clinical implications. Infections, delayed wound healing, and organ dysfunction are made more likely by hyperglycemia and insulin resistance, which also weaken the immune system, decrease leukocyte activity, raise oxidative stress, and encourage endothelial dysfunction (Duggan et al. 2017; Ceriello et al. 2020). In order to maximize surgical outcomes, these mechanistic insights offer a compelling biological justification for focused perioperative glycemic management techniques that modulate the stress response, enhance insulin sensitivity, and maintain regulated glucose levels.

8.3 Perioperative Assessment Goals of the Diabetic Patient

Perioperative evaluation with insulin resistance involves many important considerations. It is divided into three parts: pre-operative, intraoperative, and post-operative (Vogt and Bally 2020).

- The American Diabetes Association (ADA) recommends a blood glucose level (BGL) of 140–180 ml/dL for critically ill patients and 80–180 mg/dL during the perioperative period.
- According to the Society of Ambulatory Association, maintaining a BGL of <180 mg/dL is recommended for patients experiencing ambulatory surgery.
- Additionally, for critical patients with a BGL of >150 mg/dL, the Society of Critical Care Medicine (SCCM) recommends starting insulin therapy.
- The American College of Physicians, however, recommends a BGL between 140 and 200 mg/dL rather than starting rigorous insulin therapy.
- In addition, the Society of Thoracic Surgeons advocates for BGLs <180 mg/dL and, in turn, for BGLs <110 mg/dL during fasting or before meals.
- Additionally, for non-critical hospitalized patients, the Endocrine Society recommends fasting or pre-meal targets <140 mg/dL and random glucose levels <180 mg/dL.
- It also emphasizes that in people who are not critically ill, a higher aim of 200 mg/dL is acceptable.
- The Joint British Diabetes Societies also recommend a BGL of 108 to 180 mg/dL, with an acceptable range of 72 to 216 mg/dL (Dogra et al. 2024).

Table 8.1 Blood glucose target for perioperative management

Organization	Recommended blood glucose target (mg/dL)	Population	Reference
American Diabetes Association	80–180 (perioperative) 140–180 (critical patients)	General standard for most patients	Committee et al. (2024)
Society for Ambulatory Anesthesia	<180	For day-care (ambulatory) surgery	Joshi et al. (2010)
Society of Critical Care Medicine	Start insulin if >150	Focus on ICU patients	Jacobi et al. (2012)
American College of Physicians	140–200	Avoids very strict control	Qaseem et al. (2011)
Society of Thoracic Surgeons	<180 (general) <110 (fasting/pre-meal)	Stricter fasting targets	Lazar et al. (2009)
Endocrine Society	<140 (fasting) <180 (random) up to 200 acceptable	For non-critical hospitalized patients	Umpierrez et al. (2021)
Joint British Diabetes Societies	108–180 (target) 72–216 (acceptable range)	Allows a wider safety range	Dhatariya et al. (2011)

The above-mentioned organizational recommendations have been compiled in Table 8.1 for comparison.

8.4 Perioperative Management

Irregular perioperative fasting schedule, potentially hazardous administration of intravenous insulin and medications, and physiological stress may result in adverse effects. These complications may also increase the expenses related to healthcare. In order to avoid such complications, there are numerous guidelines available for perioperative management for glucose management (Crowley et al. 2023). Figure 8.2 suggests the compilation guidelines for management of perioperative care. It is well noted that poor perioperative management may lead to adverse outcomes, such as the risk of hypoglycemia during fasting. Higher BGLs are linked with complications regardless of whether patients have diabetes or insulin resistance. However, the surgical patients having high BGLs during the perioperative period have worse outcomes, particularly having a high incidence of wound infections, and an HbA1c level of 7% or higher. The recovery process is significantly impacted by blood glucose levels on the first day following surgery (Australian Diabetes Society 2022).

The perioperative pathway for people with insulin resistance undergoing elective surgery includes standardized referral with HbA1c (within 3 months), control conditions of co-existing morbidities, and a list of all supportive medications. Furthermore, an individualized care plan should be developed, covering medication changes pre-surgery and post-surgery (Berhe et al. 2017; Hulst 2022).

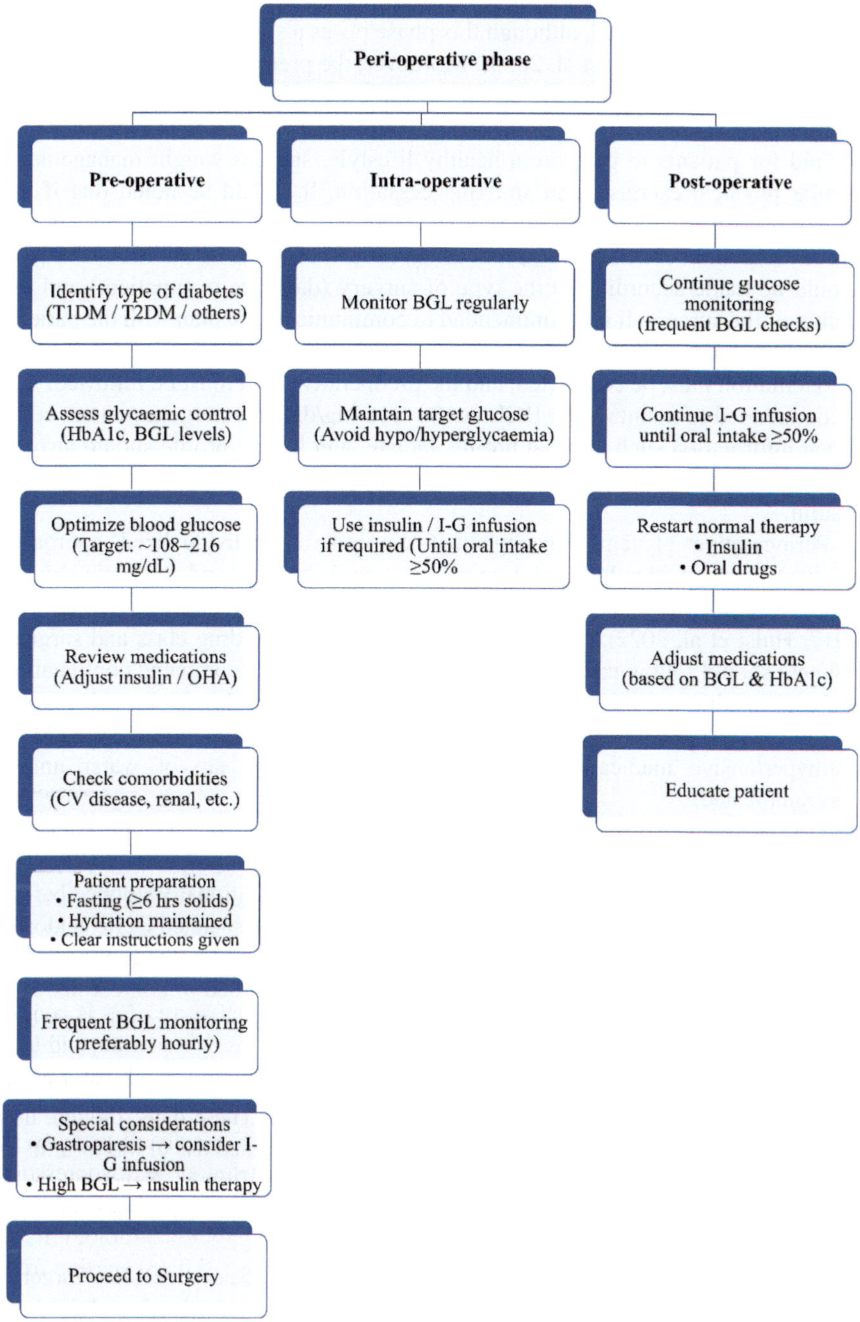

Fig. 8.2 Guidelines for perioperative management. (Created using Microsoft Word)

Preoperative administration of patients with insulin resistance and diabetes is frequently underestimated, although this phase poses a significant risk for this vulnerable group. (Crowley et al. 2023). Moreover, the preoperative stage of surgery, glucose monitoring, and associated comorbidities should be carefully assessed and optimized. A shared decision of the patient is essential. This stage is a useful teaching aid for patients to promote a healthy lifestyle, such as weight management, regular physical exercise, and smoking cessation. It should be noted that if the patient has HbA1c more than 8.5% or 69 mmol/mol (197 mg/dL), further optimization is recommended before proceeding toward surgery. In addition, the plan should be made according to the type of surgery (day care or inpatient) and the timing of the surgery. It is recommended to communicate the plan with the patient, general practitioner, and healthcare team. On admission of the patient, medication reconciliation must be completed, and the preoperative plan must be followed. It is recommended to maintain the BGL at 108–216 mg/dL. In emergency cases, additional information such as renal profile, lactate, and ketone profile should also be recorded. Additionally, patients with type 1 diabetes must continue receiving insulin.

Perioperative glycemic management requires an individualized approach. Studies suggest withholding oral agents in type 2 diabetes and modifying short-acting insulin in type 1 diabetes with frequent glucose monitoring (Berhe et al. 2017; Hulst et al. 2022)*;* however, management varies by drug class and surgical risk and should follow institutional protocols. Guidelines recommend continuation of basal insulin and maintaining controlled blood glucose levels through regular monitoring (American Diabetes Association, 2024; Umpierrez et al. 2022). Most antihypertensive medications can be continued with a sip of water unless contraindicated.

It is documented that providing similar care to type 1 diabetic and type 2 diabetic patients results in poorer short-term and long-term outcomes, especially in type 1, as well as a high risk of hypoglycemia. Metformin was traditionally stopped before surgery for type 2 diabetes, due to the risk of metformin-associated lactic acidosis. Though nowadays, the risk is considered minimal, which supports the continued use of metformin. The continuation of metformin is recommended in non-cardiac surgery. Nevertheless, it does not increase lactate levels to clinically significant levels or enhance blood glucose regulation (Hulst 2022).

Because of the possibility of metformin-associated lactic acidosis, metformin was traditionally stopped before type 2 diabetes surgery. These days, though, this danger is thought to be minimal, which supports the continued use of metformin. In non-cardiac surgery, it is advised to continue taking metformin. Nevertheless, it does not increase lactate levels to clinically significant levels or enhance blood glucose regulation.

Intraoperative management includes ESAR (Enhanced Recovery After Surgery) insulin infusion protocol, which can be computerized by incorporating algorithms that direct healthcare staff to adjust insulin infusion rates (Vogt and Bally 2020). During surgery, focus on minimizing the fasting period and maintaining BGL within

140–180 mg/dL (7.8–10.0 mmol/L) as per institutional protocol. (Berhe et al. 2017; Hulst 2022).

Postoperative ward care, i.e., after surgery care, includes medication adjustment after review. Early recovery measures include early oral intake and mobilization per ERAS protocols, often described as DREAMing (Drinking, Eating, and Mobilizing), which should be encouraged. (Berhe et al. 2017; Hulst 2022). Moreover, BGLs must be regularly monitored and maintained in the targeted range. Also, patients with Type 1 Diabetes must continue receiving insulin. If necessary, the patient must be referred to a diabetes specialized team. Moreover, at the time of discharge, clear communication with the patient must be maintained to avoid complications and to ensure the future diabetes care plan (Grant et al. 2022).

8.5 Adjuvant Drugs

8.5.1 Metformin (Biguanide)

Metformin mainly decreases the amount of glucose produced by the liver and increases peripheral insulin sensitivity. It also decreases the amount of glucose assembled in the liver and the total amount of glucose absorbed by tissues. It has good oral bioavailability and has minimal protein binding. It helps to improve lipid profile, endothelial function, and support weight loss. In addition, it helps to reduce macro and microvascular complications. Also, it is safe to consume with antidiabetic drugs and insulin (Bagry et al. 2008). Furthermore, the Intake does not affect or worsen renal function. It can be continued for minor surgeries. However, in major surgeries, metformin must be stopped on the day of surgery and restarted after 24 h if the kidney function is stable. and is only recommended if serum creatinine levels do not worsen the postoperative condition. In addition, metformin must be stopped in case of renal impairment, as it is associated with lactic acidosis (Dogra et al. 2024). Prolonged cessation of metformin may deteriorate glycemic control (Australian Diabetes Society 2022).

8.5.2 Thiazolidinediones

Thiazolidinediones (TZDs) are PPAR-γ agonists. It works through activation of PPAR—γ receptors and thereby improves glucose uptake by peripheral tissues. Moreover, it reduces insulin resistance in muscles and fat, reduces hepatic glucose production, promotes the expression of insulin-sensitive glucose transporter GLUT-4, promotes fat redistribution, and decreases visceral fat. It helps to reduce inflammatory markers (CRP, TNF- α, IL-6). However, it must be avoided in severe cases to avoid the risk of heart failure (Bagry et al. 2008).

8.5.3 Sulfonylureas and Glinides

They stimulate insulin release from pancreatic beta-cells by closing K_{ATP} (potassium) channels, causing cell depolarization. These channels are present in the heart, pancreas, and blood vessels. Different drugs have varying sensitivity towards the heart and pancreas. The older drugs, such as glimepiride, are more sensitive to the pancreas. Whereas newer drugs such as glibenclamide have greater pancreatic β-cell selectivity. The cardiac K_{ATP} is important for heart protection in ischemia. However, it is associated with hypoglycemia and is less effective in stress-induced insulin resistance (Dogra et al. 2024; Bagry et al. 2008).

8.5.4 Dexamethasone

Dexamethasone is most commonly given in surgical procedures. Nausea and vomiting post-surgery may worsen glucose control and result in ketoacidosis. Hence, it helps prevent postoperative nausea and vomiting and thus is added in post-operative procedures. Some studies indicated that a low dose of 4–8 mg does not impact blood glucose. Whereas the higher dose may raise BGLs, generally in type 2 DM (Crowley et al. 2023).

8.5.5 Magnesium Sulphate

Magnesium can help in reducing high BGLs in blood glucose levels and enhance insulin receptor sensitivity. It helps to improve insulin binding to target tissue and increase insulin secretion from the pancreas. Moreover, it enhances insulin-mediated glucose uptake and helps to regulate stored glucose breakdown. It reduces glucose production in the liver and stress hormones. Overall, it plays a pivotal role in glucose metabolism. In patients undergoing surgery, a dosage of 15 mg/kg/hour should be started 20 min before anesthesia and must be continued for 24 h postoperatively (Crowley et al. 2023). However, the role of magnesium supplementation requires further clinical validation, and its use should be guided by institutional protocols and individual patient considerations.

8.5.6 Glucagon-Like Peptide-1 and GIP-Based Drug

They are an incretin hormonal drug. That helps to regulate blood sugar. It is recommended to continue this drug in the pre-operative stage as well as in the post-operative stage if advised. Furthermore, glucose-dependent insulinotropic peptide is useful in intraoperative glucose lowering and provides more stable blood glucose (Dogra et al. 2024; Crowley et al. 2023; Hulst 2022; Australian Diabetes Society 2022).

8.6 Nutrition and Fasting Strategies

Surgical procedures cause stress, which leads to insulin resistance, which triggers a hormonal response and activates inflammatory pathways, and this condition further results in a catabolic state. To promote anabolism, preoperative carbohydrate loading is recommended, typically involving 12.5–50 g of a clear carbohydrate beverage administered 2–3 h before surgery in accordance with ERAS (Enhanced Recovery After Surgery) protocols. Fasting is an extreme state causing adverse effects on glucose and protein depletion. It is a state of nutritional stress resulting in fat-producing energy. In addition, it increases the risk of infection and oxidative stress by impairing the mononuclear phagocytic system. Animal studies have demonstrated that eating before acute injury conserves energy supplies and preserves bacterial homeostasis in the gut and immune function. Preoperative oral glucose intake is a part of the Enhanced Recovery After Surgery protocol that aims to improve patient recovery after surgery. One of the vital constituents of the ERAS protocol is the administration of oral glucose before 2 h of surgical procedures. Preoperative carbohydrate intake maintains insulin sensitivity, reduces nitrogen losses, supports protein synthesis, reduces thirst, fatigue, hunger, malaise, and anxiety (Ismy et al. 2021; Bagry et al. 2008).

Furthermore, during fasting, prandial insulin is withheld, which increases the risk of low blood sugar. However, if glucose rises, correlational insulin and subcutaneous injections should be administered. For that, the hospital should use the standard insulin scale for accurate results (Rushakoff 2015). In case of minor surgery, the patient can resume normal eating soon due to less stress. However, in major surgeries, normal eating can be resumed after 24 h. Begin with intravenous infusion of 5–10% dextrose; glucose solution (500 ml bag) over 5 h continuously to prevent low blood sugar. In addition, add potassium chloride and insulin to each bag. Also, change the bag as per the blood glucose requirement. Add five units of insulin if the blood glucose level is between 72 and 108 mg/dL; 10 units if the blood glucose level is between 109 and 180 mg/dL; 15 units if the blood glucose level is between 81 and 360 mg/dL; and 20 units if the blood glucose level is greater than 360 mg/dL. Similarly, add 20 mmol/L of potassium chloride if it is less than 3 mmol/L, add 10 mmol/L if it is between 3 and 5 mmol/L, and do not add potassium if it is more than 5 mmol/L (Berhe et al. 2017).

For enteral nutrition, preferably, low carbs and high-monounsaturated diet is recommended. Correlation between basal, nutritional, and insulin should all be included in the subcutaneous insulin protocol. Basal insulin is administered once or twice a day at a typical daily dose (TTD) of 30–50%. Nutritional insulin makes up the remaining 50–70% of TTD. An alternate method for calculating insulin intake is 1 unit of insulin per 10–15 g of carbohydrates, which can be applied for each bolus fed every 24 h. For continuous tube feeding, rapid insulin every 4 h and regular insulin every 6 h is recommended. For total parenteral nutrition (TPN), IV is given separately or mixed with TPN and can be started initially. The starting dose is 1 unit of insulin per 10 g of dextrose, which can be adjusted every one to two days as per glucose levels. Once managed, the dose can be increased to 80–100% to maintain the target glycemic range (A. D. A., 2014, 2018; Guillermo et al. 2009; Elia et al. 2005; Pichardo-Lowden et al. 2010).

8.7 Bowel Preparation in Insulin Resistance

Bowel preparation in patients with insulin resistance should be carefully planned to ensure effective intestinal cleansing while maintaining metabolic stability. The primary goals include adequate bowel emptying, prevention of electrolyte imbalance, and maintenance of stable blood glucose levels throughout the perioperative period (Gustafsson et al. 2019). Furthermore, dietary preparation generally involves a low-residue diet followed by clear fluids with controlled carbohydrate content to minimize glycemic fluctuations (Chirila et al. 2023; Agha et al. 2021).

Continuous monitoring of blood glucose and appropriate adjustment of antihyperglycemic therapy are essential to reduce the risk of hypoglycemia and hyperglycemia (Hochberg et al. 2019). Moreover, adequate hydration is important to prevent dehydration and electrolyte disturbances during bowel preparation (Kurz et al. 2018). Following surgery, gradual reintroduction of diet, restoration of bowel function, and ongoing glycemic monitoring are important for recovery and prevention of complications (Gustafsson et al. 2019). The Australian Diabetes Society (2022) has suggested the following guidelines for bowel preparation in individuals with insulin resistance:

- The insulin doses need to be lowered.
- Omit the short-acting insulin and oral anti-diabetics.
- Increase the intake of glucose-containing clear fluids, especially during bowel surgery. (not purely diet drinks or diet jelly).
- A diet with added glucose is recommended if BGL falls under 5.0 mmol/L.
- A diet with less glucose is recommended if BGL exceeds 10 mmol/L (e.g., broths and diet drinks.
- Regular BGL monitoring.
- Unstable insulin patients must use insulin-glucose infusion.
- Seek medical help if BGL fluctuates.
- Admit high-risk patients for insulin-glucose infusion.
- If the patient is on insulin, modify the insulin regimen by adding short-acting insulin with meals and glargine, or detemir/isophane twice a day, or at night only, and add premix-insulin or an insulin pump (Australian Diabetes Society 2022).

8.8 Conclusion

Insulin resistance and diabetes are most common in surgical procedures. It is associated to higher rates of morbidity and mortality. Effective perioperative glycemic management is important for improving surgical outcomes, decreasing complications, and reducing hospital stays. In clinical practice, this requires careful monitoring and timely adjustment of insulin and other glucose-lowering therapies before, during, and after surgery. Instead of counting on a single standard procedure, management techniques must be customized individually because patient responses vary greatly based on the type of diabetes, surgical stress, and related comorbidities. Despite available guidelines, uncertainties remain regarding optimal glucose targets, medication adjustments, and the balance between intensive and conventional control. Therefore, a coordinated, multidisciplinary approach along with continued research is essential to refine protocols and ensure safe, patient-centered care in the perioperative period.

References

Agha OQ, Alsayid M, Brown MD. Bowel preparation in diabetic patients undergoing colonoscopy. Ann Gastroenterol. 2021;34(3):310. https://doi.org/10.20524/aog.2021.0599.

American Diabetes Association. Standards of Medical Care in Diabetes—2014. Diabetes Care. 2014;37(Supplement_1):S14–80. https://doi.org/10.2337/dc14-s014.

American Diabetes Association. Diabetes care in the hospital: Standards of Medical Care in Diabetes—2018. Diabetes Care. 2018;41(Supplement_1):S144–51. https://doi.org/10.2337/dc18-S014.

Angelidi AM, Filippaios A, Mantzoros CS. Severe insulin resistance syndromes. J Clin Invest. 2021;131(4) https://doi.org/10.1172/jci142245.

Australian Diabetes Society (2022) ADS-ANZCA perioperative diabetes and hyperglycaemia guidelines (adults). https://www.diabetessociety.com.au/wp-content/uploads/2023/03/ADS-ANZCA-Perioperative-Diabetes-and-Hyperglycaemia-Guidelines-Adults-November-2022-v2-Final.pdf.

Bagry HS, Raghavendran S, Carli F, Warner DS, Warner MA. Metabolic syndrome and insulin resistance. Anesthesiology. 2008;108(3):506–23. https://doi.org/10.1097/aln.0b013e3181649314.

Berhe YW, Gebregzi AH, Endalew NS. Guideline on peri-operative glycemic control for adult patient with diabetic mellitus: resource limited areas. Int J Surg Open. 2017;9:1–6. https://doi.org/10.1016/j.ijso.2017.07.001.

Blonde L, Umpierrez GE, Reddy SS, McGill JB, Berga SL, Bush M, Weber SL. American Association of Clinical Endocrinology clinical practice guideline: developing a diabetes mellitus comprehensive care plan—2022 update. Endocrine Practice; 2022;28(10):923–1049. https://doi.org/10.1016/j.eprac.2022.08.002.

Ceriello A, De Nigris V, Prattichizzo F. Why is hyperglycaemia worsening COVID -19 and its prognosis? Diabetes Obes Metab. 2020;22(10):1951–2. https://doi.org/10.1111/dom.14098.

Chirila A, Nguyen ME, Tinmouth J, Halperin IJ. Preparing for colonoscopy in people with diabetes: a review with suggestions for clinical practice. J Canad Assoc Gastroenterol. 2023;6(1):26–36. https://doi.org/10.1093/jcag/gwac035.

Committee, A. D. A. P. P, ElSayed NA, Aleppo G, Bannuru RR, Beverly EA, Bruemmer D, Collins BS, Cusi K, Darville A, Das SR, Ekhlaspour L, Fleming TK, Gaglia JL, Galindo RJ, Gibbons CH, Giurini JM, Hassanein M, Hilliard ME, Johnson EL, et al. Introduction and methodology: standards of care in diabetes—2024. Diabetes Care. 2024;47(Supplement_1):S1–4. https://doi.org/10.2337/dc24-SINT.

Crowley K, Scanaill PÓ, Hermanides J, Buggy DJ. Current practice in the perioperative management of patients with diabetes mellitus: a narrative review. Br J Anaesth. 2023;131(2):242–52. https://doi.org/10.1016/j.bja.2023.02.039.

Desborough JP. The stress response to trauma and surgery. Br J Anaesth. 2000;85(1):109–17. https://doi.org/10.1093/bja/85.1.109.

Dhatariya K. Management of adults with diabetes undergoing surgery and elective procedures: improving standards. NHS Diabetes. 2011; https://www.profketandhatariya.com/publications/original_articles/JBDS_-_peri-op_guidelines.pdf

Dogra P, Anastasopoulou C, Jialal I. Diabetic perioperative management. In StatPearls Publishing. 2024; https://pubmed.ncbi.nlm.nih.gov/31082009/

Duggan EW, Carlson K, Umpierrez GE. Perioperative hyperglycemia management: an update. Anesthesiology. 2017;126(3):547–60. https://doi.org/10.1097/ALN.0000000000001515.

Elia M, Ceriello A, Laube H, Sinclair AJ, Engfer M, Stratton RJ. Enteral nutritional support and use of diabetes-specific formulas for patients with diabetes: a systematic review and meta-analysis. Diabetes Care. 2005;28(9):2267–79. https://doi.org/10.2337/diacare.28.9.2267.

Finfer S, Chittock DR, Su SY, Blair D, Foster D, Dhingra V, et al. Intensive versus conventional glucose control in critically ill patients. N Engl J Med. 2009;360(13):1283–97. https://doi.org/10.1056/nejmoa0810625.

Finney SJ. Glucose control and mortality in critically ill patients. JAMA. 2003;290(15):2041. https://doi.org/10.1001/jama.290.15.2041.

Gandhi GY, Nuttall GA, Abel MD, Mullany CJ, Schaff HV, O'Brien PC, Johnson MG, Williams AR, Cutshall SM, Mundy LM, Rizza RA, McMahon MM. Intensive intraoperative insulin therapy versus conventional glucose management during cardiac surgery. Ann Intern Med. 2007;146(4):233–43. https://doi.org/10.7326/0003-4819-146-4-200702200-00002.

Grant B, Chowdhury TA. New guidance on the perioperative management of diabetes. Clin Med. 2022;22(1):41–4. https://doi.org/10.7861/clinmed.2021-0355.

Guillermo EU. Basal versus sliding-scale regular insulin in hospitalized patients with hyperglycemia during enteral nutrition therapy. Diabetes Care 2009;32(4):751–753. https://doi.org/10.2337/dc08-2257.

Gustafsson UO, Scott MJ, Hubner M, Nygren J, Demartines N, Francis N, et al. Guidelines for perioperative care in elective colorectal surgery: enhanced recovery after surgery (ERAS®) society recommendations: 2018. World J Surg. 2019;43(3):659–95. https://doi.org/10.1007/s00268-018-4844-y.

Hochberg I, Segol O, Shental R, Shimoni P, Eldor R. Antihyperglycemic therapy during colonoscopy preparation: A review and suggestions for practical recommendations. United European Gastroenterol J. 2019;7(6):735–40. https://doi.org/10.1177/2050640619846365.

Hulst A. Glucose control therapies in the perioperative period. Abraham Hendrikus Hulst. 2022; https://hdl.handle.net/11245.1/9f8b3eed-fbd4-4d84-96aa-593b390f447c

International Diabetes Federation (2025) India diabetes statistics and health data | diabetes Atlas. https://diabetesatlas.org/data-by-location/country/india/.

Ismy J, Wisesa I, Yusuf M, Naufal I, Hidayat I, Muslim. The effect of oral glucose administration before surgery based on Enhanced Recovery After Surgery (ERAS) protocol on preventing insulin resistance and patient's quality of life. J Int Surg Clin Med. 2021;1(2):32–4. https://doi.org/10.51559/jiscm.v1i2.17.

Jacobi J, Bircher N, Krinsley J, Agus M, Braithwaite SS, Deutschman C, Freire AX, Geehan D, Kohl B, Nasraway SA, Rigby M, Sands K, Schallom L, Taylor B, Umpierrez G, Mazuski J, Schunemann H. Guidelines for the use of an insulin infusion for the management of hyperglycemia in critically ill patients. Crit Care Med. 2012;40(12):3251–76. https://doi.org/10.1097/CCM.0b013e3182653269.

Joshi GP, Chung F, Vann MA, Ahmad S, Gan TJ, Goulson DT, Merrill DG, Twersky R. Society for Ambulatory Anesthesia Consensus Statement on Perioperative Blood glucose management in diabetic patients undergoing ambulatory surgery. Anesth Analg. 2010;111(6):1378–87. https://doi.org/10.1213/ane.0b013e3181f9c288.

Kurz A, Kopyeva T, Suliman I, Podolyak A, You J, Lewis B, Sessler DI. Supplemental oxygen and surgical-site infections: an alternating intervention controlled trial. British journal of anaesthesia ; 2018;120(1):117–126. https://doi.org/10.1016/j.bja.2017.11.003.

Lazar HL, McDonnell M, Chipkin SR, Furnary AP, Engelman RM, Sadhu AR, Bridges CR, Haan CK, Svedjeholm R, Taegtmeyer H, Shemin RJ. The society of thoracic surgeons practice

guideline series: blood glucose management during adult cardiac surgery. Ann Thorac Surg. 2009;87(2):663–9. https://doi.org/10.1016/j.athoracsur.2008.11.011.
Lipshutz AKM, Gropper MA, Warner DS, Warner MA. Perioperative glycemic control. Anesthesiology. 2009;110(2):408–21. https://doi.org/10.1097/aln.0b013e3181948a80.
McGirt MJ, Woodworth GF, Brooke BS, Coon AL, Jain S, Buck D, et al. Hyperglycemia independently increases the risk of perioperative stroke, myocardial infarction, and death after carotid endarterectomy. Neurosurgery. 2006;58(6):1066–73. https://doi.org/10.1227/01.NEU.0000215887.59922.36.
Petersen MC, Shulman GI. Mechanisms of insulin action and insulin resistance. Physiol Rev. 2018;98(4):2133–223. https://doi.org/10.1152/physrev.00063.2017.
Pichardo-Lowden AR, Fan CY, Gabbay RA. Management of hyperglycemia in the non-intensive care patient: featuring subcutaneous insulin protocols. Endocr Pract. 2010;17(2):249–60. https://doi.org/10.4158/ep10220.ra.
Qaseem A, Humphrey LL, Chou R, Snow V, Shekelle P. Use of intensive insulin therapy for the management of glycemic control in hospitalized patients: a clinical practice guideline from the American college of physicians. 2011;154(4):260–7. https://doi.org/10.7326/0003-4819-154-4-201102150-00007.
Rushakoff R. Inpatient diabetes management. Europe PMC. 2015; https://europepmc.org/article/nbk/nbk278972
Thorell A, Nygren J, Ljungqvist O. Insulin resistance: a marker of surgical stress. Curr Opin Clinic Nutr Metab Care. 1999;2(1):69–78. https://doi.org/10.1097/00075197-199901000-00012.
Umpierrez GE, Pasquel FJ. Management of inpatient hyperglycemia and diabetes. Lancet Diabetes Endocrinol. 2021;9(3):174–88. https://doi.org/10.1016/S2213-8587(20)30381-8.
Van den Berghe G, Wouters P, Weekers F, Verwaest C, Bruyninckx F, Schetz M, et al. Intensive insulin therapy in critically ill patients. N Engl J Med. 2001;345(19):1359–67. https://doi.org/10.1056/NEJMoa011300.
Van den Berghe G, Wouters PJ, Bouillon R, Weekers F, Verwaest C, Schetz M, et al. Outcome benefit of intensive insulin therapy in the critically ill: insulin dose versus glycemic control. Crit Care Med. 2003;31(2):359–66. https://doi.org/10.1097/01.CCM.0000045568.12881.10.
Van den Berghe G, Wilmer A, Hermans G, Meersseman W, Wouters PJ, Milants I, et al. Intensive insulin therapy in the medical ICU. N Engl J Med. 2006;354(5):449–61. https://doi.org/10.1056/NEJMoa052521.
Vogt AP, Bally L. Perioperative glucose management: current status and future directions. Best Pract Res Clin Anaesthesiol. 2020;34(2):213–24. https://doi.org/10.1016/j.bpa.2020.04.015.
World Health Organization: WHO & World Health Organization: WHO. (2024, November 14). Diabetes https://www.who.int/news-room/fact-sheets/detail/diabetes

Nutritional Support in High-Risk Surgical Patients

9

Dhananjay Sharma, Luxita Sharma, Mansi Joon, and Shashi Soni

Abstract

High-risk surgical patients are highly susceptible to several infectious diseases, and the nutritional support plays a critical role in this management, specifically those who are malnourished or have susceptible medical complications. The low nutritional status is directly linked with increased postoperative complications, long stay, higher mortality rate, and delayed wound healing. This chapter highlights the improvised and clinical strategies that need to be included for the effective nutritional support of patients who are planning to undergo major or high-risk surgical procedures. Prominence is placed on categorizing the patients who need specialized nutritional intervention and selecting the most appropriate feeding methods. Both advanced feeding practices, such as enteral and parenteral nutrition tactics, are discussed, including their potential complications, advantages, and indications. Enteral feeding is highly recommended when the gastrointestinal tract of the patient is properly functional, as it preserves gut integrity and immune defence, whereas parenteral nutrition is recommended only when the patient is on a serious medical complication and enteral feeding is not feasible for that patient at that time. The chapter also explores the recent trends and updates that can be adopted in perioperative nutritional care, including personalized nutrition planning, tactics to be adapted to reduce the risk of infection, and improved monitoring techniques such as artificial nutritional support. Proper attention is planned for giving the balance benefits of a nutritional approach with potential complications such as catheter-related infections and metabolic disturbance. Generally, the chapter focuses on the evidence-based approaches to

D. Sharma · L. Sharma · M. Joon · S. Soni (✉)
Department of Dietetics and Applied Nutrition, Amity Medical School, Amity University Haryana, Gurugram, Haryana, India
e-mail: lshrama@ggn.amity.edu; ssoni@ggn.amity.edu

P. K. Bhattacharyya et al. (eds.), *Integrated Anesthesia and Nutrition Approaches to Enhanced Recovery after Surgery*,
https://doi.org/10.1007/978-981-92-3294-9_9

enhance the nutritional care in high-risk surgical patients to advance the recovery, minimize the complications, and improve the overall surgical outcomes.

Keywords

Nutritional support · Surgical patients · Enteral nutrition · Parenteral nutrition · Malnutrition

9.1 Overview of High-Risk Surgical Patients

High-risk surgical patients are those who do not have a good health status, and are likely to experience complications during or after the surgery. This can include patients with long-term medical issues, who are poorly nourished and are in an acute stage of disease. They often experience reduced physiological reserves, and it becomes more difficult to absorb the stress of surgery, anesthesia, and recuperation. Owing to this, even common surgeries may be tricky, and this should be carefully planned, observed, and supported to avoid the occurrence of negative results (Boyd and Jackson 2005).

The nutritional status of those at high-risk who need surgical procedures can essentially impact the ability of patients to heal and recover effectively, and their immunity and healing. The combination of malnutrition and underlying illnesses with infections and prolonged hospital stay impairs the body's defence system and slows tissue repair. To ensure safer and more effective treatment outcomes, high-risk patients have to be managed not only by treating the surgical issue but also by improving their general health with proper dietary support and pre-operative assessment, as well as multi-disciplinary care (Keerio et al. 2024).

9.1.1 Characteristics of High-Risk Patients

A high-risk surgery patient is one whose general health condition predisposes him or her to complications after the operation. Such patients often experience serious diseases, chronic diseases, or poor nutrition, all of which reduce the ability of the body to cope with the stress of surgery. Since they already have weakened physiological reserves, the perioperative period, which involves the time before, during, and after surgery, is critical to these individuals. They therefore require special dietary treatment to meet their metabolic requirements and improve their output (Schwarze et al. 2015).

More susceptible are patients with serious illnesses like advanced infections, organ failure, or severe trauma of any kind, as their bodies are already under excessive stress. Immunity is often weakened in this case, and the ability of the body to maintain normal metabolic processes is impaired. The body's ability to react appropriately may be overwhelmed when surgery is included in an already stressful situation. In a similar vein, those who suffer from long-term conditions like diabetes, cancer, heart disease, or renal illness have more difficulties. Such disorders often do not coincide with the normal metabolism, suppress the process of healing and expose individuals to infections. An example of this is that since diabetes affects blood circulation and immunological response, it is associated with poor wound healing and high chances of infection (Chávez-Reyes et al. 2021).

Malnutrition is another outstanding characteristic of high-risk patients and greatly affects the outcome of surgery. It may be brought about by chronic illness, deficiency in food intake, or high metabolic requirements not met by the available nutrients. Typical signs of malnutrition include weight loss, muscle atrophy, and a lack of important nutrients, such as proteins, different vitamins, and minerals. The malabsorption impairs the ability to repair tissues and the immune system, and reduces the muscle strength of the body. Such people cannot meet the increased nutritional requirements of the body during the perioperative period, which deteriorates their condition (Saunders and Smith 2010; Tappenden et al. 2013).

High-risk patients need careful dietary evaluation and management prior to surgery because of these considerations. Specialized perioperative nutritional therapy may include oral nutritional supplements, enteral nutrition through tubes, or intravenous parenteral nutrition. The aim is to boost the immunity of the patient, nutritionally optimize them, and prepare their body to cope with the surgical stress. Nutritional assistance should be monitored and modified to achieve the most favorable outcomes (Weimann et al. 2025).

9.1.2 Impact of Malnutrition on Surgical Outcomes

One of the most noteworthy risk factors that can be altered during surgical treatment due to its profound and profound impact on surgical outcomes is malnutrition. The malnourished patients have a higher likelihood of infection and slow wound healing, as well as long hospitalization during and after surgery. These problems increase the chances of death and healthcare costs, besides hampering recovery (Williams et al. 2019).

Malnutrition has several consequences, one of them being an increased susceptibility to infections. A healthy diet is essential to having a strong immune system, and a lack of certain vital nutrients, such as vitamins, minerals, and protein, can impair the immune system. The malnourished individuals thus become more prone to postoperative infections and cannot resist infections. These may entail urinary tract infections, pneumonia, surgical site infections, and, in the worst scenario, sepsis. Illnesses aggravate the health of the patient, complicate the healing process, and may require an increased stay in the hospital or other medication such as antibiotics (Morales et al. 2023).

Delayed wound healing is another important consequence of malnutrition. Wound healing requires enough protein to build collagen and vitamins and minerals that aid in tissue regeneration and repair. Such nutrients are often not available in undernourished people, and thus surgery wounds take longer to heal. This can result in complications like wound dehiscence, where the surgical incision re-opens, or the

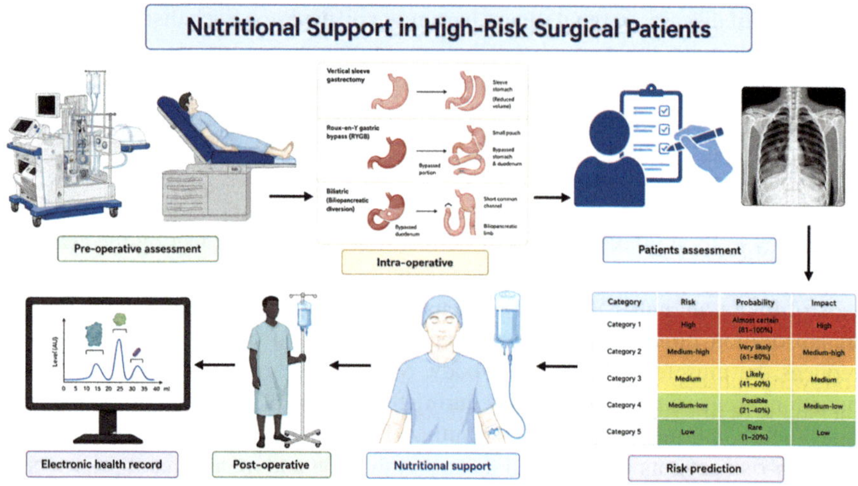

Fig. 9.1 Nutritional support in high-risk surgical patients. (Created using PowerPoint 2021)

formation of non-healing wounds that do not heal. Besides increasing the recovery period, slow healing increases the risk of infection and other complications (Seth et al. 2024).

Longer hospital stays are also a result of malnutrition. People who are malnourished often require extended medical treatment and observation as they take longer to recover and are more prone to issues. Hospital occupancies in the long run create an additional drain to the medical facilities and an increased risk of hospital-acquired diseases. Additionally, the long hospitalization can negatively affect the physical and mental health of a patient, which leads to a poorer quality of life (Gebregziabher et al. 2024). Figure 9.1 illustrates the continuum of perioperative nutritional care in high-risk surgical patients, starting from preoperative assessment through intraoperative management to postoperative nutritional support. It highlights the role of risk prediction and patient evaluation in guiding appropriate nutrition strategies. Integration with electronic health records and monitoring systems ensures personalized, safe, and effective patient management.

Functional deterioration and muscle weakness can also be caused by malnutrition. Loss of muscle mass, especially the respiratory muscles, may cause difficulties in breathing and an increased need for ventilatory support after the operation. The danger of problems like blood clots and pressure ulcers is further increased by decreased mobility. Moreover, malnutrition can affect the metabolism and efficacy of drugs and thus complicate the process of pain, infections, or other postoperative issues management (Nagano et al. 2021). Malnutrition influences the general results of surgery in a major and far-reaching manner. Nutritional deficiency can be improved by addressing it early through diagnosis and proper intervention in order to enhance recovery, reduce complications, and improve the overall outcome of surgical therapy.

9.2 Enteral Nutrition in High-Risk Patients

Nutritional support is highly needed to improve the nutritional status, clinical outcomes, and quality of life of high-risk patients. It is also associated with reduced length of hospital stay and reduced morbidity. Surgical patients who are unable to take nutrition from the oral route are directed to take nutrition from other life-sustaining procedures, in which Enteral and Parenteral nutrition (EN and PN) are the most crucial ones. The most clinically appropriate selection between EN and PN for perioperative patients depends on the physical condition and duration of nutritional therapy to be provided (Waitzberg et al. 2000).

Enteral nutrition (EN) is described as the administration of nutrients directly into the gastrointestinal tract with the help of a feeding tube. In surgical patients, development of post-operative ileus (temporary damage to peristalsis movement) leads to malnutrition as the individual is unable to take nutrition through the oral route. Thus, EN is preferred as the best nutritional support in high-risk patients. In comparison to parenteral nutrition, EN has been proven to have better clinical outcomes, reduced complications and a cost-effective technique for long term (Chen et al. 2011).

Patients of intensive care units (ICUs), severe trauma, sepsis, burns, chronic illnesses, or major surgeries are categorized under high-risk conditions. Due to hypermetabolic conditions, inflammation, and decreased food intake via the oral route, these patients are at higher risk of malnutrition. Various studies have evidenced the best outcomes of early initiation of EN, usually within 24–48 h of hospital admission or ICU stay, to preserve gut integrity, support immune function, and reduce stress response (Singer et al. 2019).

9.2.1 Indications and Benefits

Typically, for high-risk patients, EN is recommended only when the gut integrity is responsive, but the oral route gets hampered due to ileus, and nutritional requirements are not fulfilled. Both acute and chronic care settings can provide EN. Major indications for the provision of EN are: *Inadequate oral intake* due to anorexia, prolonged fasting after surgery, or severe illness, leading to malnutrition is the general and foremost indication for the commencement of enteral nutrition following the GI tract (McClave et al. 2016); *Gastrointestinal disorders with functional gut* occur in many conditions like as inflammatory bowel disease, pancreatitis or short bowel syndrome in perioperative patients which may require sufficient supply of nutrients through enteral nutrition, and; *Severe malnutrition* occurred in post-operative surgical patients with significant weight loss, prolonged hospitalization and chronic illness are benefited from EN with replenished nutrient balance and complication prevention (Debaveye and Van den Berghe 2006).

Enteral nutrition is associated with several health benefits and primarily helps maintain the structural and functional integrity of the gut. EN also helps to reduce bacterial translocation and prevents muscular atrophy, thus the risk of infection and sepsis decreases. Moreover, it plays a crucial role in immune defence by supporting gut-associated lymphoid tissue (GALT) (McClave et al. 2016).

Perioperative EN has two benefits: better wound healing and a decreased incidence of surgical infections and sequelae (Peev et al. 2015). Furthermore, there would be fewer potentially fatal surgical side effects, including superficial or deep fascial surgical site infections, delayed stomach emptying, anastomotic stenosis or leak, and recurrent nerve palsy. EN has been shown to be cost-effective by reducing hospital stays. These effects are thought to be caused by EN's capacity to reduce the body's response to stress, prevent villous atrophy by preserving the integrity of the GI, and maintain immunocompetency by secreting IgA (Beattie et al. 2000).

EN is contraindicated in a few situations, including intestinal blockage, malabsorption, numerous fistulas with high output, intestinal ischemia, severe shock with diminished splanchnic perfusion, and fulminant sepsis (Wobith and Weimann 2021). The three main types of EN issues are metabolic, mechanical, and gastrointestinal. It is normal to experience symptoms of gastrointestinal intolerance, such as nausea, vomiting, diarrhea, and excessive gastric residual volumes. To reduce these issues, careful observation and modest feeding rate advancement are crucial. When stomach feeding is not accepted, post-pyloric feeding (such as through nasojejunal tubes) may be necessary.

The possibility of aspiration pneumonia is another issue for high-risk individuals, especially those who have trouble swallowing or are unconscious. Elevating the head of the bed, employing prokinetic drugs, and routinely checking tube placement are methods to lower this risk (Boullata et al. 2017). Another critical side effect of starting nutrition in people who are extremely malnourished is refeeding syndrome. Electrolyte abnormalities, especially hypophosphatemia, which can cause respiratory and cardiac problems, are its defining feature. As a result, nutrition should be started carefully, with modest increases in calories and careful electrolyte monitoring (da Silva et al. 2020).

In clinical practice, the guidelines of EN are not closely followed, but early intervention of EN in mechanically ventilated critically ill post-operative patients has been proven to be more beneficial. However, personalized nutrition should be followed considering the metabolic need of the individuals. Haines et al. (2023) compared the outcomes of early EN, within 3 days after intubation, and late EN, after 3 days of intubation. The result of the regression analysis showed that lower mortality, reduced hospital stays, cost-effective and fewer MV days in the early EN group in comparison to the late EN group. Saluja et al. (2002) conducted a study on 60 malnourished patients undergoing major abdominal surgery and categorized them according to nutritional risk index into severely (SM), moderately (MM), and borderline (BM) malnourished. Further, the patients were randomly subdivided into treatment (TG) and control (CG) groups. Anthropometric, biochemical, hematological, and complication rates of these two groups were compared after intervening in the TG patients with oral sip feed (500 kcal and 16.66 g protein). Significant improvement in TG patients of the SM category was noted with reduced weight loss and maximum reduction in complications or risk factors. McCartt et al. (2022) proved that the implementation of a multidisciplinary nutrition enhancement protocol (EP) improves the delivery of EN in surgical and critically ill trauma patients. Comparison of the prior to implementation of protocol (PP) group and EP group in 256 and 232 patients, respectively, evidenced that implementation of EP improved the nutritional delivery in surgical patients with 69.9% improvement in the PP vs. 78.7% improvement in the EP group. The result achieved compliance with American Society for Parenteral and Enteral Nutrition and Society of Critical Care Medicine guidelines. Ward (2003) also suggests the benefits of EN in reducing postoperative infectious complications, along with improved response in the wound healing process, alteration in antigen exposure, and influence on oxygenation of gut mucosa.

9.2.2 Methods and Delivery Routes

Suitable method of delivery is the utmost important for EN supply. It should be selected according to the aspiration risk, gastrointestinal anatomy, and estimated duration for which enteral feeding must be provided. Small intestine function resumes about 6–8 h following surgery. Contrary to earlier beliefs, a moderate amount of absorptive capacity is present even in the absence of peristalsis. Therefore, EN is both safe and advantageous in the early postoperative phase. The functioning condition of the gut determines whether EN should be started after surgery or not. However, a window of around 5 days is appropriate, and EN is not recommended in a well-nourished postoperative patient (Schattner 2003). Preoperative nutrition for 7–10 days may be necessary for patients who are clinically malnourished, as was previously indicated (Delsoglio et al. 2020). The enteral route is favoured over the parenteral route if the patient can tolerate the feeding and the gut is functional. There are a total of 6 methods for the administration of EN as listed below:

1. *Continuous feeding* method involves the administration of formula slowly and steadily over 16–24 h with the help of an infusion pump. It is basically used for critically ill patients, those who cannot tolerate a large quantity of feed at one time, which ultimately improves the absorption of nutrients and reduces the adverse symptoms like diarrhea and vomiting due to gastrointestinal intolerance (McClave et al. 2016).
2. *Intermittent feeding* method is selected when feed must be provided for a shorter duration (20–60 min), several times a day, like every 4–6 h, which imitates the normal meal pattern. Stable patients are advised more for this EN method instead of patients with poor gastric tolerance.
3. *Bolus feeding* method provides a larger quantity of formula administration with the use of a syringe i.e., about 200–400 ml for a short period, approximately 10–20 min. For high-risk patients, this method is generally not recommended as it may cause aspiration or gastrointestinal discomfort (Boullata et al. 2017).
4. *Cyclic feeding* method is a variation of continuous feeding. The difference is only in the duration for which the feed needs to be given. In cyclic feeding, usually for 8–16 h a day, overnight feed is administered. This method is more fea-

sible for high-risk patients as there is more independence and mobility during the daytime. Often, this method is preferred for long-term or home-based EN.

According to the functionality and duration of feeding, the delivery route for EN is selected (Harvey et al. 2014). There are two major categories for EN delivery, which are further divided into subcategories and are listed below:

1. Short-term provision: When EN needs to be supplied only for a short duration, generally for 4–6 weeks, then it is termed as short-term provision. There are various routes for the delivery of short-term EN:
   (a) *Nasogastric tube (NG) feeding:* This is the most often used and simplest route of delivery for short-term EN. A feeding tube is inserted via the nose into the stomach, which is suitable for patients with normal gastric emptying, but the risk of aspiration is high in this method.
   (b) *Nasojejunal tube (NJ) feeding:* This route is often used for patients with delayed gastric emptying, severe reflux, or high aspiration risk. The tube is inserted from the nose and extended to the jejunum. Better tolerance in critically ill patients has been evidenced, and this route also allows post-pyloric feeding.
   (c) *Nasoduodenal tube feeding:* In this route, the feeding tube is inserted from the nose and extended up to the duodenum. This is the less commonly used route but serves as an alternative when gastric feeding is not feasible.
2. Long-term provision: When EN needs to be provided for a longer duration that is greater than 4–6 weeks. There are basically two routes for long-term EN provision.
   (a) *Percutaneous Endoscopic Gastrostomy (PEG):* This route of EN delivery allows the feeding tube to be inserted through the abdominal wall directly to the stomach and supports long-term supply of EN in patients suffering from chronic neurological disorders. This method avoids nasal irritation (Singer et al. 2019).
   (b) *Percutaneous Endoscopic Jejunostomy (PEJ):* This route of delivery allows the feeding tube to be inserted from the abdominal wall to the jejunum. After major gastric surgeries or high aspiration risk or gastric dysfunction, this method is preferred for long-term access to nutrition.

Several factors determine the selection of method and route of provision of EN, such as the ability of the patient to swallow food and the neurological condition of the patient; the risk of aspiration; the functioning of the gut and peristalsis movement; the duration for which nutritional support is to be provided; and any other medical conditions underlying the surgical condition. Every factor should be considered at the individual level according to the clinical status and needs of the patient (Heyland et al. 2010). In high-risk patients, continuous feeding and post-pyloric routes are preferred due to their long-term effects.

9.3 Parenteral Nutrition Support

Total parenteral nutrition (TPN) is provided through the catheterization using the central nervous system when the GI tract is unable to absorb the nutrients due to several reasons. Provision of TPN is only restricted to patients with high-risk conditions or severely malnourished post-operative patients because it imparts many adverse effects like pneumothorax, subclavian vein thrombosis, and septicemia. TPN provided in the central venous system with added trace elements and vitamins quickly improves nitrogen balance, infectious and non-infectious problems through faster lymphocyte recovery and better wound healing. It is a life-saving intervention in clinical conditions for non-functioning GI systems (Singer et al. 2019). TPN provided in a heterogenous group of perioperative multi-centre clinical trial patients showed no benefits in mild malnutrition conditions. Thus, it should be limited only to the severely malnourished patients, and significant improvement in infectious and non-infectious complications was observed (Ward 2003).

9.3.1 Indications for Parenteral Nutrition

Parenteral nutrition is an important component for nutritional needs in high-risk surgical patients when EN is not sufficient or not feasible. Metabolic stress, post-operative complications, inflammation, and pre-existing nutritional deficiency in surgical patients often increase the risk of malnutrition. In such conditions, PN serves a crucial role in maintaining nutritional balance and reducing morbidity and mortality.

Non-functional GI tract, where nutrient absorption is difficult, is the key indication for the provision of PN. Paralytic ileus, bowel obstruction, or severe gastrointestinal dysmotility after surgery are few conditions that come under non-functional GI tract (McClave et al. 2016). *Prolonged post-operative ileus is* formed in patients, after GI surgery or major abdominal surgery, who may feel that delayed bowel function needs PN because EN does not provide nutritional support in this situation. *Severely malnourished* patients who cannot utilize the enteral route require PN to prevent further nutritional deficiency. *High-output enterocutaneous fistula* patients may lose a large amount of nutrients along with fluid loss. This condition is also an indication for using PN for bypassing GI tract and allowing bowel rest (Singer et al. 2019). *Short bowel syndrome,* characterized by insufficient intestinal surface area for nutrient absorption, is another indication for the provision of PN. *Severe GI complications* such as anastomotic leaks, severe pancreatitis, and intra-abdominal sepsis may require avoidance of EN and preference for PN. *Pre-operative support in malnourished patients*, PN may be suggested for patients before surgery if they are severely malnourished and require better surgical outcomes and improved nutritional status. PN may reduce post-operative complications but cannot reduce morbidity or mortality (Boullata et al. 2017).

It is still unclear whether and how perioperative TPN should be administered to surgical patients based on the material that has been published thus far. According to a meta-analysis of perioperative TPN by Heyland et al. (2001), research before 1988 indicates a lower death rate when TPN was utilized, but findings are still conflicting. Except for the Veterans Affairs study, research released after 1989 does not show an advantage. Therefore, it's critical to weigh the relative benefits of TPN against other nutrition support options for postoperative patients. Tables 9.1 and 9.2 explain the enteral vs parenteral nutrition in surgical cases.

Table 9.1 Enteral vs parenteral nutrition

Parameter	Enteral nutrition (EN)	Parenteral nutrition (PN)	References
Definition	Nutrition via GI tract (oral/tube)	IV nutrition bypassing GI tract	Singer et al. (2019)
Preferred use	Functional GI tract	Non-functional GI tract	Weimann et al. (2017); Singer et al. (2019)
Energy requirement	25–30 kcal/kg/day	25–30 kcal/kg/day	Singer et al. (2019)
Protein requirement	1.2–2.0 g/kg/day; up to 2.5 g/kg in ICU	1.2–2.5 g/kg/day	McClave et al. (2016)
Carbohydrates	50–60% of total calories	3–5 mg/kg/min glucose infusion	Weimann et al. (2017); Singer et al. (2019)
Fat (lipids)	20–30% of total calories	0.7–1.5 g/kg/day lipids	Weimann et al. (2017); Singer et al. (2019)
Fluids	25–35 mL/kg/day	25–35 mL/kg/day	McClave et al. (2016)
Micronutrients	Provided in formula	Must be supplemented daily	Weimann et al. (2017); Singer et al. (2019)
Timing	Within 24–48 hrs post-surgery	Start after 3–7 days if EN not feasible	Weimann et al. (2017); McClave et al. (2016)
Indications	ICU patients with functional gut	Ileus, obstruction, malabsorption	Singer et al. (2019); McClave et al. (2016)
Advantages	Maintains gut integrity, ↓ infections	Useful when EN is contraindicated	Singer et al. (2019); Weimann et al. (2017)
Complications	Diarrhea, aspiration	Infection, hyperglycemia	Casaer and Van den Berghe (2014); McClave et al. (2016)
Combined approach	Preferred first-line	Supplemental PN if EN <60% needs	Singer et al. (2019); Weimann et al. (2017)

Table 9.2 Condition-based requirements of parenteral and enteral nutrition

Condition	Energy	Protein	Notes	References
Critical illness	25–30 kcal/kg	1.5–2.5 g/kg	Avoid overfeeding	Singer et al. (2019); McClave et al. (2016)
Sepsis	20–25 kcal/kg	1.5–2.0 g/kg	Monitor glucose	Singer et al. (2019)
Burns/trauma	30–35 kcal/kg	2.0–2.5 g/kg	High protein demand	Weimann et al. (2017)
Renal failure	20–25 kcal/kg	0.8–1.5 g/kg	Adjust electrolytes	McClave et al. (2016)
Liver disease	25–30 kcal/kg	1.0–1.5 g/kg	Monitor ammonia	Weimann et al. (2017)

9.3.2 Monitoring and Complication Prevention

Several serious hazards of TPN have been noticed despite its advantages. Negative consequences could occur if hyperglycemia and its metabolic implications are not managed. Moreover, volume overload may cause respiratory compromise, particularly in those with insufficient cardiac reserve (Braga et al. 2009). Hyperglycemia is also associated with impaired immunological response. The anomalies include granulocyte adhesion, chemotaxis, phagocytosis, respiratory burst function, complement function, and intracellular killing. Consequently, it is not unexpected that Senkal et al. (2021) were able to demonstrate that stringent glucose control reduced infection complications and death in TPN-using ICU patients. Overfeeding is another problem with TPN, especially in very young or very obese patients. Overfeeding can cause metabolic acidosis, hypertonic dehydration, and azotemia (Smith and Elia 2006). Excessive carbohydrate infusion results in hyperglycemia, hypertriglyceridemia, and hepatic steatosis. High lipid infusions can cause hypertriglyceridemia and fat-overload syndrome. Hypercapnia and refeeding syndrome may result from aggressive feeding (Dudrick and Pimiento 2011).

Strict aseptic technique during catheter insertion and handling, regular dressing changes using sterile procedures, minimizing catheter manipulation, and using dedicated lines for PN administration are some techniques for infection prevention. Gradual initiation and advancement of PN, careful monitoring and correction of electrolyte imbalances, maintaining appropriate glucose control using insulin if necessary, monitoring for refeeding syndrome, especially in malnourished patients, adjusting fluid volume based on patient needs, monitoring intake-output balance closely, individualizing electrolyte composition of PN solutions, avoiding overfeeding, especially excess carbohydrates, including lipid emulsions appropriately, cycling PN (intermittent infusion) in long-term patients, proper insertion techniques by trained personnel, confirming catheter placement radiologically, regular inspection and maintenance of the catheter are some steps for prevention of fluid and electrolyte imbalance, prevention of hepatic complications and prevention of mechanical complications (Boullata et al. 2017). Figure 9.2 outlines a clinical decision algorithm for perioperative nutrition management, guiding whether to continue tube feeding (TF), oral diet (PO), or

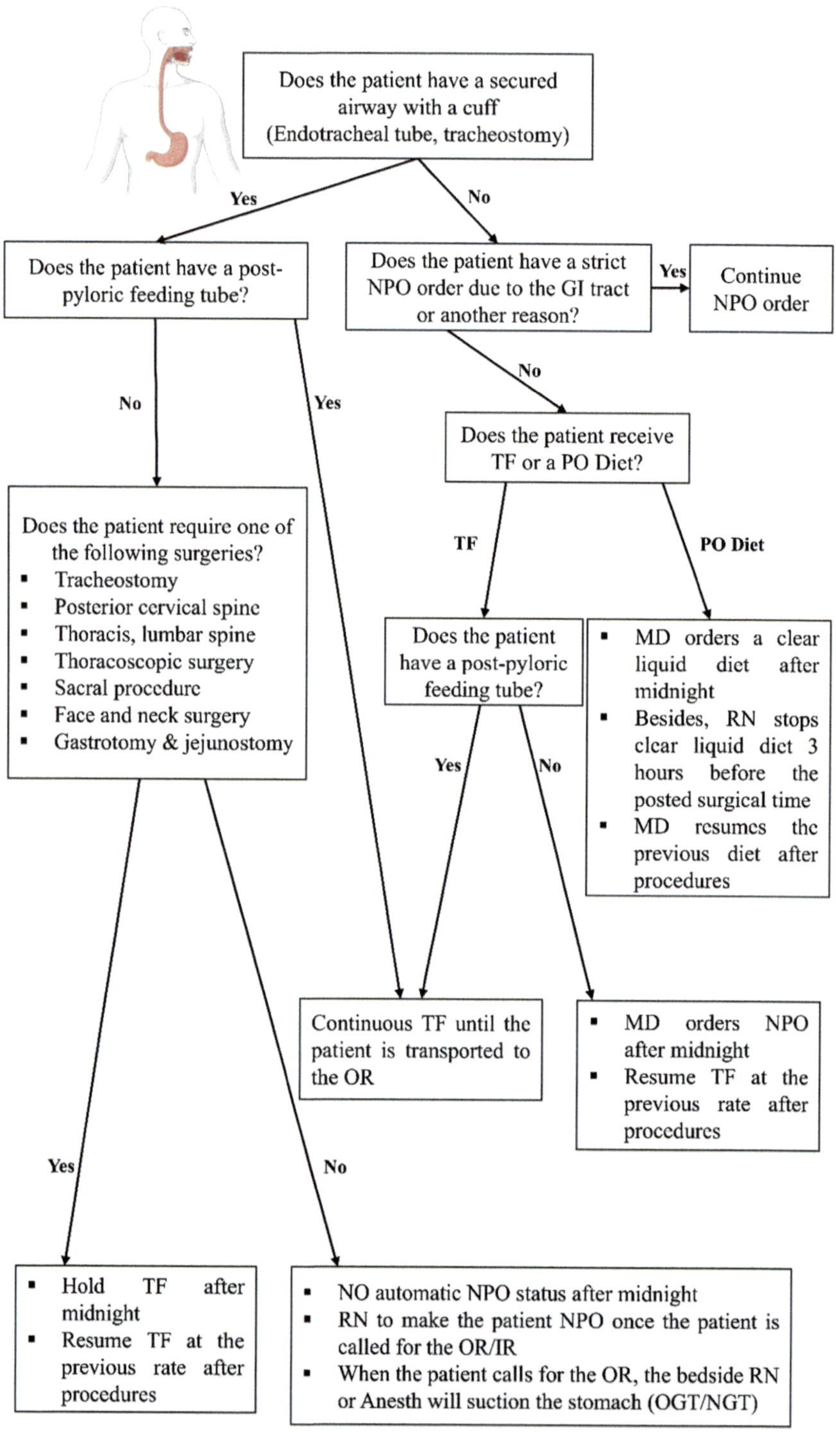
Does the patient have a secured airway with a cuff (Endotracheal tube, tracheostomy)
Yes
No
Does the patient have a post-pyloric feeding tube?
Does the patient have a strict NPO order due to the GI tract or another reason?
Yes
Continue NPO order
No
Yes
No
Does the patient receive TF or a PO Diet?
TF
PO Diet
Does the patient require one of the following surgeries?
Tracheostomy
Posterior cervical spine
Thoracis, lumbar spine
Thoracoscopic surgery
Sacral procedure
Face and neck surgery
Gastrotomy & jejunostomy
Does the patient have a post-pyloric feeding tube?
MD orders a clear liquid diet after midnight
Besides, RN stops clear liquid diet 3 hours before the posted surgical time
MD resumes the previous diet after procedures
Yes
No
Continuous TF until the patient is transported to the OR
MD orders NPO after midnight
Resume TF at the previous rate after procedures
Yes
No
Hold TF after midnight
Resume TF at the previous rate after procedures
NO automatic NPO status after midnight
RN to make the patient NPO once the patient is called for the OR/IR
When the patient calls for the OR, the bedside RN or Anesth will suction the stomach (OGT/NGT)

Fig. 9.2 Perioperative nutritional management algorithm on decision-making for enteral feeding and Npo status based on airway security and surgical risk. ET Tube Endotracheal Tube, TF Tube Feeding, PO Diet Per Oral Diet, NPO Nil Per Os, OR Operating Room, GI Tract Gastrointestinal Tract, MD medical doctor, RN Registered Nurse, Anesth Anesthesiologist, OGT Orogastric tube, NGT Nasogastric tube. (Created by author using MS Word 2021)

maintain NPO status. It considers factors such as airway security, type of feeding route, surgical risk, and GI conditions. The goal is to ensure safe feeding practices while minimizing aspiration risk and optimizing patient care before surgery.

9.4 Recent Advances in Perioperative Nutritional Support

The patients having high-risk surgical management, especially in cancer, severe malnutrition, geriatric, and severely ill, require perioperative nutritional support, and these advancements have significantly evolved in recent years. These patients are more prone to postoperative complications due to muscle wasting (sarcopenia), inflammation, low immunity, and increased metabolic stress (Prema et al. 2025). The recent trends and advancements emphasize highly focusing on malnutrition, as it is not only a comorbidity but also an associated risk factor, and the studies showed that the rate of complications and mortality is three times higher in these cases. So, shifting the patients from common nutritional protocol to advanced, precision-based, patient-centric approaches improves the medication system. These advancements optimize metabolic signals, reduce complications, enhanced recovery after surgery (ERAS) (Norman et al. 2021; Moningi et al. 2019).

9.4.1 Personalized Nutrition Strategies

This strategy presents one of the most recent advances in perioperative care. Where the traditional approaches are based only on standardized caloric and protein targets, the emerging evidence focuses on individual variability in metabolism, surgical stress strategies, and disease severity, which promotes the modified nutritional plans (Li and Zhang 2025). Modern treatment begins with a comprehensive nutritional assessment, including anthropometric, biochemical markers, clinical history, and functional parameters such as muscle mass composition and strength. Several tools, such as mNUTRIC, MUST, and NRS-2002 score, are used strategically based on nutritional risk. These evaluations help clinicians to prepare and start the strategies on individual intervention that address the specific deficiencies, such as protein-energy malnutrition or micronutrient deficiencies (Serón-Arbeloa et al. 2022).

An important component of personalized nutrition is maintaining heterogeneity among patients' risk factors. For example, cancer patients mostly face cachexia, whereas geriatric patients mostly suffer from sarcopenia. Most of the critically ill patients express hypermetabolism. As per this understanding, each case requires a different nutritional management. Therefore, personalized strategies are not limited only to the quantity variation but also to the constituents of the nutrients, including the fat profile, protein level, and micronutrient supplementation (Wang et al. 2025). Recent studies focus on the importance of pre-habilitation, which combines the strategic management of nutritional, physical activity, and psychological counseling before surgery. This trimodal approach has been reported to be beneficial in improving the muscle mass, functional activity, and postoperative outcomes. This prehabilitation approach is productive for the severely ill patients, as it enhances the physio-psychological resilience to the surgical stress (Popescu et al. 2025).

Another bridge-gaping recent trend emerging is the immunonutrition therapy, which helps to supplement with highly demanding nutrients such as omega-3 fatty acids, nucleotides, and essential amino acids (glutamine and arginine). These nutrients facilitate the immune function and inflammatory responses, which reduce the infection and complications in the postoperative cases. So, this management seems beneficial in high-risk surgical patients (Dalimunthe et al. 2026).

The advances in the technologies are further increased the demand of personalization treatment in perioperative nutrition. Nowadays, artificial intelligence (AI) and machine learning play a crucial role in analyzing patients' data and planning the diet. For instance, current findings have demonstrated that tailoring the enteral nutrition based on the current status of the physiological parameters of the patients. These advanced technologies also adjust and modify the caloric intake, protein needs, and fluid balance as per the data input, and also give many suggestions regarding these. Another most attaining approach is the metabolomics and nutrigenomics. In this, the metabolic profile, the physicians can assess the specific nutrient deficiencies and focus on more targeted interventions (Agrawal et al. 2025). Such as evaluating the inflammatory biomarkers, nitrogen balance, and insulin resistance, they plan more accurately the energy and protein requirements for the patients. Additionally, the other most strategically personalized intervention that used is route administration and timing. In this, the clinicians planned the enteral and parenteral nutrition based on the functionality of the gastrointestinal tract, tolerance, and risk of complications. In several cases, both strategies are needed, and combined treatments are to be supported, such as enteral and parenteral nutrition to meet the nutritional goal effectively (Stoian et al. 2025). Figure 9.3 highlights recent advances in perioperative nutritional support, emphasizing improved monitoring systems and safety measures, including the use of AI-based predictive models over traditional approaches. It also showcases personalized nutrition strategies based on metabolomics, nutrigenomics, microbiome analysis, and biochemical assessment. Together, these innovations enable tailored, data-driven nutrition care to improve surgical outcomes and recovery.

In conclusion to this context, the study says the personalized nutrition approaches are mobilizing the perioperative treatments from a uniform protocol to individualized, data-driven interventions. By setting up tailored nutrition support to individual patients' clinical and metabolic profiles, these approaches improve the surgical outcomes, enhance the recovery, and reduce the complications. Table 9.3 explains the personalized nutrition strategies in the operative cases.

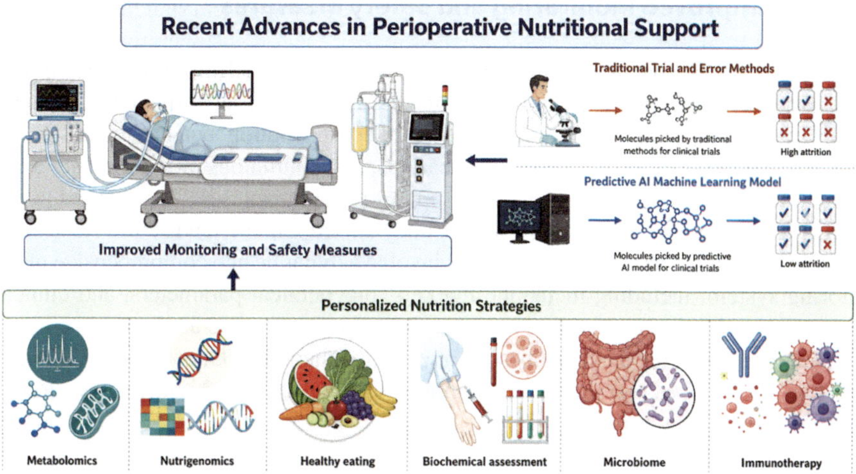

Fig. 9.3 Recent advances in perioperative nutritional support of the peri-and postoperative patient. (Created using MS PowerPoint 2021)

Table 9.3 Personalized nutrition strategies

Aspect	Description	References
Definition	Tailoring nutritional support based on individual patient needs, risk, and metabolic status	Serón-Arbeloa et al. (2022); Clemente-Suárez et al. (2024)
Basis of personalization	Nutritional risk scores (NRS-2002, MUST), metabolic profile, disease condition	Serón-Arbeloa et al. (2022)
Target population	High-risk patients (cancer, elderly, ICU, malnourished)	Clemente-Suárez et al. (2024)
Nutritional components	Customized calories, high-protein diet, micronutrients	Roman et al. (2024); Serón-Arbeloa et al. (2022)
Disease-specific approach	Cachexia (cancer), sarcopenia (elderly), hypermetabolism (ICU)	Serón-Arbeloa et al. (2022)
Prehabilitation	Nutrition + exercise + psychological support before surgery	Roman et al. (2024); Serón-Arbeloa et al. (2022)
Immunonutrition	Arginine, glutamine, omega-3 fatty acids to improve immunity	Serón-Arbeloa et al. (2022); Clemente-Suárez et al. (2024)
Route of nutrition	Individualized choice: enteral (EN), parenteral (PN), or combination	Clemente-Suárez et al. (2024)
Technological advances	AI-based nutrition planning, machine learning models	Stoian et al. (2025)
Biomarker use	CRP, albumin, insulin resistance, nitrogen balance	Stoian et al. (2025); Clemente-Suárez et al. (2024)
Recent trend	Precision medicine and metabolomics-based nutrition	Serón-Arbeloa et al. (2022); Clemente-Suárez et al. (2024)
Clinical outcome	Reduced complications, improved recovery, shorter hospital stay	Clemente-Suárez et al. (2024)

9.4.2 Improved Monitoring and Safety Measures

Enhanced safety and monitoring measures present another fruitful management in the perioperative nutritional approach. In the high-risk surgical patients, efficient nutritional management not only apposite the prescription but also their timely adjustment, early detection, risk complications, and continuous monitoring are evaluated. In the beginning, the nutritional support management was very limited to the general parameters such as fluid balance, body anthropometric and serum electrolyte profile. Moreover, the recent approaches involve a dynamic and comprehensive monitoring system, including metabolic markers, biochemical parameters, and clinical indicators. These advancements improve the more appropriate assessment of nutritional assessment for the patients and for effective therapies (Gazouli et al. 2024).

One of the most significant developments is the use of multidimensional monitoring, which includes:

- Biochemical parameters (albumin, prealbumin, CRP, glucose)
- Metabolic indicators (energy expenditure, nitrogen balance)
- Functional measures (muscle strength, mobility)
- Clinical outcomes (infection rates, wound healing)

This integrated strategy provides a holistic approach to early detection of complications and patients' status, such as metabolic imbalance, under-or overfeeding. Current guidelines focus on not feeding over, because it leads to many health complications such as high serum glucose, liver dysfunction, and elevated carbon dioxide. Appropriate application of dietary caloric intake and metabolic response is an important assessment specially in critically ill patients. The advancements in technology have significantly improved the monitoring scales. Indirect calorimetry is commonly used for accurate energy expenditure calculation, and glucose monitoring machines help to assess the real-time tracking of blood glucose, which improves the blood glucose control and helps manage glycemic surges and after impact (Dhondge et al. 2024; Cehan et al. 2025).

Another important strategy is to use the computerized nutrition protocol and the smart infusion system. These systems avoid human error, safeguard the correct delivery of the nutrients, and enable real-time adjustments based on the patient's parameters. Aligned with the electronic health records later on, enhanced decisions can be made to improve the patient's health and for healthcare providers to assess the later complications. The safety concern is increase specially on those patients who receive parenteral nutrition, as the chance of infection may raise on such patients. Advances in clinical setups, such as aseptic techniques, catheter care, and monitoring protocol, significantly reduce the chance of bloodstream-related infections, so in this case, strict adherence to the standard protocol is the key component (Kirkendall et al. 2020; Alamer et al. 2023).

Early detection in the clinical setting is one of the best strategies. For example, feeding problem specially intolerance in enteral nutrition, are manifested as nausea, vomiting, and abdominal distension. Similarly, electrolyte imbalance and refeeding syndrome can be prevented by careful monitoring and gradual initiation of nutrition therapy. Recent studies also focus on the role of digital health technologies and predictive analytics in improvising the patient safety. Machine learning is used in large amounts for the early detection and prediction of complications prior to surgery, which allows for proactive intervention and increased patient outcomes. Another emerging trend is the inclusion of remote and telemedicine monitoring, particularly in post-operative and long-term care management. These advancements enable the improve the patients' compliance, follow-up, and plan the intervention for the complications (Martinez-Esteban et al. 2026; Reignier et al. 2025; Dixon et al. 2024).

So, a multidisciplinary approach and collaboration are the milestone achievements in patient monitoring and safety. Clinical experts such as pharmacists, dietitians, anesthesiologists, surgeons, and others work together to ensure optimal nutritional management. This collaborative approach not only enhances communication but also improves the patient's outcome, reduces errors, and ensures strict adherence to the medical protocol. Table 9.4 explains the improved monitoring and safety measures in the operative condition.

Table 9.4 Improved monitoring and safety measures

Aspect	Description	References
Goal	Ensure safe, effective, and complication-free nutritional therapy	Ayalew et al. (2025); Altman et al. (2019)
Monitoring parameters	Weight, intake-output, glucose, electrolytes, albumin	Ayalew et al. (2025)
Advanced monitoring	Indirect calorimetry, nitrogen balance, inflammatory markers	Pisu et al. (2024); Ayalew et al. (2025)
Glucose monitoring	Continuous glucose monitoring systems (CGMS)	Altman et al. (2019); Jeerangsapasuk et al. (2025)
Avoiding overfeeding	Prevent hyperglycemia, liver dysfunction, CO_2 excess	Pisu et al. (2024); Jeerangsapasuk et al. (2025)
Feeding tolerance	Monitor nausea, vomiting, abdominal distension	Jeerangsapasuk et al. (2025); Ayalew et al. (2025)
Complication prevention	Refeeding syndrome, electrolyte imbalance	Altman et al. (2019)
Infection control	Aseptic catheter care in PN	Pisu et al. (2024); Altman et al. (2019)
Technology use	Smart infusion pumps, computerized protocols	Pisu et al. (2024); Ayalew et al. (2025)
Digital health	Telemedicine, remote monitoring systems	Altman et al. (2019)
Predictive tools	AI-based risk prediction and early complication detection	Jeerangsapasuk et al. (2025)
Multidisciplinary approach	Surgeons + dietitians + nurses + pharmacists	Altman et al. (2019)
Integration with ERAS	Supports early feeding and faster recovery	Jeerangsapasuk et al. (2025)
Clinical outcome	Reduced complications, improved safety, better outcomes	Altman et al. (2019); Altman et al. (2019)

9.5 Risk Management and Multidisciplinary Care

The high-risk patients undergoing surgery are more likely to experience complications because of their frail physical and metabolic states, and thus, they need a proactive and well-coordinated mode of treatment. When this occurs, risk management is more of discovering what can go wrong and putting countermeasures to stop this instead of handling the problems once the fact is realized (Mistry et al. 2017). This will involve a comprehensive pre-operative evaluation, constant check-up of the treatment and appropriate care after surgery. Safety of patients during all the steps of this process is an essential consideration, especially when nutrition support is provided. Due to the need for enteral or parenteral nutrition of numerous high-risk patients, even minor errors or oversight of cleanliness and observation may have significant repercussions. To achieve better outcomes and reduce risks, it will be instrumental to maintain high clinical standards and follow evidence-based practices (Mulatie Zewudie et al. 2023).

9.5.1 Infection Prevention and Clinical Safety

Prevention of infection is the most essential aspect of high-risk surgical patient care, as they are prone to having compromised immunity. The aseptic principles should be observed at all times when dealing with feeding tubes, intravenous lines, or surgical wounds. These involve maintaining a clean environment when carrying out the processes, using sterile equipment, and practicing good hand hygiene. Lack of proper procedures increases the risk of contamination in cases of nutritional support, especially via enteral or parenteral routes. As an example, improper handling of feeding formulae or infusion systems may lead to infections due to the entry of harmful germs into the body. Routine observation of the patient status is also very important as it can help to early identify signs, such as fever, inflammation, or alterations of test outcomes that can indicate an infection (Andersen 2019).

Another element of clinical safety is careful observation of the reaction of the patient to nutritional treatment. To avoid complications such as refeeding syndrome or electrolyte imbalances, healthcare experts should monitor blood sugar levels, electrolyte state, and fluid status. Upon this understanding, it is possible to prevent minor issues from forming into larger ones by utilizing the available information in a timely manner. Early movement, keeping clean, and wound care are other measures that reduce the chances of infections and enhance healing. Overall, effective infection control and patient safety emphasize providing a stable environment that grants efficient healing (Khan et al. 2011; Persaud-Sharma et al. 2020).

9.5.2 Role of the Multidisciplinary Team

The care of high-risk surgical patients is carried out through surgery, nutrition, critical care, and rehabilitation, just to mention a few, which even a single healthcare provider cannot control. This is an area where the role of a multidisciplinary team can be critical. A great number of professionals interrelate and share their experience to provide the complete treatment, which is patient-specific. To ensure the mitigation of surgical stress whilst being mindful of the overall state of the patient, the surgeon has to plan and carry out the surgery. Dietitians are necessary when it comes to assessment of nutritional status and coming up with appropriate diet plans that help one heal and recover. They make sure that the patient receives the proper balance of nutrients at the right moment by means of oral consumption or special feeding techniques (Lasithiotakis et al. 2025).

Critical care professionals handle patients requiring close attention, and especially those who have severe conditions or complications. They focus on maintaining essential processes, organ support, and addressing any possible crises. Nurses are the most vital part of patient care, and they also administer treatment, attend to patients round the clock, and ensure that the treatment undertaken is closely adhered to. They also have a great impact on infection prevention and maintenance of hygiene. Since other professionals are involved in offering the necessary treatment to help a patient regain his strength and mobility, such as pharmacists and physiotherapists, they also assist (Aamodt et al. 2025).

All team members need to coordinate and communicate effectively to achieve successful results. Each person is in agreement with the care plan of a patient because of constant discussions, collaborative decision-making, and frequent updates. Multidisciplinary care is a critical component of high-risk surgery patient care as it not only enhances clinical outcomes but also the overall patient recovery experience (O'Daniel and Rosenstein 2008; Curşeu et al. 2025).

9.6 Conclusion

The malnourished and highly susceptible patients are more prone to infectious diseases while undergoing a surgical operation. Inappropriate nutrition or a lack of nutrition is directly linked with postoperative complications and has a high rate of mortality and fatal outcomes. Proper clinical strategies and nutritional management can mitigate these complications. The advanced feeding practices, such as enteral and parenteral approaches, can minimize these complications and reduce patient complications. The enteral feeding is supported when the gastrointestinal tract is functioning; when it's not, then parenteral feeding is advised so that the later complications can be handled properly. Recent updates, such as metabolomics, nutrigenomics, immunotherapy, microbiome, and various testing, help in early detection and its management in both peri and post-operative conditions and help to provide more appropriate and personalized dietary recommendations.

References

Aamodt IT, Stubberud DG, Eikeland A, Sunde KW, Petersen FJJ, Hammer SK, Halvorsen K. Critical care nurses role and scope of practice during a global crisis: a qualitative study. BMC Nurs. 2025;24(1):242. https://doi.org/10.1186/s12912-025-02872-w.

Agrawal K, Goktas P, Kumar N, Leung MF. Artificial intelligence in personalized nutrition and food manufacturing: a comprehensive review of methods, applications, and future directions. Front Nutr. 2025;12:1636980. https://doi.org/10.3389/fnut.2025.1636980.

Alamer F, Alanazi AT, Al Alkhaibari E. The impact of smart pump technology in the healthcare system: a scope review. Cureus. 2023;15(3) https://doi.org/10.7759/cureus.36007.

Altman AD, Helpman L, McGee J, Samouëlian V, Auclair MH, Brar H, Nelson GS. Enhanced recovery after surgery: implementing a new standard of surgical care. CMAJ. 2019;191(17):E469–75. https://doi.org/10.1503/cmaj.180635.

Andersen BM. Prevention of postoperative wound infections. In: Prevention and control of infections in hospitals: practice and theory. Cham: Springer; 2019. p. 377–437. https://doi.org/10.1007/978-3-319-99921-0_33.

Ayalew AF, Delie AM, Fornah L, Shimbre MS, Ma W. Understanding safety measure practices and improvement strategies among health professionals in resource-limited health care settings in the Awi Zone, Amhara, Ethiopia: a qualitative study. BMJ Open. 2025;15(12):e107492. https://doi.org/10.1136/bmjopen-2025-107492.

Beattie AH, Prach AT, Baxter JP, Pennington CR. A randomised controlled trial evaluating the use of enteral nutritional supplements postoperatively in malnourished surgical patients. Gut. 2000;46(6):813–8. https://doi.org/10.1136/gut.46.6.813.

Boullata JI, Carrera AL, Harvey L, Escuro AA, Hudson L, Mays A, McGinnis C, Wessel JJ, American Society for Parenteral and Enteral Nutrition (ASPEN). ASPEN safe practices for enteral nutrition therapy. J Parenter Enter Nutr. 2017;41(1):15–103. https://doi.org/10.1177/0148607116673053.

Boyd O, Jackson N. Clinical review: how is risk defined in high-risk surgical patient management? Crit Care. 2005;9(4):390. https://doi.org/10.1186/cc3057.

Braga MARCO, Ljungqvist O, Soeters P, Fearon K, Weimann A, Bozzetti F. ESPEN guidelines on parenteral nutrition: surgery. Clin Nutr. 2009;28(4):378–86.

Casaer MP, Van den Berghe G. Nutrition in the acute phase of critical illness. N Engl J Med. 2014;370(13):1227–36. https://doi.org/10.1056/nejmra1304623.

Cehan VD, Cehan AR, Pui MC, Lazar A. A new perspective on overfeeding in the intensive care unit (ICU): challenges, dangers and prevention methods. Life. 2025;15(5):828. https://doi.org/10.3390/life15050828.

Chávez-Reyes J, Escárcega-González CE, Chavira-Suárez E, León-Buitimea A, Vázquez-León P, Morones-Ramírez JR, et al. Susceptibility for some infectious diseases in patients with diabetes: the key role of glycemia. Front Public Health. 2021;9:559595. https://doi.org/10.3389/fpubh.2021.559595.

Chen Y, Liu BL, Shang B, Chen AS, Liu SQ, Sun W, Su Q. Nutrition support in surgical patients with colorectal cancer. World J Gastroenterol: WJG. 2011;17(13):1779. https://doi.org/10.3748/wjg.v17.i13.1779.

Clemente-Suárez VJ, Peris-Ramos HC, Redondo-Flórez L, Beltrán-Velasco AI, Martín-Rodríguez A, David-Fernandez S, et al. Personalizing nutrition strategies: bridging research and public health. J Pers Med. 2024;14(3):305. https://doi.org/10.3390/jpm14030305.

Curşeu PL, van Rijswijk J, Schruijer SG. Collaborative and shared leadership dynamics in healthcare action teams: a systematic literature review. J Healthc Leadersh. 2025;877–899 https://doi.org/10.2147/JHL.S520534.

da Silva JSV, Seres DS, Sabino K, Adams SC, Berdahl GJ, Citty SW, Cober MP, Evans DC, Greaves JR, Gura KM, et al. ASPEN consensus recommendations for refeeding syndrome. Nutr Clin Pract. 2020;35(2):178–95. https://doi.org/10.1002/ncp.10474.

Dalimunthe A, Tan MW, Lu FC, Angiosaki Y, Usman AN, Nugraha SE, et al. Immunonutrients as modulators of inflammation, barrier integrity, and immune regulation: toward precision nutrition. J Funct Foods. 2026;136:107119.

Debaveye Y, Van den Berghe G. Risks and benefits of nutritional support during critical illness. Annu Rev Nutr. 2006;26(1):513–38. https://doi.org/10.1146/annurev.nutr.26.061505.111307.

Delsoglio M, Pichard C, Singer P. How to choose the best route of feeding during critical illness. Clin Nutr ESPEN. 2020;37:247–54. https://doi.org/10.1016/j.clnesp.2020.03.019.

Dhondge RH, Agrawal S, Patil R, Kadu A, Kothari M. A comprehensive review of metabolic syndrome and its role in cardiovascular disease and type 2 diabetes mellitus: mechanisms, risk factors, and management. Cureus. 2024;16(8) https://doi.org/10.7759/cureus.67428.

Dixon D, Sattar H, Moros N, Kesireddy SR, Ahsan H, Lakkimsetti M, et al. Unveiling the influence of AI predictive analytics on patient outcomes: a comprehensive narrative review. Cureus. 2024;16(5):e59954. https://doi.org/10.7759/cureus.59954.

Dudrick SJ, Pimiento JM. Parenteral nutrition and nutritional support of surgical patients: reflections, controversies, and challenges. Surg Clin. 2011;91(3):675–92. https://doi.org/10.1016/j.suc.2011.04.001.

Gazouli A, Georgiou K, Frountzas M, Tsourouflis G, Boyanov N, Nikiteas N, et al. Perioperative nutritional assessment and management of patients undergoing gastrointestinal surgery. Annals of Gastroenterology. 2024;37(2):142. https://doi.org/10.20524/aog.2024.0867.

Gebregziabher Z, Nane D, Dake SK, Handiso YH. Effect of malnutrition at admission on length of hospital stay among adult surgical patients in Wolaita Sodo University Comprehensive Specialized Hospital, South Ethiopia: prospective cohort study. Front Nutr. 2024;11:1451463. https://doi.org/10.3389/fnut.2024.1451463.

Haines KL, Ohnuma T, Grisel B, Krishnamoorthy V, Raghunathan K, Sulo S, Wischmeyer PE. Early enteral nutrition is associated with improved outcomes in critically ill mechanically ventilated medical and surgical patients. Clin Nutr ESPEN. 2023;57:311–7. https://doi.org/10.1016/j.clnesp.2023.07.001.

Harvey SE, Parrott F, Harrison DA, Bear DE, Segaran E, Beale R, Rowan KM. Trial of the route of early nutritional support in critically ill adults. N Engl J Med. 2014;371(18):1673–84. https://doi.org/10.1056/nejmoa1409860.

Heyland DK, Montalvo M, MacDonald S, Keefe L, Su XY, Drover JW. Total parenteral nutrition in the surgical patient: a meta-analysis. Can J Surg. 2001 Apr;44(2):102-11. PMID: 11308231. https://pubmed.ncbi.nlm.nih.gov/11308231/.

Heyland DK, Cahill NE, Dhaliwal R, Sun X, Day AG, McClave SA. Impact of enteral feeding protocols on enteral nutrition delivery: results of a multicenter observational study. J Parenter Enter Nutr. 2010;34(6):675–84. https://doi.org/10.1177/0148607110364843.

Jeerangsapasuk W, Hongmeng W, Traitanon O, Chatkrailert A. Indirect calorimetry and nitrogen balance guided nutrition therapy in ICU patients with acute kidney injury. Sci Rep. 2025;15(1):12558. https://doi.org/10.1038/s41598-025-97443-z.

Keerio RB, Ali M, Shah KA, Iqbal A, Mehmood A, Iqbal S. Evaluating the impact of preoperative nutritional status on surgical outcomes and public health implications in general surgery patients. Cureus. 2024;16(12) https://doi.org/10.7759/cureus.76633.

Khan LU, Ahmed J, Khan S, MacFie J. Refeeding syndrome: a literature review. Gastroenterol Res Pract. 2011;2011(1):410971. https://doi.org/10.1155/2011/410971.

Kirkendall ES, Timmons K, Huth H, Walsh K, Melton K. Human-based errors involving smart infusion pumps: a catalog of error types and prevention strategies. Drug Saf. 2020;43(11):1073–87. https://doi.org/10.1007/s40264-020-00986-5.

Lasithiotakis K, Andreou A, Migdadi H, Kritsotakis EI. Malnutrition and perioperative nutritional rehabilitation in major operations. Eur Surg. 2025;57(5):188–203. https://doi.org/10.1007/s10353-025-00863-4.

Li Y, Zhang T. Advances in perioperative nutritional management in metabolic and bariatric surgery. In: Diabetes, metabolic syndrome and obesity; 2025. p. 2191–202. https://doi.org/10.2147/DMSO.S518912.

Martinez-Esteban A, Peña-Solórzano S, Sanchez-Saavedra EP, Rojas-Evaristo MM, de la Puente-Diaz VM, Rojas-Evaristo ME, De la Puente-Diaz VM. Assessment of electrolyte imbalances as an early manifestation of refeeding syndrome in critically ill patients receiving total parenteral nutrition at a Tertiary Hospital in Mexico City. Cureus. 2026;18(1) https://doi.org/10.7759/cureus.101608.

McCartt J, Loszko A, Backes K, Cunningham K, Evans S, Draughon M, Sachdev G. Improving enteral nutrition delivery in the critically ill trauma and surgical population. J Parenter Enter Nutr. 2022;46(5):1191–7. https://doi.org/10.1002/jpen.2353.

McClave SA, Taylor BE, Martindale RG, Warren MM, Johnson DR, Braunschweig C, McCarthy MS, Davanos E, Rice TW, Cresci GA, et al. Guidelines for the provision and assessment of nutrition support therapy in the adult critically ill patient. J Parenter Enter Nutr. 2016;40(2):159–211. https://doi.org/10.1177/0148607115621863.

Mistry PK, Gaunay GS, Hoenig DM. Prediction of surgical complications in the elderly: can we improve outcomes? Asian J Urol. 2017;4(1):44–9. https://doi.org/10.1016/j.ajur.2016.07.001.

Moningi S, Patki A, Padhy N, Ramachandran G. Enhanced recovery after surgery: an anesthesiologist's perspective. J Anaesthesiol Clin Pharmacol. 2019;35(Suppl 1):S5–S13. https://doi.org/10.4103/joacp.joacp_238_16.

Morales F, Montserrat-De la Paz S, Leon MJ, Rivero-Pino F. Effects of malnutrition on the immune system and infection and the role of nutritional strategies regarding improvements in children's health status: a literature review. Nutrients. 2023;16(1):1. https://doi.org/10.3390/nu16010001.

Mulatie Zewudie M, Yaregal Melesse D, Dereje Filatie T, Getahun AB, Adie Admass B. Perioperative nutrition support for elective surgical cancer patients: a narrative review. Open Access Surg. 2023;33-45 https://doi.org/10.2147/OAS.S405799.

Nagano A, Wakabayashi H, Maeda K, Kokura Y, Miyazaki S, Mori T, Fujiwara D. Respiratory sarcopenia and sarcopenic respiratory disability: concepts, diagnosis, and treatment. J Nutr Health Aging. 2021;25(4):507–15. https://doi.org/10.1007/s12603-021-1587-5.

Norman K, Haß U, Pirlich M. Malnutrition in older adults—recent advances and remaining challenges. Nutrients. 2021;13(8):2764. https://doi.org/10.3390/nu13082764.

O'Daniel M, Rosenstein AH. Professional communication and team collaboration. In: Patient safety and quality: an evidence-based handbook for nurses; 2008.

Peev MP, Yeh DD, Quraishi SA, Osler P, Chang Y, Gillis E, Velmahos GC. Causes and consequences of interrupted enteral nutrition: a prospective observational study in critically ill surgical patients. J Parenter Enter Nutr. 2015;39(1):21–7. https://doi.org/10.1177/0148607114526887.

Persaud-Sharma D, Saha S, Trippensee AW. Refeeding syndrome; 2020.

Pisu A, Elia N, Pompianu L, Barchi F, Acquaviva A, Carta S. Enhancing workplace safety: a flexible approach for personal protective equipment monitoring. Expert Syst Appl. 2024;238:122285. https://doi.org/10.1016/j.eswa.2023.122285.

Popescu GA, Minca DG, Jafal NM, Toma CV, Alexandrescu ST, Costea RV, Vasilescu C. Multimodal prehabilitation in major abdominal surgery—rationale, modalities, results and limitations. Medicina. 2025;61(5):908. https://doi.org/10.3390/medicina61050908.

Prema SS, Ganapathy D, Shanmugamprema D. Prehabilitation strategies: enhancing surgical resilience with a focus on nutritional optimization and multimodal interventions. Adv Nutr. 2025;16(4):100392. https://doi.org/10.1016/j.advnut.2025.100392.

Reignier J, Gaillard-Le Roux B, Dequin PF, Maluf VAB, Bohe J, Casaer MP, et al. Expert consensus-based clinical practice guidelines for nutritional support in the intensive care unit: the French Intensive Care Society (SRLF) and the French-Speaking Group of Pediatric Emergency Physicians and Intensivists (GFRUP). Ann Intensive Care. 2025;15(1):99. https://doi.org/10.1186/s13613-025-01509-0.

Roman S, Campos-Medina L, Leal-Mercado L. Personalized nutrition: the end of the one-diet-fits-all era. Front Nutr. 2024;11:1370595. https://doi.org/10.3389/fnut.2024.1370595.

Saluja SS, Kaur N, Shrivastava UK. Enteral nutrition in surgical patients. Surg Today. 2002;32(8):672–8. https://doi.org/10.1007/s005950200125.

Saunders J, Smith T. Malnutrition: causes and consequences. Clin Med. 2010;10(6):624–7. https://doi.org/10.7861/clinmedicine.10-6-624.

Schattner M. Enteral nutritional support of the patient with cancer: route and role. J Clin Gastroenterol. 2003;36(4):297–302. https://doi.org/10.1097/00004836-200304000-00004.

Schwarze ML, Barnato AE, Rathouz PJ, Zhao Q, Neuman HB, Winslow ER, et al. Development of a list of high-risk operations for patients 65 years and older. JAMA Surg. 2015;150(4):325–31. https://doi.org/10.1001/jamasurg.2014.1819.

Senkal M, Bonavina L, Reith B, Caruso R, Matern U, Duran M. Perioperative peripheral parenteral nutrition to support major gastrointestinal surgery: expert opinion on treating the right patients at the right time. Clin Nutr ESPEN. 2021;43:16–24. https://doi.org/10.1016/j.clnesp.2021.04.006.

Serón-Arbeloa C, Labarta-Monzón L, Puzo-Foncillas J, Mallor-Bonet T, Lafita-López A, Bueno-Vidales N, Montoro-Huguet M. Malnutrition screening and assessment. Nutrients. 2022;14(12):2392. https://doi.org/10.3390/nu14122392.

Seth I, Lim B, Cevik J, Gracias D, Chua M, Kenney PS, et al. Impact of nutrition on skin wound healing and aesthetic outcomes: a comprehensive narrative review. JPRAS Open. 2024;39:291–302. https://doi.org/10.1016/j.jpra.2024.01.006.

Singer P, Blaser AR, Berger MM, Alhazzani W, Calder PC, Casaer MP, Hiesmayr M, Mayer K, Montejo JC, Pichard C, et al. ESPEN guideline on clinical nutrition in the intensive care unit. Clin Nutr. 2019;38(1):48–79. https://doi.org/10.1016/j.clnu.2018.08.037.

Smith T, Elia M. Artificial nutrition support in hospital: indications and complications. Clin Med. 2006;6(5):457. https://doi.org/10.7861/clinmedicine.6-5-457.

Stoian M, Andone A, Bândilă SR, Onişor D, Babă DF, Niculescu R, et al. Personalized nutrition strategies for patients in the intensive care unit: a narrative review on the future of critical care nutrition. Nutrients. 2025;17(10):1659. https://doi.org/10.3390/nu17101659.

Tappenden KA, Quatrara B, Parkhurst ML, Malone AM, Fanjiang G, Ziegler TR. Critical role of nutrition in improving quality of care: an interdisciplinary call to action to address adult hospital malnutrition. J Acad Nutr Diet. 2013;113(9):1219–37. https://doi.org/10.1016/j.jand.2013.05.015.

Waitzberg DL, Plopper C, Terra RM. Access routes for nutritional therapy. World J Surg. 2000;24(12):1468–76. https://doi.org/10.1007/s002680010264.

Wang T, Zhou D, Hong Z. Sarcopenia and cachexia: molecular mechanisms and therapeutic interventions. MedComm. 2025;6(1):e70030. https://doi.org/10.1002/mco2.70030.

Ward N. Nutrition support to patients undergoing gastrointestinal surgery. Nutr J. 2003;2(1):18. https://doi.org/10.1186/1475-2891-2-18.

Weimann A, Bezmarevic M, Braga M, Correia MIT, Funk-Debleds P, Gianotti L, et al. ESPEN guideline on clinical nutrition in surgery–update 2025. Clin Nutr. 2025;53:222–61. https://doi.org/10.1016/j.clnu.2025.08.029.

Weimann A, Braga M, Carli F, Higashiguchi T, Hübner M, Klek S, et al. ESPEN guideline: clinical nutrition in surgery. Clin Nutr. 2017;36(3):623–50. https://doi.org/10.1016/j.clnu.2017.02.013.

Williams DG, Molinger J, Wischmeyer PE. The malnourished surgery patient: a silent epidemic in perioperative outcomes? Curr Opin Anesthesiol. 2019;32(3):405–11. https://doi.org/10.1097/ACO.0000000000000722.

Wobith M, Weimann A. Oral nutritional supplements and enteral nutrition in patients with gastrointestinal surgery. Nutrients. 2021;13(8):2655. https://doi.org/10.3390/nu13082655.

Synergistic Anaesthesia and Nutrition Protocols in Colorectal Surgery

10

Mudit Gambhir, Nandini Kamkolam, and Pawan Manohar Lokhande

Abstract

Colorectal surgery leads to an identifiable stress reaction which is mainly physiological in nature, involving metabolic, neuro-endocrine pathways, and inflammation, having impact on the recovery period during the post-operative phase. The protocols of ERAS revolutionized perioperative care through a multidisciplinary strategy where inclusion of nutrition and anaesthesia has been identified to improve postoperative care. Modern anaesthetic strategies concentrate on limiting the stress of surgery through the use of opioid-sparing, multimodal analgesia and GDFT, thereby achieving metabolic stability and early mobilization. Likewise, optimal nutrition during the perioperative period maintains metabolic homeostasis, boosts the immune system, and decreases catabolism.

The critical strategies include assessment of nutrition before operation, carbohydrate loading, immunonutrition, and early nutrition. Nutritional state, systemic inflammation, and sarcopenia are the critical factors of suboptimal result of operation of colon and rectum. The combined effect of nutritional state and anaesthesia is an essential part of ERAS, since adequate pain relief and early introduction of nutrition support fast postoperative recovery. This chapter covers the ERAS principles, body's reactions on stress, and methods of combining nutrition and anaesthesia.

M. Gambhir
Department of General Surgery, Medline Hospital, Karnal, Haryana, India

N. Kamkolam
Symbiosis Institute of Health Sciences, Symbiosis International (Deemed University), Lavale (Hill Base), Pune, Maharashtra, India

P. M. Lokhande (✉)
Department of Anaesthesia & Operation Theatre Technology, Dr. D.Y. Patil Vidyapeeth, Pimpri-Chinchwad, Maharashtra, India

P. K. Bhattacharyya et al. (eds.), *Integrated Anesthesia and Nutrition Approaches to Enhanced Recovery after Surgery*,
https://doi.org/10.1007/978-981-92-3294-9_10

Keywords

ERAS · Colorectal surgery · Peri-operative care · Anaesthetic techniques · Nutritional therapy · Malnutrition

10.1 Introduction

Postoperative complications are important considerations in the setting of colorectal surgery pathways due to their direct effect on outcome measures associated with postoperative ileus, delayed ability to tolerate oral intake, increased length of stay, and problems with mobility (Greco et al. 2014; Zhuang et al. 2013). The incidence of complications following surgery has been reported to be between 20% to 40%, while the occurrence of malnutrition among patients with colorectal cancer has been noted to occur in 30–50% of patients; this elevated incidence is associated with impaired wound healing, infection, ileus, and prolonged hospital stay (Waitzberg et al. 2006; GlobalSurg Collaborative and NIHR Global Health Unit on Global Surgery 2023).

The ERAS protocol implementation during colorectal surgery has been specifically designed for addressing several important issues of patient recovery, namely, a decrease in the body's stress reaction and gastrointestinal complications associated with stress caused by surgery (Ljungqvist et al. 2017; Gustafsson et al. 2019). Such methods as early mobilization, cautious use of analgesics such as opioids, and GDFT are used not only to enhance recovery but also to avoid the development of ileus and early acceptance of oral nutrition (Feldheiser et al. 2016; Zorrilla-Vaca et al. 2021).

Stress induced by the surgery and the condition of the body of the patient is of special significance during colorectal surgery because restoring gastrointestinal functions represents one of the major tasks during the procedure (Scott et al. 2015; Awad et al. 2013). The effects of stress cause metabolic changes in the body due to increased metabolism and catabolic reactions, including protein catabolism, resulting in decreased motility of the gut and ileus. Providing enteral nutrition from an early period helps to maintain intestinal mucosal barrier integrity, avoid bacterial migration, and regulate inflammatory processes in the gut (Smith et al. 2014; Lewis et al. 2009).

Nutritional support can include the use of immunonutrition, such as the administration of omega-3 fatty acids and arginine, which contribute to enhancing immunity and lowering the risk of infection following surgery (Moya et al. 2016; Song et al. 2015). Anaesthesiology is one of the most important elements of the recovery process after colorectal surgery because the type of anaesthetic used has a direct effect on the recovery process by influencing gastrointestinal mobility and stress reactions (Feldheiser et al. 2016; White et al. 2007).

Additionally, the physiological stabilization of the patient during surgery, particularly the maintenance of normothermia and optimal haemodynamic, is essential for reducing metabolic stress and ensuring proper blood supply to tissues, which plays a crucial role in both recovery and further nutritional support (Wijnberge et al. 2021; Feldheiser et al. 2016). The relationship between anaesthesia and nutrition is evident in the ERAS program for colorectal surgery since the anaesthetic regimen affects the opportunity for early enteral nutrition, while nutrition promotes recovery from gastrointestinal motility and metabolism disorders (Gillis and Carli 2015; Gustafsson et al. 2019).

Undoubtedly, the use of anaesthetic techniques in combination with nutrition therapy using early feeding is a win-win situation for both parties, since the primary factors affecting the postoperative recovery period following colorectal surgery include delayed bowel motility and feeding, lack of physical activity, and extended hospital stays (Greco et al. 2014; Hübner et al. 2015).

10.2 Physiological Stress Response to Colorectal Surgery

The surgical procedure affecting the colon and rectum activates a range of physiological responses, such as the neuroendocrine response, systemic inflammation, catabolic state, and increased oxidative stress (Scott et al. 2015; Awad et al. 2013). As shown in Fig. 10.1, such physiological responses include the neuroendocrine response, inflammatory response, metabolic state, and oxidative stress. Although the above physiological responses can be considered as a protective mechanism, their excessive activation leads to complications, impaired recovery, and worse outcomes after surgery. The purpose of ERAS programs is to minimize the adverse effects of excessive physiological responses (Ljungqvist et al. 2017; Gustafsson et al. 2019).

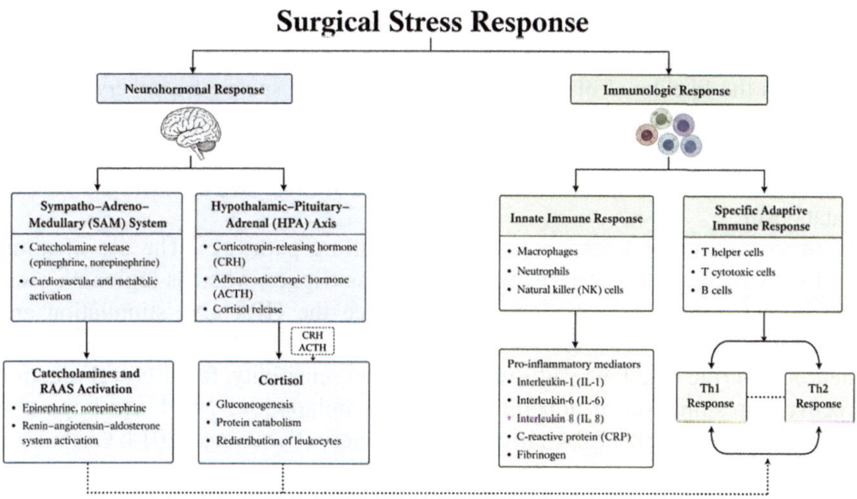

Fig. 10.1 Physiology of stress response. (Created by author using PowerPoint 2021)

Advanced anaesthetic and regional anaesthesia methods minimize the activation of neuroendocrine pathways, which include spikes in levels of corticosteroids and catecholamines, leading to decreased insulin resistance and immune suppression (White et al. 2007; Feldheiser et al. 2016). Minimally invasive surgery and fluid and electrolyte management are effective tools that enable limiting the inflammatory response, release of cytokines, and tissue injury (Greco et al. 2014; Ripollés et al. 2019). To mitigate postoperative catabolism, it is effective to begin enteral feeding since it prevents intestinal mucosa injury, promotes protein balance, and avoids muscle atrophy (Smith et al. 2014; Yu et al. 2017). Mobilization helps accelerate physiological recovery, increase insulin sensitivity, promote better lung function, and improve inflammatory profile, thus creating the basis for successful ERAS programs in colorectal surgery associated with a reduced risk of adverse events, shorter length of stay in hospital, and postoperative inflammatory response (Mathiasen et al. 2021; van Rooijen et al. 2019).

10.2.1 Neuroendocrine Response to Surgical Stress

The activation of the neuroendocrine system caused by stress associated with surgery mainly happens through the hypothalamus-pituitary-adrenal (HPA) axis and sympathetic nervous system (Scott et al. 2015). As a result of tissue injury, afferent neural stimulation results in the production of cortisol and catecholamines. The degree of hormone production depends on the extent of injury, and it affects postoperative healing directly (Kehlet and Wilmore 2002). The increased concentration of cortisol causes enhanced gluconeogenesis and increases the rate of protein and fat decomposition, whereas catecholamines increase the cardiac and metabolic demands.

The persistent activation of the neuroendocrine system during colonic surgery results in various complications related to the implementation of the Enhanced Recovery after Surgery (ERAS) strategy. Insulin resistance caused by cortisol increases the likelihood of infections and reduces the speed of recovery, whereas stimulation of the sympathetic system and opioids negatively affect gut peristalsis, causing postoperative ileus (Scott et al. 2015; Wijnberge et al. 2021). Additionally, they cause a loss of appetite and delayed oral intake. Fatigue facilitates muscle catabolism.

Interventions for ERAS target these signalling pathways. The use of minimally invasive surgery reduces the initial stress trigger, whereas regional anaesthesia and opioid-sparing pain control reduce the HPA axis stimulation and sympathetic activity (Feldheiser et al. 2016; White et al. 2007). Inhibition of the neuroendocrine reaction results in better insulin sensitivity, faster bowel function recovery, resumption of appetite, and faster ambulation, which are important clinical markers for the ERAS in colorectal surgery (Greco et al. 2014; Gustafsson et al. 2019).

10.2.2 Inflammatory Response and Cytokine Activation

Traumatic injury during surgery initiates an innate immune response, marked by the secretion of cytokines that include IL-6, TNF-α, and IL-1β (Scott et al. 2015). A summary of the primary inflammatory cytokines, highlighting their types and functions, is illustrated in Table 10.1. Out of all the listed cytokines, IL-6 is the most correlated with surgical trauma, and its level acts as a predictor for the occurrence of postoperative morbidity. The dysfunction of the intestinal barrier can cause sepsis and infections through increased translocation of bacteria and cytokines production.

Higher levels of cytokines contribute to ileus in postoperative patients, since inflammation-induced motility disturbance affects the gut; high capillary permeability causes fluid retention; fatigue and catabolic state decrease physical activity (Vather et al. 2014). On one hand, inflammation may negatively impact wound recovery and increase risks of developing anastomosis complications, whereas on the other hand, anti-inflammatory response leads to temporary immunodeficiency after surgery.

The ERAS protocol seeks to counteract the above-mentioned effects of inflammation by adopting specific strategies during the period before and after the surgical procedure. Invasive surgery is reduced to minimize tissue damage and cytokine generation, while GDFT will decrease tissue swelling and ensure microcirculatory flow (Zorrilla-Vaca et al. 2021; Ripollés et al. 2019). Early introduction of enteral nutrition will help maintain the integrity of the gut barrier to avoid any bacterial translocation (Smith et al. 2014; Yu et al. 2017). The lack of unnecessary tubes and drains will contribute to avoiding additional sources of inflammation.

Table 10.1 Inflammatory response and activation of cytokines

S.No	Mediators	Type	Action	References
1	IL-1, TNF- α	Pro inflammatory	Pyrexia, activation of leukocytes	Weber et al. (2010), Bradley (2008)
2	IL-6	Pro inflammatory	Acute phase responses	Tanaka et al. (2014)
3	IL-10, TGF- β	Anti inflammatory	Inhibits inflammation	Shimabukuro-Vornhagen et al. (2012)
4	Prostaglandins	Mediator of lipid	Vasodilation and pain	Ricciotti and FitzGerald (2011)
5	Chemokine	Signals proteins	Recruitment of leukocyte	Hughes and Nibbs (2018)

10.2.3 Body's Reaction and Breaking Down State

Surgery for colorectal diseases causes major metabolic disturbances, such as hypermetabolism and catabolism, which result from stress hormones and inflammatory markers (Scott et al. 2015; Awad et al. 2013). These disturbances have adverse effects on the recovery goals that are proposed by ERAS protocols, including early gastrointestinal recovery, low chances of infection, and enhanced functional ability.

Insulin Resistance Insulin resistance is one of the core features of the stress reaction resulting from surgery. Insulin resistance interferes with glucose metabolism and results in a catabolic condition; for example, during colorectal surgery, insulin resistance contributes to slow recovery from the operation, higher infection rates, poor wound healing, and slow restoration of oral feeding (Ljungqvist et al. 2017; Kwon et al. 2013). The use of carbohydrate loading before surgery and shorter periods of fasting are among ERAS techniques that can prevent the onset of insulin resistance and restore normal nutrition earlier (Smith et al. 2014).

Hyperglycaemia Hyperglycaemia following surgery occurs due to high glucose production by the liver and low glucose utilization by peripheral tissues. Patients with postoperative hyperglycaemia have increased incidences of surgical site infections, anastomosis complications, and hospitalization time (Kwon et al. 2013). In the ERAS pathway, glycemic control via insulin treatment together with stress reduction is crucial for avoiding complications and achieving recovery milestones (Ljungqvist et al. 2017; Kwon et al. 2013).

Protein Catabolism The process of protein degradation after surgical intervention may result in the loss of lean body mass due to muscle breakdown. This leads to higher metabolic requirements and plays an important role in contributing to fatigue, impaired respiratory performance, and delayed mobilization. Consequently, recovery objectives become more difficult to achieve when following ERAS principles in colorectal surgery patients (GlobalSurg Collaborative and NIHR Global Health Unit on Global Surgery 2023; van Rooijen et al. 2019). Sufficient protein consumption through enteral nutrition, according to ERAS recommendations, aids in reducing muscle wastage and facilitating mobilization (Weimann et al. 2017, 2021).

Negative Nitrogen Balance The imbalance between protein breakdown and synthesis results in a negative nitrogen balance, which is characterized by poor wound healing, infection, and delayed recovery (Waitzberg et al. 2006). The provision of early nutritional support following colorectal surgery plays an important role in maintaining nitrogen balance, muscle maintenance, and early recovery, which includes mobility and discharge (Smith et al. 2014; Weimann et al. 2021).

10.2.4 Oxidative Stress and Cellular Injury

Oxidative stress has come to be recognized as an important part of the body's reaction to surgical stress. Trauma and decreased perfusion cause the formation of reactive oxygen species, leading to lipid, protein, and DNA damage, and impairing normal cell functions by inducing cell death through apoptosis (Awad et al. 2013; Braga et al. 2002). Oxidative stress exacerbates inflammation and immune activation, thus forming a vicious cycle involving cell injury and immune response. Minimal-invasive surgeries, where injury and reduced perfusion are less pronounced, as well as optimization of perfusion, help in preventing oxidative stress (Greco et al. 2014; Ripollés et al. 2019). Furthermore, perioperative nutritional approach, involving administration of antioxidants and omega-3 fatty acids, could play an important role in controlling oxidative stress (Song et al. 2015; Braga et al. 2002).

10.2.5 What Surgical Stress Means for Patients

Clinical implications of enhanced stress responses are vital, influencing the recovery process following surgery. A heightened stress response is related to increased complications, prolonged recovery and hospitalization time, infection risk, impaired wound healing, and diminished muscle strength with low functionality (Scott et al. 2015; GlobalSurg Collaborative and NIHR Global Health Unit on Global Surgery 2023).

Research indicates that a reduction in surgical stress responses via the application of ERAS programs results in a decrease in complications and faster patient discharge (Greco et al. 2014; Song et al. 2015; Lau and Chamberlain 2017). For instance, a meta analysis of colorectal ERAS programs reveals decreased hospital stays by several days without raising re-admission or mortality rates (Greco et al. 2014; Song et al. 2015).

10.2.6 How Food Affects Surgical Stress

Perioperative nutrition plays a significant role in determining the extent and impact of surgical stress. Providing proper nutrition prior to surgery prevents the occurrence of surgical problems among nutritionally vulnerable individuals (Weimann et al. 2021; GlobalSurg Collaborative and NIHR Global Health Unit on Global Surgery 2023). Preoperative carbohydrate loading increases insulin sensitivity and comfort for patients (Smith et al. 2014; Ljungqvist et al. 2017).

Some nutrients, such as arginine, omega-3 fatty acids, and glutamine, can increase immune response and regulate inflammatory reactions; immunonutrition during the perioperative period may be related to decreased infections following gastrointestinal surgery (Moya et al. 2016; Braga et al. 1999; Song et al. 2015). Postoperative nutrition is an essential component of the ERAS process and helps in maintaining gut barrier integrity, decreasing bacterial translocation, improving nutritional balance, and facilitating functional recovery (Smith et al. 2014; Yu et al. 2017; Lewis et al. 2009). Protein supplementation is critical for preventing catabolic conditions, healing wounds, and promoting recovery (Weimann et al. 2021; Weimann et al. 2017).

10.2.7 Role of Anaesthesia in Modulating Stress Response

The use of anaesthetics greatly impacts the stress response of the human body during surgery. Modern approaches seek to minimize neuroendocrine and inflammatory activation and metabolic stability (Feldheiser et al. 2016; White et al. 2007). General anaesthesia ensures hypnosis and analgesia, but it is an incomplete blocker of the stress response, unlike regional anaesthesia, which blocks nociception better and releases fewer stress hormones (Feldheiser et al. 2016; Hamid et al. 2020).

Multi-modal analgesia and opioid-sparing practices are essential for ERAS principles and are associated with better patient outcomes and fewer adverse events (Elsarrag et al. 2019; Gedda et al. 2023). The stress response elicited by surgery involves sympathetic activation and the activation of the HPA axis, leading to cortisol and catecholamine elevation. The former is suppressed, and the latter is reduced by general and regional anaesthesia, respectively, whereas total intravenous anaesthesia and carefully administered opioids decrease inflammation and sympathetic activation (Kehlet and Wilmore 2002; Feldheiser et al. 2016). The details of how each of these anaesthetics affect the stress response are described in Table 10.2.

10.2.8 Negative Nitrogen Balance

With proper anaesthesia, there will be decreased stress and hormones that prevent muscle protein breakdown; hence, a proper balance of nitrogen can be achieved (Scott et al. 2015; Gillis and Carli 2015). Together with early post-operative food intake, it leads to a faster recovery of physical performance and quicker discharge, which means that anaesthesia and nutrition work together in promoting a positive outcome following surgery (Ljungqvist et al. 2017; Gustafsson et al. 2019).

Table 10.2 Anaesthetic modulation of stress response

Technique	Mechanism	Effect	References
General anaesthesia	CNS suppression	Partial attenuation of the neuroendocrine response	Kim (2023)
Epidural anaesthesia	Blocks afferent pathways	Reduced cortisol, improved recovery	Han et al. (2024), Zhao et al. (2024)
Multimodal analgesia	Opioid-sparing, anti-inflammatory	Reduced complications, enhanced recovery (2,6)	Elsarrag et al. (2019), Elnour et al. (2025)

10.3 Nutritional Optimization in the Preoperative Period

Nutrition optimization is another key component in ERAS programs when dealing with colorectal surgery. This is done by targeting malnutrition that poses risks to patients by being a major determinant of postoperative infections, delayed wound healing, prolonged hospital stay, and increased morbidity (Weimann et al. 2021; GlobalSurg Collaborative and NIHR Global Health Unit on Global Surgery 2023). Every patient who needs elective colorectal surgery must undergo a preoperative nutritional evaluation based on BMI, recent weight loss, laboratory tests, and screening tools (Weimann et al. 2021; van Rooijen et al. 2019).

Any patient who is at risk of malnutrition should be intervened using oral nutritional supplements and diets such as protein-rich and energy-dense regimens (Weimann et al. 2021; Waitzberg et al. 2006). Contemporary ERAS programs also suggest limiting preoperative fasting and giving carbohydrate beverages within 2–3 hours before the administration of anaesthesia to avoid developing insulin resistance (Smith et al. 2014; Ljungqvist et al. 2017). Through nutrition optimization, health professionals will be able to reduce metabolic and inflammatory responses as well as body mass loss in the perioperative phase (Gillis and Carli 2015; Weimann et al. 2017).

10.3.1 Nutritional Assessment

Nutrition assessment before colorectal surgery is another essential element of the ERAS approach, as poor nutrition increases the risk of complications and negatively affects postoperative recovery (Weimann et al. 2021; GlobalSurg Collaborative and NIHR Global Health Unit on Global Surgery 2023). The tools that assess the patient's nutritional status include the Malnutrition Universal Screening Tool (MUST), Nutritional Risk Screening 2002 (NRS-2002), and Subjective Global Assessment (SGA). These tools consider BMI, weight loss, intake, and severity of disease to determine the presence of nutritional risk (Weimann et al. 2021). Table 10.3 provides an overview of popular tools for nutritional screening and assessment, along with the main elements and practical application of each.

The findings of nutritional assessment will affect ERAS-based treatment: the patients who have high-risk scores will need additional nutritional therapy, possibly supplemented by prehabilitation, while those with lower risk scores may follow regular protocols (van Rooijen et al. 2019). Screening is usually included in multimodal prehabilitation programs that aim to improve physical function before surgery (van Rooijen et al. 2019).

Table 10.3 Nutrition assessment tools

Assessment tool	Target population	Key components	Risk interpretation	ERAS-based clinical action
SGA (Subjective Global Assessment)	Adult	Nutrition intake, weight loss, GI symptoms, functional status Physical examination	Well-nourished/ Moderately malnourished/ Severely malnourished	Moderate–severe risk → initiate nutritional support; consider delaying elective surgery for optimization
MNA (Mini Nutritional Assessment)	Geriatrics	Body Mass Index, mobility, diet, and psychological stress	Normal/At risk/ Malnourished	At risk → start oral supplements; Malnourished → structured nutritional therapy + prehabilitation
MUST (Malnutrition Universal Screening Tool)	Adult (hospitalized)	Evaluated Body Mass Index, weight loss, acute disease effect	Rapid screening Score 0 (low), 1 (medium), ≥2 (high risk)	Medium risk → nutritional monitoring + supplements; High risk → intensive nutritional support before surgery
NRS 2002 (Nutritional Risk Screening 2002)	Adult	Used for hospitalized patients, detects disease severity & nutritional status	Score < 3 (low risk), ≥3 (high risk)	≥3 → Initiate nutritional therapy; consider postponing surgery if severe risk
PG-SGA(patient-generated SGA)	Cancer patients	Symptoms, loss of weight, intake, functional capacity	Score-based severity grading	High score → aggressive nutritional intervention and oncology-specific nutritional care

10.3.2 Prehabilitation

Multidimensional prehabilitation before colorectal surgery is an approach to increase physiological reserve and optimize recovery post-surgery (Gillis et al. 2014). The multidimensional approach to prehabilitation includes nutrition optimization, exercises, anaemia treatment, and smoking cessation.

Protein and caloric nutrition before surgery ensure muscle mass and immune system function (Gillis and Carli 2015; van Rooijen et al. 2019). Exercise programs ensure improved cardiopulmonary endurance and muscular strength, allowing for earlier mobilization without increased fatigue (Gillis et al. 2014). Treatment of anaemia increases the amount of oxygen transport to organs and systems, and stopping smoking decreases the risk of pulmonary problems. Combined with the ERAS protocol, prehabilitation programs can positively affect bowel recovery and mobility (Gillis et al. 2014; van Rooijen et al. 2019).

10.3.3 Carbohydrate Loading

Carbohydrate loading before surgery is another essential metabolic measure in ERAS protocols used in colorectal surgery (Smith et al. 2014; Ljungqvist et al. 2017). Instead of fasting before surgery, patients consume carbohydrate-containing fluids 2–3 hours prior to surgery.

The use of carbohydrate loading allows for preventing insulin resistance perioperatively due to sufficient glycogen storage and reduced catabolic response to surgery (Smith et al. 2014; Awad et al. 2013). It ensures maintenance of lean body mass and stabilizes metabolism during postoperative recovery. The procedure provides patients with better physical and psychological conditions because it eliminates discomfort related to hunger, thirst, and stress during preoperative preparation (Ljungqvist et al. 2017). The use of carbohydrate loading in colorectal ERAS protocols was recognized as an indispensable part of metabolic management and was found to reduce postoperative nitrogen losses (Smith et al. 2014).

10.3.4 Avoidance of Prolonged Fasting

Instead of traditional prolonged fasting, evidence-based guidelines are used that help ensure metabolic stability during the ERAS protocol. Patients may eat solids up to 6 hours prior and clear carbohydrates up to 2 hours prior to anaesthetic induction (Smith et al. 2014; Ljungqvist et al. 2017).

The practice of prolonged fasting leads to the depletion of glycogen stores, insulin resistance, dehydration, and metabolic imbalance under stress conditions, leading to lean body mass loss, poor glucose control, and slower recovery (Awad et al. 2013). Prolonged fasting rules, along with carbohydrate loading, help stay hydrated, keep the metabolism balanced, and minimize the patient's suffering from dehydration and postoperative nausea and vomiting (Smith et al. 2014; Ljungqvist et al. 2017).

10.4 Anaesthesia Strategies in ERAS During Intra-operative Care

10.4.1 Intra-operative Management: ERAS Anaesthesia Bundle

The anaesthesia used during surgery in ERAS should be administered according to an evidence-based approach, which goes further than the induction and emergence phase. With respect to colorectal surgery, the aim of this bundle is to achieve low levels of surgical stress, physiological stability, and enhanced recovery profiles

(Feldheiser et al. 2016; White et al. 2007). Some clinically important objectives to attain are reduced postoperative pain, avoidance of opioid administration, reduction of PONV, and early gastrointestinal recovery with tolerance to feeding (Elsarrag et al. 2019; Gedda et al. 2023).

These include haemodynamic stabilization, the avoidance of excessive deep anaesthesia, opioids' sparing, as well as maintaining normothermia (Feldheiser et al. 2016; Wijnberge et al. 2021). This strategy decreases the neuroendocrine stimulation while enhancing blood flow to tissues leading to improved recovery of functions like anastomosis healing. Anaesthesiologists play a major role by choosing rapid-acting and titrable agents, performing regional anaesthesia, and managing perioperative physiology as part of the ERAS process (White et al. 2007; Feldheiser et al. 2016).

10.4.2 Principles of ERAS Anesthesia

The main ERAS anaesthesia techniques include three major concepts: maintaining homeostasis, procedure-oriented anaesthesia, and opioid-sparing analgesia (Feldheiser et al. 2016; White et al. 2007). Maintaining homeostasis includes sufficient oxygenation, perfusion, normothermia, and euvolemia, as well as avoiding hypotension, hypoxia, hypothermia, and fluid overload (Wijnberge et al. 2021; Zorrilla-Vaca et al. 2021).

It is crucial to minimize the use of opioids during anaesthesia since opioids cause respiratory depression, ileus, nausea, vomiting, urinal retention, and delays in food intake (Gedda et al. 2023; Beverly et al. 2017). Minimization of opioid use leads to faster postoperative recovery, better tolerance of food intake, and shorter hospitalization periods. Procedure-oriented anaesthesia implies adapting the anaesthesia method to the complexity of the procedure, anticipated pain, and patient comorbid conditions. For example, minimal access surgery favours light general anaesthesia with regional blocks, and for open surgeries, neuroaxis anaesthesia is more beneficial (Feldheiser et al. 2016; Hamid et al. 2020).

10.4.3 Multimodal Analgesia

Multimodal analgesia is an essential element of the ERAS approach, involving the use of different medications acting on peripheral, spinal, and supraspinal levels for the provision of synergic analgesia with reduced opioid consumption (Feldheiser et al. 2016; Elsarrag et al. 2019). Paracetamol and NSAIDs, local anaesthetics, regional blockade, ketamine, and dexmedetomidine are often employed as non-opioid analgesics (Vigneault et al. 2011; Rizk et al. 2021).

Multimodal analgesia helps prevent central sensitization and reduces the stress response induced by surgical interventions, thus contributing to better pain management and overall recovery after colorectal surgery (Elsarrag et al. 2019; White et al. 2007). This approach was linked to decreased pain, reduced opioid-related adverse effects (PONV and ileus, among others), and earlier restoration of bowel function, early intake of oral food, and ambulation (Gedda et al. 2023; Beverly et al. 2017).

10.4.4 Regional Anaesthetic Techniques

It is important to use regional anaesthesia in ERAS because it minimizes the nociceptive afferent activity, reducing the stress reaction. Regional anaesthesia techniques like neuraxial and abdominal wall blocks can reduce opioid consumption, promote gastrointestinal motility, decrease PONV occurrence, and promote early mobilization (Feldheiser et al. 2016; Hamid et al. 2020).

US-guided neuraxial and fascia plane blocks (such as transversus abdominis plane block) increase safety and effectiveness (Hain et al. 2018; Wu et al. 2025). ERAS does not imply that all surgical patients receive regional anaesthesia. On the contrary, it recommends using regional techniques selectively based on the nature of the operation and its anticipated pain intensity. Too much motor blockade or cardiovascular instability may prevent early mobility and oral feeding. Thus, regional anaesthesia should be used prudently (White et al. 2007; Feldheiser et al. 2016).

10.4.5 Epidural Analgesia

Thoracic epidural analgesia is well-known to be used during open colorectal and thoracoabdominal surgery, resulting in excellent somatic and visceral anaesthesia with suppression of the surgical stress response (Feldheiser et al. 2016; Hamid et al. 2020). This analgesic method improves respiratory mechanics and decreases postoperative pain, making it beneficial for certain patients' recovery.

However, epidural analgesia can result in hypotension, motor paralysis, and urinary retention, which may interfere with early mobilization and enteral nutrition. Therefore, according to the recommendations of the ERAS program, epidural analgesia is preferred for open surgery, as there will be a great amount of pain (Feldheiser et al. 2016; Gustafsson et al. 2019).

10.4.6 TAP Block

In laparoscopic colorectal surgery under ERAS protocols, the TAP block is being widely used because it is able to offer sufficient somatic analgesia with minimal systemic effect (Hain et al. 2018; Wu et al. 2025). TAP block reduces opioid requirement, lowers PONV incidence, helps early mobilization, and ensures early acceptance of oral feeding (Hain et al. 2018).

Nevertheless, the TAP block cannot effectively address visceral pain; hence, it is more efficient when used together with other analgesics as part of a multimodal approach (Vigneault et al. 2011; Rizk et al. 2021). In laparoscopic colorectal

Table 10.4 Comparison of epidural vs TAP block in open vs laparoscopic procedures

	Epidural analgesia		TAP-block	
	Open procedure	Laparoscopic	Open procedure	Laparoscopic
Efficacy of the analgesic	Provides superior and visceral analgesia	Exceeded requirement of analgesia	Balanced	Somatic pain control
Pain control (visceral)	Excellent	Not needed	Constrained	Constrained
Effects on hemodynamic	Hypotension, prolonged immobilization	Hypotension, prolonged immobilization	Limited	Limited

surgery, the TAP block helps in achieving rapid recovery and early discharge since it allows for adequate pain relief without compromising mobilization. The comparative analysis between epidural analgesia and TAP block in open and laparoscopic surgery can be found in Table 10.4.

10.4.7 Pharmacological Adjuncts in ERAS

Use of pharmacological agents in ERAS helps with recovery through modulation of the stress response and decreasing the use of opioids. As an NMDA receptor blocker, ketamine lowers central sensitization and facilitates pain management, early mobility, and gastrointestinal function (Vigneault et al. 2011). Lidocaine infusion offers analgesia, anti-inflammatory, and anti-hyperalgesic properties, and may lead to lower post-operative ileus after colonic surgery (Rizk et al. 2021).

The α2-adrenergic agonist dexmedetomidine decreases sympathetic activation and provides sedation along with decreased requirements for opioids and PONV, while careful cardiovascular assessment is required due to the risk of bradycardia and hypotension (Vigneault et al. 2011). The use of gabapentinoids in ERAS may be effective for lowering central sensitization and opioid requirements, but their sedating effect delays mobilization (Beverly et al. 2017).

10.4.8 Goal-Directed Fluid Therapy (GDFT)

The GDFT customizes intraoperative fluid therapy by employing haemodynamic parameters like stroke volume and cardiac output (Zorrilla-Vaca et al. 2021). The technique makes sure that adequate intravascular volume is achieved without inducing hypovolaemia and volume excess.

Effective fluid resuscitation contributes to favourable results following colorectal procedures by promoting tissue perfusion, preventing surgical site injuries, minimizing postoperative ileus, and sustaining cardiovascular and respiratory functions (Zorrilla-Vaca et al. 2021; Ripollés et al. 2019). Exclusion of volume excess is vital within the ERAS framework since excess volume impairs gastrointestinal function and extends hospital stays (Feldheiser et al. 2016; Gustafsson et al. 2019).

10.4.9 Minimally Invasive and Robotic Surgery

MIS and robotically-assisted operations have proven to be well suited to ERAS protocols because they minimize operative trauma, the inflammatory reaction, and pain after surgery (Greco et al. 2014; Prete et al. 2018). This leads to decreased opioid consumption, earlier restoration of gut function, faster mobilization, reduced hospitalization time, and faster resumption of eating by mouth (Ripollés et al. 2019; Prete et al. 2018).

Success depends upon proper patient selection, surgeon skill, and strict adherence to the ERAS protocol elements, although the costs involved may restrict its use widely (Kahokehr et al. 2009; Cavallaro and Bordeianou 2019).

10.4.10 Temperature Management

Normothermia during surgery is vital for ERAS since anaesthetic administration affects thermal regulation and leads to the possibility of hypothermia. Hypothermia causes a higher probability of developing coagulopathy, wound infections, delayed medication absorption, and slow recovery (Feldheiser et al. 2016).

Warming procedures and temperature control minimize metabolic stress, increase patient comfort, and facilitate postoperative mobilization and readiness for discharge. Consequently, normothermia is an important objective of ERAS-compatible perioperative management (Feldheiser et al. 2016; Scott et al. 2015).

10.5 Nutritional Strategies in the Post-operative Period

Nutritional therapy after the procedure in the case of ERAS-colorectal surgery is timely and well-organized, with emphasis on starting oral and enteral nutrition on the day following surgery (Smith et al. 2014; Gustafsson et al. 2019; Weimann et al. 2021). This will fast-track the process of healing and reduce the risk of adverse events.

Postoperative Day (POD) 0–1 Patients are motivated to initiate enteral intake early postoperatively, starting with clear liquids and moving up as appropriate (Smith et al. 2014; Lassen et al. 2008). Early enteral nutrition aids in preventing ileus by triggering enteric reflexes and gut hormones, especially in combination with opioid-sparing analgesia and proper fluid balance (Greco et al. 2014; Yu et al. 2017).

POD 1–3 Energy and protein intake should be adequate enough to compensate for hypermetabolism and catabolism. According to the ERAS and ESPEN protocols, it is advisable to have a high-protein diet and nutritional supplements that will help avoid negative nitrogen balance and loss of lean body mass, particularly among high-risk and malnourished patients (Weimann et al. 2021; Lewis et al. 2009). Transitioning to a regular diet will depend on tolerance, which can also be an indication of the healing of the gastrointestinal tract.

Monitoring of intake, digestion, and nutrition is important. For patients who have inadequate oral intake, it becomes imperative to increase the enteral feeds through nasogastric/jejunal tubes in order to prevent energy-protein deficits (Weimann et al. 2021; Yu et al. 2017).

10.5.1 Early Enteral Nutrition (EEN)

Early enteral nutrition within 24–48 hours after surgery is a critical ERAS guideline, replacing conventional prolonged fasting protocols after surgery (Smith et al. 2014; Weimann et al. 2021). Early enteral nutrition ensures the maintenance of intestinal motility, preserves the intestinal epithelial lining, and prevents infections (Yu et al. 2017; Lewis et al. 2009).

Through early stimulation of the gastrointestinal system, enteral nutrition hastens gastrointestinal recovery and ensures tolerance to feeding, minimizing reliance on parenteral nutrition (Smith et al. 2014; Lassen et al. 2008). Enteral nutrition is more physiologically appropriate than parenteral feeding due to its health benefits, reduced infection rates, and economic advantages (Weimann et al. 2021; Yu et al. 2017).

10.5.2 Protein and Energy Requirements

Postoperatively, proteins play an important role in tissue healing, immune system functioning, and muscle mass maintenance. The protein requirement is around 1.2–2.0 grams per kilogram per day, taking into account the degree of surgical stress and individual status (Weimann et al. 2017, 2021). Protein-rich formulas containing leucine and amino acid mixtures can facilitate muscle protein synthesis and improve muscle strength, especially in older and sarcopenic individuals (Weimann et al. 2017; van Rooijen et al. 2019).

The amount of energy needed is higher after the procedure due to increased energy consumption. Common values are from 25 to 30 kilocalories per kilogram per day, depending on patient age, comorbidity, and surgical complexity (Weimann et al. 2021; Awad et al. 2013). Carbohydrates act as the main energy source, with lipids, including omega-3 fatty acids, providing extra energy and anti-inflammatory properties (Song et al. 2015).

10.5.3 Immunonutrition

Immunonutrition utilizes certain nutrients, including arginine, glutamine, and omega-3 fatty acids, to modify immune reactions and inflammation. Specifically, arginine aids T cell responses, glutamine provides metabolic energy for immune cells and enterocytes, and omega-3 fatty acids play a role in the biosynthesis of eicosanoids and inflammation (Moya et al. 2016; Braga et al. 1999; Song et al. 2015).

Numerous randomized studies and systematic reviews have demonstrated the efficacy of perioperative immunonutrition on the prevention of postoperative infections and complications following gastrointestinal operations, particularly in malnourished/high-risk individuals (Moya et al. 2016; Braga et al. 1999; Song et al. 2015). Nevertheless, immunonutrition is still considered beneficial in selected colorectal ERAS patients as per existing guidelines (Weimann et al. 2021, 2025).

10.5.4 Glycaemic Control

Postoperative hyperglycaemia is often encountered as a consequence of the stress response and counter-regulatory hormones, including cortisol and glucagon, resulting in insulin resistance (Kwon et al. 2013). Hyperglycaemia can negatively affect immunity, wound healing, and susceptibility to infections. All ERAS guidelines target maintaining blood glucose under 180 mg/dL without inducing hypoglycaemia through monitoring and proper management of glucose levels with insulin (Kwon et al. 2013; Ljungqvist et al. 2017).

Sufficient hydration, minimal use of dextrose-containing solutions, and early ambulation are some measures that help in achieving steady glucose metabolism (Kwon et al. 2013). As the delayed start of nutrition after surgery is often associated with postoperative ileus and opioid-induced side effects, opioid-sparing techniques and early feeding have become essential for maintaining metabolic stability (Gedda et al. 2023; Yu et al. 2017).

10.5.5 Monitoring of Nutritional Status

A continuous assessment of the patient's nutritional state before and following surgery is necessary for ensuring proper nutrition and detecting any deficiencies (Weimann et al. 2021). The parameters to monitor include weight, body mass index, food intake, serum protein levels (e.g., albumin, prealbumin), nitrogen balance, and glucose metabolism. For patients with high risk, assessment of their body composition and physical function may prove beneficial (GlobalSurg Collaborative and NIHR Global Health Unit on Global Surgery 2023; van Rooijen et al. 2019).

Periodic monitoring is linked to better treatment efficacy, less complication rate, shorter hospitalization time, and successful rehabilitation (Weimann et al. 2021; Waitzberg et al. 2006).

10.6 Synergistic Interaction Between Anaesthesia and Nutrition

In ERAS, a concept of synergy is used whereby anaesthesia and nutrition work together to prevent surgical stress. The pre-existing malnutrition, increased fasting duration, excessive opioid utilization, pain not being controlled, fluid overloading, and delayed nutrition all contribute to stress, resulting in insulin resistance, protein catabolism, fluid retention, and delayed healing (Ljungqvist et al. 2017; GlobalSurg Collaborative and NIHR Global Health Unit on Global Surgery 2023).

In order to reduce catabolism, the ERAS approach utilizes short-acting anaesthesia, normothermia, multimodal opioid-sparing analgesia, PONV prevention measures, early nutrition, minimized fasting, carbohydrate drinks before surgery, and high-protein nutrition within the first hours after surgery (Feldheiser et al. 2016; Weimann et al. 2021). Together, these components optimize pain relief, nutrition and minimize nausea, allowing the patient to be mobilized quickly; hence, ERAS operates on a synergy of anaesthesia and nutrition (Ljungqvist et al. 2017; Gustafsson et al. 2019).

10.6.1 Anaesthesia, Nutrition, and ERAS in Colorectal Surgery

ERAS has shifted the process of perioperative care for colorectal surgeries from separate procedures to systematic recovery processes (Ljungqvist et al. 2017; Gustafsson et al. 2019). Effective recovery is not only dependent upon the surgical technique but also upon factors such as metabolic balance, bowel movement, mobility, oral intake, and prevention of infections (Greco et al. 2014; Ripollés et al. 2019).

The combination of anaesthesia and nutritional elements has the potential to minimize surgical stress and maintain an efficient immune system, facilitate healing, and aid in digestive health (Gillis and Carli 2015; Feldheiser et al. 2016). The implementation of the ERAS protocol has shown improved results with respect to lower levels of insulin resistance, infections, ileus, and hospitalization periods (Greco et al. 2014; Zhuang et al. 2013; Lau and Chamberlain 2017).

10.6.2 Reduced Surgical Stress

Modern anaesthesia for colorectal surgery seeks to minimize stress while not delaying awakening. Short-acting drugs, proper depth control, multimodal pain management, heating, and balanced fluid therapy help prevent side effects (Feldheiser et al. 2016; White et al. 2007). Non-opioid anaesthesia is preferred to avoid vomiting, ileus, sedation, and delayed ambulation (Gedda et al. 2023; Beverly et al. 2017).

Nutritional interventions like selective fasting, clear liquids up to 2 hours prior to surgery, and carbohydrate solutions further minimize dehydration and insulin resistance (Smith et al. 2014; Ljungqvist et al. 2017). Nutrients consumed orally that ensure sufficient caloric intake and protein promote healing, especially in malnutrition cases (Weimann et al. 2021; Waitzberg et al. 2006).

10.6.3 Improved Gut Function

Successful recovery from surgery requires the restoration of gut functions. Several factors can cause postoperative ileus, and these include opioids, sympathetic stimulation, manipulation of the bowels, hypoperfusion, fluid overload, and fasting (Vather et al. 2014; Yu et al. 2017). Anaesthesia guided by ERAS principles (stable haemodynamic, opioid-sparing pain relief, prophylactic treatment of PONV and fluid restriction) contributes to early gut recovery (Feldheiser et al. 2016; Greco et al. 2014). Minimally invasive procedures help reduce inflammation and encourage early ambulation (Ripollés et al. 2019; Prete et al. 2018).

Various nutritional interventions like reduced preoperative fasting and early initiation of oral nutrition stimulate the production of gut hormones and facilitate movement in the intestine (Smith et al. 2014; Yu et al. 2017). Stepwise advancement in diet is recommended depending on tolerance levels. Research provides recent evidence for an effective combination of nutrition with appropriate protein intake for malnutrition patients (Weimann et al. 2017, 2021).

10.6.4 Enhanced Immune Function

A key aspect of immune efficiency in colorectal surgery is nutritional state. Poor nutrition, including protein-calorie malnutrition, sarcopenia, and unintentional weight loss from the disease, impairs immunity, collagen formation, and the ability to fight infections (GlobalSurg Collaborative and NIHR Global Health Unit on Global Surgery 2023; van Rooijen et al. 2019). Proper surgical techniques and avoidance of hypothermia, hypoxemia, and hyperglycaemia will help overcome further immune impairment (Scott et al. 2015; Kwon et al. 2013).

Several studies have found that immunonutrition may reduce the incidence of complications and infection in gastrointestinal surgeries (Moya et al. 2016; Braga et al. 1999; Song et al. 2015). If combined with efficient anaesthesia, immunonutrition improves overall patient recovery and health.

10.6.5 Faster Functional Recovery

The perioperative period is measured based on functional recovery. Quick recovery depends on maintained muscle strength, effective pain management, timely bowel movement, adequate nutrition, mobility, and minimal nausea (Ljungqvist et al. 2017; Mathiasen et al. 2021). Both anaesthesia and nutrition play significant roles in achieving these goals; multimodal and opioid-free anaesthetic techniques aid in early mobilization, whereas adequate protein and energy intake help maintain muscle bulk and physiotherapy engagement (Beverly et al. 2017; Weimann et al. 2017). The avoidance of PONV and excess fluids allows for early ingestion. Proper pain management, timely food intake, and mobility help to hasten functional recovery and subsequent hospital discharge (Greco et al. 2014; Song et al. 2015).

10.7 Enhanced Recovery After Surgery Protocols in Colorectal Procedures

ERAS for colorectal surgery is an established protocol that reduces the impact of surgery on physiology, ensures proper physiological functioning, and expedites recovery through a series of interventions grounded in scientific evidence (Ljungqvist et al. 2017; Gustafsson et al. 2019). This involves the use of perioperative optimization procedures, intraoperative procedures, and postoperative protocols that contribute to minimizing complications, improving results, and reducing length of stay, resulting in reduced costs of healthcare delivery (Greco et al. 2014; Zhuang et al. 2013; Ripollés et al. 2019). The relationship between anaesthesia and nutrition is a key factor in ERAS.

10.7.1 Preoperative Phase

Preoperative risk stratification and optimization are especially crucial in colorectal surgery, given that nutrition-related issues such as cancer-induced malnutrition and functional decline are prevalent (GlobalSurg Collaborative and NIHR Global Health Unit on Global Surgery 2023; van Rooijen et al. 2019). Nutritional assessment through MUST, NRS-2002, SGA, PG-SGA, and MNA helps identify those who would need intervention (Weimann et al. 2021).

Interventions for high-risk patients include perioperative protein-calorie supplementation, immunonutrition, and a combination of physical exercise training and anaemia correction (Gillis et al. 2014). In terms of metabolic optimization, preoperative carbohydrate intake and the avoidance of prolonged fasting help maintain proper glycogen stores and insulin resistance (Smith et al. 2014; Ljungqvist et al. 2017). Education of the patient about expectations and the ERAS pathway itself is also helpful (Kahokehr et al. 2009; Cavallaro and Bordeianou 2019).

10.7.2 Intraoperative Phase

The intraoperative components of ERAS aim at stabilizing physiology and reducing stress from surgery. The use of short-acting aesthetic agents, depth of anaesthesia monitoring, multimodal pain management including regional anaesthesia, and GDFT are essential components (Feldheiser et al. 2016; Zorrilla-Vaca et al. 2021). The use of regional anaesthesia through epidural blocks or TAP blocks helps reduce pain and speeds up gastrointestinal recovery (Hain et al. 2018; Hamid et al. 2020; Wu et al. 2025).

GDFT helps achieve normovolemia and organ perfusion by avoiding both hypovolemia and excessive fluid administration, which delays the return of bowel function (Zorrilla-Vaca et al. 2021; Ripollés et al. 2019). Other components involve lung-protective ventilation, active patient warming, PONV prevention, and minimally invasive surgical techniques when possible (Greco et al. 2014; Prete et al. 2018). The use of a nasogastric tube and drains should be avoided to maintain splanchnic perfusion and facilitate early oral intake (Gustafsson et al. 2019).

10.7.3 Postoperative Phase

Postoperative management entails planned rehabilitation regimens. Early feeding, which should preferably be initiated within 24 hours, is an integral part of the process even without bowel sounds because it helps in maintaining the health of the mucosa, increases motility, and prevents muscle wasting (Smith et al. 2014; Yu et al. 2017; Lewis et al. 2009).

Nutritional support through oral supplements or enteral feeding through a tube becomes necessary when oral intake falls short, with the provision continuing post-discharge to avoid sarcopenia (Weimann et al. 2017, 2021). Multimodal opioid-sparing analgesia for better respiration, coughing, and mobilization, and regional anaesthesia to decrease opioid-induced ileus and PONV constitute other important measures (Beverly et al. 2017; Gedda et al. 2023). All these aspects together constitute the holistic approach shown in Fig. 10.2 below.

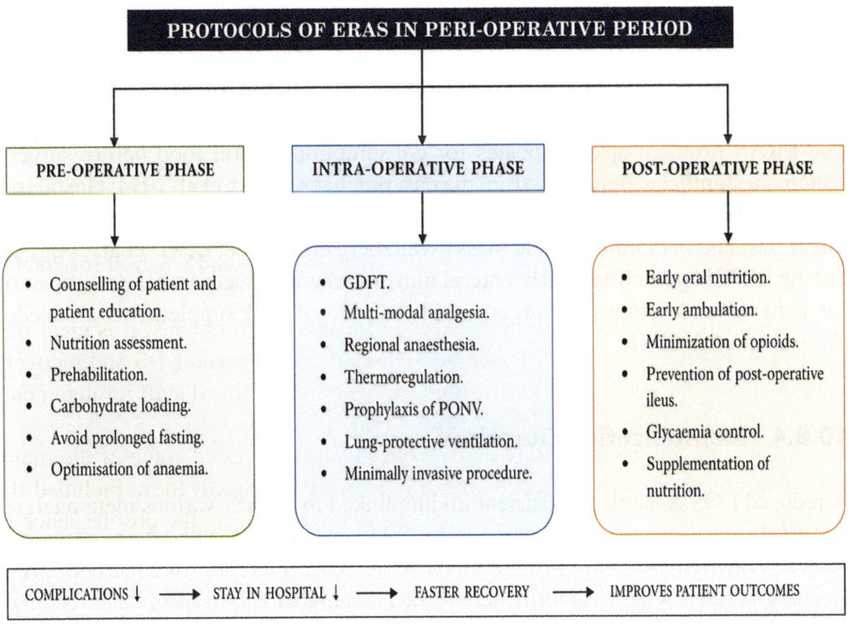

Fig. 10.2 ERAS protocols in the perioperative phase. (Created by author using PowerPoint 2021)

10.8 Clinical Outcomes and Evidence

10.8.1 ERAS Implementation in Colorectal Surgery: Endpoint-Based Review

ERAS has proven to make significant improvements in surgical outcome parameters since its application in colorectal surgery. Instead of focusing on vague assertions, it would be wise to evaluate the evidence based on concrete parameters like gastrointestinal function, complications, duration of hospitalization, readmission rate, and mortality rate (Greco et al. 2014; Zhuang et al. 2013; Lau and Chamberlain 2017).

10.8.2 Postoperative Ileus and Gastrointestinal Recovery

Ileus following surgery plays an important role in determining recovery following colorectal surgeries. Ileus can be minimized and prevented from occurring due to various factors, including early enteral nutrition, opioid-sparing analgesic technique, optimal fluid management, and early mobilization (Greco et al. 2014; Zhuang et al. 2013; Yu et al. 2017). Various studies indicate that patients who underwent ERAS had a quicker flatus passage and gastrointestinal recovery than patients undergoing conventional treatment procedures (Greco et al. 2014; Zhuang et al. 2013).

10.8.3 First Postoperative Oral Intake and Nutritional Recovery

The ERAS protocol also advocates for consumption of oral food before surgery, which is a significant departure from the past practices (Smith et al. 2014; Gustafsson et al. 2019). Consumption of oral foods improves nitrogen balance, helps prevent infections, and maintains muscle mass (Waitzberg et al. 2006; Lewis et al. 2009). As per the ESPEN guidelines, early enteral nutrition therapy needs to become the norm for patients undergoing GI surgery, with the use of oral supplements as needed (Weimann et al. 2021, 2025).

10.8.4 Hospitalization Duration

A reduced LOS is another consistent finding linked to ERAS. Various meta-analyses and RCTs have reported a decrease in LOS by several days without an increase in readmissions (Greco et al. 2014; Zhuang et al. 2013; Lau and Chamberlain 2017). Registry-based research has further confirmed that higher ERAS compliance is linked to reduced LOS in actual clinical practice (Hübner et al. 2015; Ripollés et al. 2019).

10.8.5 Postoperative Complications

The implementation of ERAS decreases morbidity after surgery, which includes infections and cardiopulmonary complications (Greco et al. 2014; Zhuang et al. 2013; Ripollés et al. 2019). As a result, ERAS decreases the inflammatory response by preventing systemic stress to maintain the physiological balance. Lower risks of surgical wound infection, pulmonary complications, and cardiovascular incidents were noted when ERAS was practiced (Waitzberg et al. 2006; GlobalSurg Collaborative and NIHR Global Health Unit on Global Surgery 2023; Ripollés et al. 2019).

10.8.6 Opioid Usage and Pain Management

ERAS focuses on opioid-sparing analgesic therapy, which facilitates recovery and minimizes adverse effects. Research has shown that ERAS patients exhibit decreased opioid usage, effective pain management, and enhanced functional recovery when compared to patients undergoing traditional treatment methods (Gedda et al. 2023; Elsarrag et al. 2019). Decreased opioid usage results in decreased ileus, early mobilization, and quicker gastrointestinal recovery (Beverly et al. 2017; Hain et al. 2018).

10.8.7 Rate of Readmissions and Patient Safety

Even though early discharges can cause apprehensions about re-admissions, findings have shown that there is no link between ERAS and high risks of re-admission or re-operation when this approach is applied properly (Greco et al. 2014; Zhuang et al. 2013; Yip et al. 2016). Selection and follow-up are important for safety.

10.8.8 Mortality Risk and Vulnerable Groups

Mortality in elective colon surgery is relatively low, although ERAS is linked to a reduction, especially for older patients and those with comorbid conditions (Bagnall et al. 2014; Greco et al. 2014; Ripollés et al. 2019). Registry analyses reveal that hospitals with high compliance with ERAS report lower rates of 30-day mortality (Ripollés et al. 2019; Hübner et al. 2015).

10.8.9 Utilization of Healthcare Services and Cost-Effectiveness

ERAS brings about significant financial gains, especially due to a decrease in morbidity rates, shorter duration of hospitalization, and optimal resource utilization (Lau and Chamberlain 2017; Cavallaro and Bordeianou 2019). Such benefits have been a contributing factor in making ERAS a benchmark for treatment in colorectal surgery based on well-organized anaesthesia and nutrition practices (Gustafsson et al. 2019; Kahokehr et al. 2009).

10.9 Challenges in Implementing ERAS

Inclusion of ERAS into colorectal surgery demands multidisciplinary collaboration, but its practical execution proves to be rather inconsistent (Kahokehr et al. 2009; Cavallaro and Bordeianou 2019). The obstacles appear on the organizational, professional, and patient sides and impact both analgesia and nutrition, as well as physical activity and ERAS compliance.

10.9.1 Institutional and Resource Barriers

The institutional factors include ineffective coordination between surgeons, anaesthetists, nurses, dietitians, and physiotherapists, and a lack of standardized perioperative pathways (Cavallaro and Bordeianou 2019; Hübner et al. 2015). Inconsistency in multimodal analgesic application may lead to increased use of opioids, delayed bowel recovery, and mobilization. The lack of systematic nutrition protocols would delay the initiation of feeding. Workforce problems and overload may also interfere with the implementation of early mobilization and continuous monitoring as part of ERAS management protocol (Kahokehr et al. 2009).

The financial aspect is another factor that could inhibit the introduction of ERAS due to its associated initial costs (Lau and Chamberlain 2017; Cavallaro and Bordeianou 2019). Recommendations for dealing with these barriers could include implementing standardized ERAS protocols, applying checklists and auditing methods to ensure consistency in their performance, educating the interdisciplinary team on opioid-sparing treatment and early feeding, and assigning perioperative care coordinators (Hübner et al. 2015; Cavallaro and Bordeianou 2019).

10.9.2 Patient-Related Factors

Patient-related barriers are equally important. Patients having sarcopenia, diabetes, and cardiovascular diseases will have reduced tolerance to early mobilization and enteral nutrition. They will also have difficulty managing their pain because these diseases make them sensitive to opioids (GlobalSurg Collaborative and NIHR Global Health Unit on Global Surgery 2023; van Rooijen et al. 2019). Other patient-related issues like low health literacy, poor awareness, and lack of adherence to prehabilitation further limit the adoption of ERAS (Kahokehr et al. 2009).

Structured prehabilitation, including nutrition, exercise, and anaemia management, along with structured preoperative counselling, can be useful in promoting patients' understanding of ERAS and encouraging its adoption (Gillis et al. 2014). Personalized analgesia in the light of comorbidities and proper educational material for patients also helps with early feeding and mobilization approaches (Yip et al. 2016; van Rooijen et al. 2019).

10.9.3 Challenges in Low- and Middle-Income Countries

Additional barriers exist in the implementation of ERAS in LMICs, such as poor infrastructural facilities, staff shortage, and limited availability of advanced technology in surgical procedures and monitoring (Kahokehr et al. 2009). Regional anaesthesia and perioperative nutritional care may not be readily available; opioids may continue to dominate the use of anaesthesia; large numbers of patients coupled with fewer staff members delay early mobilization efforts; and poor access to laparoscopic surgeries exacerbate stress reactions and recovery time (Cavallaro and Bordeianou 2019).

Limited resources, poor knowledge base, and lack of country-specific ERAS protocols pose more barriers to implementing ERAS. The pragmatic approach includes tailoring ERAS protocols according to the hospital's resources, such as prioritizing effective but inexpensive strategies like early mobilization and multimodal analgesia (Kahokehr et al. 2009; Cavallaro and Bordeianou 2019). Implementing pilot projects that incorporate ERAS elements into routine surgical protocols, supplemented by education, training, and outcome audits, proves to yield considerable improvements in patient recovery regardless of partial implementation.

10.10 Future Directions

Further evolution in colorectal ERAS pathways will emphasize more personalization, ongoing quality monitoring, and application of emerging technologies, along with sustained clinical benefits for gastrointestinal function, feeding tolerance, postoperative complications, hospital stay, and repeat admissions (Ljungqvist et al. 2017; Gustafsson et al. 2019). Noting the introduction of entirely novel ideas, advancements will build on current ERAS elements based on personalized risk stratification and scientific developments, such as those from ESPEN and ERAS Society recommendations (Weimann et al. 2025; Gustafsson et al. 2025).

10.10.1 AI in Perioperative Care

AI technology can benefit the ERAS approach for colorectal surgery through risk stratification and process optimization. AI algorithms can predict the likelihood of developing delayed gut motility, feed tolerance, or adverse outcomes, which could then guide clinicians to take proactive measures such as individualized pain management strategies, enhanced nutritional intake, and monitoring signs of ileus (Weimann et al. 2017). In addition, the implementation of AI-driven improvements in glycemic regulation and fluid administration could significantly lower the incidence of complications while meeting ERAS targets, such as prompt gut recovery and decreased lengths of stay (Kwon et al. 2013; Zorrilla-Vaca et al. 2021).

Nevertheless, the efficacy of AI solutions in clinical practice requires adequate validation, workflow integration, and the mitigation of unintended effects; human judgment should not be overlooked.

10.10.2 Precision Nutrition in ERAS

Precision nutrition is a significant milestone in the development of ERAS, where calorie and protein requirements have been tailored into personalized nutrition plans according to the metabolic state, body composition, and inflammation (Weimann et al. 2017; van Rooijen et al. 2019). Within colorectal surgery, the use of precision nutrition could aid in the retention of lean mass, facilitate oral tolerance, and minimize adverse effects, especially among patients with sarcopenia or marked malnutrition (GlobalSurg Collaborative and NIHR Global Health Unit on Global Surgery 2023; Weimann et al. 2017).

Innovative techniques that combine information obtained from diet with genomics, metabolomics, and gut microbiota analysis can reveal patient groups who would derive the greatest benefits from targeted nutrition interventions, such as immunonutrition and protein-enriched prehabilitation (Song et al. 2015; Weimann et al. 2025).

10.10.3 Biomarker-Guided Nutritional Assessment

Nutritional evaluation in the future will likely have a strong focus on biomarker assessment. Classic biomarkers like serum albumin and pre-albumin levels are affected by inflammation and do not serve as true biomarkers for nutritional status (Awad et al. 2013; Weimann et al. 2021). More sophisticated markers include C-reactive protein and the Glasgow prognostic score.

Further evaluation of nutritional status can be accomplished using metabolomics, proteomics, and body composition assessments to understand the complex relationships among malnutrition, sarcopenia, and inflammatory catabolism (GlobalSurg Collaborative and NIHR Global Health Unit on Global Surgery 2023; van Rooijen et al. 2019). Assessment of ERAS patients undergoing colorectal surgery using the above measures could enable earlier recognition of any nutritional deficiencies and lead to better tolerance and outcomes, as well as shorter lengths of stay.

10.10.4 Wearable Monitoring Systems and Telemedicine

The use of wearable devices and telemedicine is expanding ERAS out of hospitals through the use of continuous monitoring of perioperative recovery. Activity monitors, heart rate monitors, and symptom diaries can flag any deviation from normal recovery that may arise, such as low activity levels, low intake, or indicators of dehydration, infection, or ileus, in order to allow for intervention and follow-up (Mathiasen et al. 2021).

For colorectal ERAS programs, remote monitoring can facilitate adherence to mobilization and nutrition targets even after hospital discharge, preventing unnecessary return trips (Yip et al. 2016). The issues surrounding data collection, alert fatigue, technology access, and cost must be managed to implement remote monitoring efficiently.

To conclude, the future directions in colorectal ERAS include data-based personalized care, precise nutrition, biomarker-based evaluation, and digital tracking, all with the objective to improve GI function, nutrition, morbidity, and discharge procedures using sound ERAS protocols (Ljungqvist et al. 2017; Gustafsson et al. 2019; Weimann et al. 2025).

10.11 Conclusion

The evidence described in this chapter clearly demonstrates that successful recovery after surgery of the colon or rectum cannot be achieved with individual strategies, but requires a multidisciplinary approach that incorporates anaesthesiology approaches along with specific nutrition interventions in the context of ERAS guidelines. The stress reaction caused by colorectal surgery includes a variety of physiological responses that include the release of neuroendocrine hormones as part of the HPA pathway, cytokine-related inflammatory response, insulin resistance, protein degradation, and oxidative damage.

The use of modern aesthetic techniques, such as the multimodal approach involving opioids sparingly, regional anaesthesia using thoracic epidural analgesia and TAP block, goal-directed fluid administration, maintaining core temperature, and selective administration of medications like ketamine, lidocaine infusion, and dexmedetomidine, helps in reducing the impact of neuroendocrine and sympathetic elements of the surgical stress response. Alongside the application of nutritional support measures, such as preoperative nutritional evaluation, prehabilitation, carbohydrate loading, no fasting beyond 8 hours, commencement of enteral feeding in 24–48 hours after surgery, immunonutritional support using arginine, glutamine, and omega-3 fatty acids, and strict glycemic control, surgical stress can be effectively controlled metabolically and immunologically.

However, the scientific data show that following the principles of ERAS in terms of anaesthetic and nutritional management leads to fewer cases of postoperative ileus, fewer infections, lower hospital stay, but no increases in readmission or death. According to meta-analyses conducted on the ERAS protocol used in colorectal surgery, it was proven that using ERAS led to shorter stays in hospitals by a few days.

Although there is considerable scientific proof, problems still exist in terms of implementation, ranging from an institutional level to a professional one, as well as in relation to patients. This especially occurs in developing countries where the lack of funding, the lack of cooperation among different professionals, and the lack of laparoscopy and regional anaesthesia represent substantial obstacles.

Going forward, the emergence of AI in perioperative risk stratification, precision nutrition based on metabolomic and body composition assessments, nutritional evaluation based on advanced biomarkers rather than conventional serum albumin levels, and remote monitoring using wearable technology appears promising for an even more patient-specific and optimal ERAS approach. Altogether, these innovations seem capable of transforming the existing evidence-based concept into a precision-perioperative approach, where both anaesthesia and nutrition will be used not just as supporting strategies, but rather as interdependent therapeutic cornerstones of postoperative management in colorectal surgery.

References

Awad S, Varadhan KK, Ljungqvist O, Lobo DN. A meta-analysis of randomised controlled trials on preoperative oral carbohydrate treatment in elective surgery. Clin Nutr. 2013;32(1):34–44. https://doi.org/10.1016/j.clnu.2012.10.011.

Bagnall NM, Malietzis G, Kennedy RH, Athanasiou T, Faiz O, Darzi A. A systematic review of enhanced recovery care after colorectal surgery in elderly patients. Colorectal Dis. 2014;16(12):947–56. https://doi.org/10.1111/codi.12718.

Beverly A, Kaye AD, Ljungqvist O, Urman RD. Essential elements of multimodal analgesia in enhanced recovery after surgery (ERAS) guidelines. Anesthesiol Clin. 2017;35(2):e115–43. https://doi.org/10.1016/j.anclin.2017.01.018.

Bradley J. TNF-mediated inflammatory disease. J Pathol. 2008;214:149–60. https://doi.org/10.1002/path.2287.

Braga M, Gianotti L, Radaelli G, Vignali A, Mari G, Gentilini O, Di Carlo V. Perioperative immunonutrition in patients undergoing cancer surgery: results of a randomized double-blind phase 3 trial. Arch Surg. 1999;134(4):428–33. https://doi.org/10.1001/archsurg.134.4.428.

Braga M, Gianotti L, Vignali A, Carlo VD. Preoperative oral arginine and n-3 fatty acid supplementation improves the immunometabolic host response and outcome after colorectal resection for cancer. Surgery. 2002;132(5):805–14. https://doi.org/10.1067/msy.2002.128350.

Cavallaro P, Bordeianou L. Implementation of an ERAS pathway in colorectal surgery. Clin Colon Rectal Surg. 2019;32(2):102–8. https://doi.org/10.1055/s-0038-1676474.

Elnour M, Radwan Ahmed R, Elkhalifa A, et al. Optimizing postoperative recovery in colorectal surgery: a systematic review on the efficacy of enhanced recovery after surgery (ERAS) protocols. Cureus. 2025;17(8):e90087. https://doi.org/10.7759/cureus.90087.

Elsarrag M, Soldozy S, Patel P, Norat P, Sokolowski JD, Park MS, Tvrdik P, Kalani MYS, Yağmurlu K. Enhanced recovery after surgery (ERAS) protocol in gastrointestinal surgery. J Gastrointest Surg. 2019;23(2):384–93. https://doi.org/10.1007/s11605-018-4022-2.

Feldheiser A, Aziz O, Baldini G, Cox BPBW, Fearon KCH, Feldman LS, Gan TJ, Kennedy RH, Ljungqvist O, Lobo DN, Miller T, Radtke FF, Ruiz Garces T, Schricker T, Scott MJ, Thacker J, Ytrebø LM, Carli F. Enhanced Recovery After Surgery (ERAS) for gastrointestinal surgery, part 2: consensus statement for anaesthesia practice. Acta Anaesthesiol Scand. 2016;60(3):289–334. https://doi.org/10.1111/aas.12651.

Gedda C, Nygren J, Garpenbeck A, Hoffström L, Thorell A, Soop M. Multimodal analgesia bundle and postoperative opioid use among patients undergoing colorectal surgery. JAMA Netw Open. 2023;6(9):e2332408. https://doi.org/10.1001/jamanetworkopen.2023.32408.

Gillis CRD, Carli F. Promoting perioperative metabolic and nutritional care. Anesthesiology. 2015;123(6):1455–72. https://doi.org/10.1097/ALN.0000000000000795.

Gillis C, Li C, Lee L, et al. Prehabilitation versus rehabilitation: a randomized control trial in patients undergoing colorectal resection for cancer. Anesthesiology. 2014;121(5):937–47. https://doi.org/10.1097/aln.0000000000000393.

GlobalSurg Collaborative and NIHR Global Health Unit on Global Surgery. Impact of malnutrition on early outcomes after cancer surgery: an international, multicentre, prospective cohort study. Lancet Glob Health. 2023;11(3):e341–9. https://doi.org/10.1016/S2214-109X(22)00550-2.

Greco M, Capretti G, Beretta L, Gemma M, Pecorelli N, Braga M. Enhanced recovery program in colorectal surgery: a meta-analysis of randomized controlled trials. World J Surg. 2014;38(6):1531–41. https://doi.org/10.1007/s00268-013-2416-8.

Gustafsson UO, Scott MJ, Hubner M, Nygren J, Demartines N, Francis N, Rockall TA, Young-Fadok TM, Hill AG, Soop M, de Boer HD, Urman RD, Chang GJ, Fichera A, Kessler H, Grass F, Whang EE, Fawcett WJ, Carli F, Lobo DN, Rollins KE, Balfour A, Baldini G, Riedel B, Ljungqvist O. Guidelines for perioperative care in elective colorectal surgery: Enhanced Recovery After Surgery (ERAS®) Society recommendations: 2018. World J Surg. 2019;43(3):659–95. https://doi.org/10.1007/s00268-018-4844-y.

Gustafsson UO, Rockall TA, Wexner S, How KY, Emile S, Marchuk A, Fawcett WJ, Sioson M, Riedel B, Chahal R, Balfour A, Baldini G, de Groof EJ, Romagnoli S, Coca-Martinez M, Grass F, Brindle M, Hubner M. Guidelines for perioperative care in elective colorectal surgery: Enhanced Recovery After Surgery (ERAS) Society recommendations 2025. Surgery. 2025;184:109397. https://doi.org/10.1016/j.surg.2025.109397.

Hain E, Maggiori L, Prost à la Denise J, Panis Y. Transversus abdominis plane (TAP) block in laparoscopic colorectal surgery improves postoperative pain management: a meta-analysis. Color Dis. 2018;20:279–87. https://doi.org/10.1111/codi.14037.

Hamid HKS, Ahmed AY, Mohammed SH. Transversus abdominis plane block versus thoracic epidural analgesia in colorectal surgery: a systematic review and meta-analysis. Surg Endosc. 2020;34(11):4733–45. https://doi.org/10.1007/s00464-020-07599-2.

Han H, Wan R, Chen J, Fan X, Zhang L. Effects of the enhanced recovery after surgery (ERAS) protocol on the postoperative stress state and short-term complications in elderly patients with colorectal cancer. Cancer Rep (Hoboken). 2024;7(2):e1979. https://doi.org/10.1002/cnr2.1979.

Hübner M, Addor V, Slieker J, Griesser AC, Lécureux E, Blanc C, Demartines N. The impact of an enhanced recovery pathway on nursing workload: a retrospective cohort study. Int J Surg. 2015;24(Pt A):45–50. https://doi.org/10.1016/j.ijsu.2015.10.025.

Hughes CE, Nibbs RJB. A guide to chemokines and their receptors. FEBS J. 2018;285:2944–71. https://doi.org/10.1111/febs.14466.

Kahokehr A, Sammour T, Zargar-Shoshtari K, Thompson L, Hill AG. Implementation of ERAS and how to overcome the barriers. Int J Surg. 2009;7(1):16–9. https://doi.org/10.1016/j.ijsu.2008.11.006.

Kehlet H, Wilmore DW. Multimodal strategies to improve surgical outcome. Am J Surg. 2002;183(6):630–41. https://doi.org/10.1016/S0002-9610(02)00866-8.

Kim MK. The latest results and future directions of research for enhanced recovery after surgery in the field of colorectal surgery. Ewha Med J. 2023;46(Suppl 1):e23. https://doi.org/10.12771/emj.2023.e23.

Kwon S, Thompson R, Dellinger P, Yanez D, Farrohki E, Flum D. Importance of perioperative glycemic control in general surgery: a report from the Surgical Care and Outcomes Assessment Program. Ann Surg. 2013;257(1):8–14. https://doi.org/10.1097/SLA.0b013e31827b6bbc.

Lassen K, Kjaeve J, Fetveit T, Trano G, Sigurdsson HK, Horn A, Revhaug A, Norwegian Gastrointestinal Surgery Group. Allowing normal food at will after major upper gastrointestinal surgery does not increase morbidity: a randomized multicenter trial. Ann Surg. 2008;247(5):721–9. https://doi.org/10.1097/SLA.0b013e31815cca68.

Lau CS, Chamberlain RS. Enhanced recovery after surgery programs improve patient outcomes and recovery: a meta-analysis. World J Surg. 2017;41(4):899–913. https://doi.org/10.1007/s00268-016-3807-4.

Lewis SJ, Andersen HK, Thomas S. Early enteral nutrition within 24 h of intestinal surgery versus later commencement of feeding: a systematic review and meta-analysis. J Gastrointest Surg. 2009;13(3):569–75. https://doi.org/10.1007/s11605-008-0592-x.

Ljungqvist O, Scott M, Fearon KC. Enhanced recovery after surgery: a review. JAMA Surg. 2017;152(3):292–8. https://doi.org/10.1001/jamasurg.2016.4952.

Mathiasen MC, Andersen RM, Schmidt DS, Thomsen T. Early mobilisation after colorectal surgery: a qualitative study. Gastrointest Nurs. 2021;19(3):30–6. https://doi.org/10.12968/gasn.2021.19.3.30.

Moya P, Miranda E, Soriano-Irigaray L, et al. Perioperative immunonutrition in normo-nourished patients undergoing laparoscopic colorectal resection. Surg Endosc. 2016;30(11):4946–53. https://doi.org/10.1007/s00464-016-4836-7.

Prete FP, Pezzolla A, Prete F, et al. Robotic versus laparoscopic minimally invasive surgery for rectal cancer: a systematic review and meta-analysis of randomized controlled trials. Ann Surg. 2018;267(6):1034–46. https://doi.org/10.1097/sla.0000000000002523.

Ricciotti E, FitzGerald GA. Prostaglandins and inflammation. Arterioscler Thromb Vasc Biol. 2011;31(5):986–1000. https://doi.org/10.1161/ATVBAHA.110.207449.

Ripollés-Melchor J, Ramírez-Rodríguez JM, Casans-Francés R, Aldecoa C, Abad-Motos A, Logroño-Egea M, García-Erce JA, Argente-Navarro MP, González-Bris A, Garcia-Fernandez J, POWER Study Investigators Group. Association between use of enhanced recovery after surgery protocol and postoperative complications in colorectal surgery: the postoperative outcomes within enhanced recovery after surgery protocol (POWER) study. JAMA Surg. 2019;154(8):725–36. https://doi.org/10.1001/jamasurg.2019.0995.

Rizk E, Haas EM, Swan JT. Opioid-sparing effect of liposomal bupivacaine and intravenous acetaminophen in colorectal surgery. J Surg Res. 2021;259:230–41. https://doi.org/10.1016/j.jss.2020.09.002.

Scott MJ, Baldini G, Fearon KCH, Feldheiser A, Feldman LS, Gan TJ, Ljungqvist O, Lobo DN, Rockall TA, Schricker T, Carli F. Enhanced Recovery After Surgery (ERAS) for gastrointestinal surgery, part 1: pathophysiological considerations. Acta Anaesthesiol Scand. 2015;59(10):1212–31. https://doi.org/10.1111/aas.12601.

Shimabukuro-Vornhagen A, Draube A, Liebig TM, et al. The immunosuppressive factors IL-10, TGF-β, and VEGF do not affect the antigen-presenting function of CD40-activated B cells. J Exp Clin Cancer Res. 2012;31:47. https://doi.org/10.1186/1756-9966-31-47.

Smith MD, McCall J, Plank L, Herbison GP, Soop M, Nygren J. Preoperative carbohydrate treatment for enhancing recovery after elective surgery. Cochrane Database Syst Rev. 2014;2014(8):CD009161. https://doi.org/10.1002/14651858.CD009161.pub2.

Song GM, Tian X, Liang H, Yi LJ, Zhou JG, Zeng Z, Ou YX. Role of enteral immunonutrition in patients undergoing surgery for gastric cancer: a systematic review and meta-analysis of randomized controlled trials. Medicine. 2015;94(31):e1311. https://doi.org/10.1097/MD.0000000000001311.

Tanaka T, Narazaki M, Kishimoto T. IL-6 in inflammation, immunity, and disease. Cold Spring Harb Perspect Biol. 2014;6(10):a016295. https://doi.org/10.1101/cshperspect.a016295.

van Rooijen S, Carli F, Dalton S, et al. Multimodal prehabilitation in colorectal cancer patients to improve functional capacity and reduce postoperative complications: the first international randomized controlled trial for multimodal prehabilitation. BMC Cancer. 2019;19:98. https://doi.org/10.1186/s12885-018-5232-6.

Vather R, O'Grady G, Bissett IP, Dinning PG. Postoperative ileus: mechanisms and future directions for research. Clin Exp Pharmacol Physiol. 2014;41(5):358–70. https://doi.org/10.1111/1440-1681.12220.

Vigneault L, Turgeon AF, Côté D, Lauzier F, Zarychanski R, Moore L, McIntyre LA, Nicole PC, Fergusson DA. Perioperative intravenous lidocaine infusion for postoperative pain control: a meta-analysis of randomized controlled trials. Can J Anaesth. 2011;58(1):22–37. https://doi.org/10.1007/s12630-010-9407-0.

Waitzberg DL, Saito H, Plank LD, Jamieson GG, Jagannath P, Hwang TL, Mijares JM, Bihari D. Postsurgical infections are reduced with specialized nutrition support. World J Surg. 2006;30(8):1592–604. https://doi.org/10.1007/s00268-005-0657-x.

Weber A, Wasiliew P, Kracht M. Interleukin-1 (IL-1) pathway. Sci Signal. 2010;3(105):cm1. https://doi.org/10.1126/scisignal.3105cm1.

Weimann A, Braga M, Carli F, Higashiguchi T, Hübner M, Klek S, Laviano A, Ljungqvist O, Lobo DN, Martindale R, Waitzberg DL, Bischoff SC, Singer P. ESPEN guideline: clinical nutrition in surgery. Clin Nutr. 2017;36(3):623–50. https://doi.org/10.1016/j.clnu.2017.02.013.

Weimann A, Braga M, Carli F, Higashiguchi T, Hübner M, Klek S, Laviano A, Ljungqvist O, Lobo DN, Martindale RG, Waitzberg D, Bischoff SC, Singer P. ESPEN practical guideline: clinical nutrition in surgery. Clin Nutr. 2021;40(7):4745–61. https://doi.org/10.1016/j.clnu.2021.03.031.

Weimann A, Bezmarevic M, Braga M, Correia MITD, Funk-Debleds P, Gianotti L, Gillis C, Hübner M, Inciong JFB, Jahit MS, Klek S, Kori T, Laviano A, Ljungqvist O, Lobo DN, Loinaz Segurola C, Montroni I, Reddy BR, Saur NM, Schweinlin A, et al. ESPEN guideline on clinical nutrition in surgery—update 2025. Clin Nutr. 2025;53:222–61. https://doi.org/10.1016/j.clnu.2025.08.029.

White PF, Kehlet H, Neal JM, Schricker T, Carr DB, Carli F. The role of the anesthesiologist in fast-track surgery: from multimodal analgesia to perioperative medical care. Anesth Analg. 2007;104(6):1380–96. https://doi.org/10.1213/01.ane.0000263034.96885.e1.

Wijnberge M, Schenk J, Bulle E, Vlaar AP, Maheshwari K, Hollmann MW, Binnekade JM, Geerts BF, Veelo DP. Association of intraoperative hypotension with postoperative morbidity and mortality: systematic review and meta-analysis. BJS Open. 2021;5(1):zraa018. https://doi.org/10.1093/bjsopen/zraa018.

Wu Q, Liu Y, et al. From support to strategy: the evolving role of perioperative nutrition in regulating the prognosis of colorectal cancer surgery. Curr Surg Rep. 2025:100110. https://doi.org/10.1016/j.cson.2025.100110.

Yip VS, Dunne DFJ, Samuels S, Tan CY, Lacasia C, Tang J, Burston C, Malik HZ, Poston GJ, Fenwick SW. Adherence to early mobilisation: key for successful enhanced recovery after liver resection. Eur J Surg Oncol. 2016;42(10):1561–7. https://doi.org/10.1016/j.ejso.2016.07.015.

Yu HM, Ou GY, Che Y, Huang Y, Li GX, Zhuang K. Early enteral nutrition versus parenteral nutrition after resection of esophageal cancer: a retrospective analysis. Indian J Surg. 2017;79(1):13–8. https://doi.org/10.1007/s12262-015-1420-7.

Zhao X, Jin S, Peng M, Wang J. A retrospective study on the efficacy of the ERAS protocol in patients who underwent laparoscopic left and right colectomy surgeries. Front Surg. 2024;11:1395271. https://doi.org/10.3389/fsurg.2024.1395271.

Zhuang CL, Ye XZ, Zhang XD, Chen BC, Yu Z. Enhanced recovery after surgery programs versus traditional care for colorectal surgery: a meta-analysis of randomized controlled trials. Dis Colon Rectum. 2013;56(5):667–78. https://doi.org/10.1097/DCR.0b013e3182812842.

Zorrilla-Vaca A, Mena GE, Ripolles-Melchor J, Abad-Motos A, Aldecoa C, Lorente JV, Ramirez-Rodriguez JM, Grant MC. Goal-directed fluid therapy and postoperative outcomes in an enhanced recovery program for colorectal surgery: a propensity score-matched multicenter study. Am Surg. 2021;87(8):1189–95. https://doi.org/10.1177/0003134820973365.

Fast-Track Anesthesia and Early Nutrition in Cardiac ERAS

11

Dheeraj Barma and Abhinav

Abstract

The implementation of Enhanced Recovery After Surgery (ERAS) protocols has revolutionized the perioperative management process in various surgical fields, and a similar approach to Enhance Recovery After Cardiac Surgery (ERACS) is gaining increasing traction internationally. Indeed, performing cardiac surgery involves many physiological, anesthetic, and nutritional concerns related to cardiopulmonary bypass (CPB), ischemia-reperfusion injury, inflammatory response, and the presence of associated medical conditions. In this chapter, we review current research findings and clinical guidelines concerning the use of ERAS strategies for adult cardiac surgery, emphasizing anesthetics and nutrition in particular.

The topics covered include patient selection and stratification, perioperative optimization and prehabilitation, anesthesia techniques to achieve fast-track and ultra-fast extubation, multimodal opioid-sparing analgesia, hemodynamics and fluid administration, blood conservation, and early mobility. Following this, there is a comprehensive discussion of perioperative nutrition evaluation and support, which includes nutritional screening for malnutrition and sarcopenia, carbohydrate loading, early enteral nutrition, macronutrient requirements, and nutritional interventions for selected populations (e.g., frailty, obesity, diabetes,

D. Barma (✉)
Allied Health Sciences, Vivekananda Global University, Jaipur, Rajasthan, India
e-mail: Dheeraj.barma@vgu.ac.in

Abhinav
Department of Operation Theater Technology, Vivekananda Global University, Jaipur, Rajasthan, India
e-mail: abhinav.1@vgu.ac.in

P. K. Bhattacharyya et al. (eds.), *Integrated Anesthesia and Nutrition Approaches to Enhanced Recovery after Surgery*,
https://doi.org/10.1007/978-981-92-3294-9_11

and renal failure). Based on evidence generated from randomized trials, observational studies, and meta-analyses, ERACS bundles appear to shorten the duration of mechanical ventilation and ICU stay, decrease morbidity, and may improve mortality.

The practicalities involved in the process of implementation of the program, standards of quality, and auditing approaches are discussed, placing emphasis on the importance of interdisciplinary teamwork involving surgeons, anesthesiologists, intensive care physicians, nurses, dieticians, physical therapists, and pharmacists. The issues of knowledge gaps and research needs include topics such as ideal nutritional regimens, accurate hemodynamic goals, and evidence-based ERACS tailored to each individual patient's needs.

Keywords

Enhanced Recovery After Cardiac Surgery (ERACS) · Cardiac anesthesia · Perioperative nutrition · Fast-track extubation · Early enteral nutrition

11.1 Introduction

11.1.1 Evolution of ERAS and Emergence of ERACS

ERAS was initially introduced in colorectal surgery towards the end of the 1990s as a multimodal approach using evidence-based perioperative pathways with the aim of minimizing surgical stress, maintaining physiological function, and speeding up recovery (Kehlet 1997; Gustafsson et al. 2016). Research evidence from studies carried out in abdominal surgery, orthopedic surgery, thoracic surgery, and bariatric surgery shows that ERAS pathways can lower the risk of complications and hospital stays by as much as 30–50% without increasing the rate of readmissions (Gustafsson et al. 2016; Ljungqvist et al. 2017). Because of its potential benefits, the ERAS society has developed guidelines for specific procedures (ERAS Society 2021; Gustafsson et al. 2016).

Cardiac surgery had traditionally been slow in adopting ERAS strategies due to potential issues related to hemodynamic instability, lengthy mechanical ventilation, and the inherent vulnerability of patients undergoing CPB (Gunaydin et al. 2024). But recent improvements in the surgical procedure, anesthesia, myocardial preservation, and critical care management, as well as the need to enhance productivity and cost-effectiveness, have spurred innovations in ERACS programs (Navas-Blanco et al. 2024). The landmark ERAS Society consensus statement authored by Engelman and others, as well as national guidelines, like the French SFAR/SFCTCV guideline, serve as blueprints for ERACS delivery (Engelman et al. 2019; Mertes et al. 2022).

11.1.2 Rationale for Focusing on Anesthesia and Nutrition

Anesthesia and perioperative medicine are essential for ERACS since they affect almost all physiologically modifiable parameters such as cardiovascular function, neuroendocrine responses, ventilation, and pain management (Navas-Blanco et al. 2024). The implementation of fast-track and ultra-fast-track anesthesia for cardiac surgery, where the goal is extubation in 6–8 hours or even intraoperatively, is another important pillar of ERACS and relies on appropriate medication choice, anesthetic depth, and postoperative pain treatment (Cheng et al. 1996; Ender et al. 2008).

However, malnutrition, sarcopenia, and dysmetabolism are frequent in cardiac surgery patients, especially older people who have heart failure, valve diseases, or chronic kidney disease (Stoppe et al. 2017). Malnutrition correlates with higher risks for infection, increased ICU time, and mortality, but proper nutritional management will help reduce catabolism, maintain gut health, and increase positive clinical results (Hill et al. 2018). Nonetheless, nutrition has remained an underappreciated aspect of cardiac surgery (Weimann et al. 2021).

Thus, this chapter will focus on the inclusion of anesthesia and nutrition management within the ERACS framework, considering that there are two-way connections between them, such as the effect of sedation and vasopressors on gut perfusion and feeding tolerance, as well as the effect of metabolic reserves on anesthesia pharmacodynamics and extubation (Hill et al. 2018; Weimann et al. 2021).

11.2 Pathophysiology of Cardiac Surgery and Implications for ERACS

11.2.1 Surgical Stress, CPB, and Systemic Inflammation

Cardiac surgery with CPB causes significant inflammatory and neuroendocrine changes involving complement system activation, cytokine secretion, endothelial dysfunction, and capillary leakage. Hemodilution, hypothermia, ischemia-reperfusion injury, and contact between blood and non-endothelial surfaces enhance this reaction, causing dysfunction of vital organs such as the lungs, kidneys, brain, and the gut (Gunaydin et al. 2024; Hirai 2003). This physiology is relevant to several ERACS components like strict temperature control, restrictive transfusion guidelines, lung-protective ventilation, and early ambulation (Navas-Blanco et al. 2024).

11.2.2 Hemodynamic Instability and Organ Perfusion

Hemodynamic instability in cardiac surgery arises due to baseline ventricular dysfunction, myocardial stunning during the operation, vasoplegia, arrhythmia, and fluid shifts. Too much fluid infusion may cause pulmonary edema and right ventricular dysfunction, whereas inadequate volume may lead to inadequate renal and intestinal perfusion. According to the ERACS guidelines, the use of goal-directed therapy, utilizing invasive monitoring including arterial blood pressure, central venous or pulmonary artery pressures, and echocardiography, is advocated (Mertes et al. 2022; Grant et al. 2024).

This is because these changes influence the safe and optimal timing for early extubation and enteral nutrition. For instance, hemodynamically unstable individuals might not tolerate aggressive ventilatory and nutritional support withdrawal well, while stable individuals can have their breathing support withdrawn quickly and receive enteral feeding early on (Reignier et al. 2018; Weimann et al. 2021).

11.2.3 Metabolic and Nutritional Consequences

The operation causes a condition of heightened metabolism with higher energy requirement, insulin resistance, catabolism, and lipolysis (Stoppe et al. 2017). The use of CPB and fasting results in depleted glycogen stores and negative nitrogen balance, especially among patients with reduced preoperative nutritional status. Studies have reported cases of malnutrition, significant energy deficits, and protein loss in ICU stays after cardiac operations (Hill et al. 2018; Weimann et al. 2021).

Nutrition intervention within ERACS aims to counteract such consequences via pre-operative optimization (screening, supplementation, glycogen loading), as well as early post-operative provision of enteral nutrition adjusted to patients' tolerability and metabolic risk profile (Hill et al. 2018). Proper nutrition helps to promote recovery, including wound healing and immunocompetence, and contributes to respiratory muscle strengthening, issues related to anesthesia and ventilator weaning approaches (Stoppe et al. 2017; Weimann et al. 2021).

11.3 ERAS and ERACS Frameworks and Guidelines

11.3.1 ERAS Society Cardiac Surgery Recommendations

Engelman and colleagues' ERAS Society guideline represents the cornerstone of perioperative management in cardiac surgery patients. The guideline integrates evidence from meta-analyses, randomized trials, and large observational studies to develop evidence-based guidelines for pre-operative, operative, and post-operative care. Important aspects include patient education and engagement, fasting minimization, glycogen loading, standardized anesthetic regimen with multimodal pain control, lung-protective ventilatory strategy, restrictive blood transfusion policy, early extubation, early ambulation, and audits (Engelman et al. 2019).

Specifically, the guidelines identify the importance of conducting nutritional assessment, which includes pre-operative malnutrition screening (such as the Subjective Global Assessment and NRS-2002), postoperative nutrition support using enteral feeding if possible, and management of glycemia and protein energy requirements (Stoppe et al. 2017; Hill et al. 2018).

11.3.2 National and Specialty Society Guidelines

Guidelines on ERACS from France, released in 2022, support the guidelines produced by the ERAS Society through the provision of recommendations for six specific areas, namely pathway selection and education of patients, preoperative management and rehabilitation, anesthetic technique and analgesia, operative approach and coronary artery bypass grafting technique, perioperative patient blood management, and enhanced recovery after operation. The French guidelines emphasize early extubation, multimodal analgesic approach, and early nutrition as key measures in ERACS, among other important recommendations (Mertes et al. 2022).

Similar contemporary consensus guidelines from anesthetic and cardiothoracic surgical societies also emphasize the importance of perioperative medicine involving a multidisciplinary approach, incorporation of fast-track anesthesia, and use of care bundles to minimize variation (Grant et al. 2024; Wainwright et al. 2019). Many institutions have incorporated such guidelines in their own set of order templates/checklist procedures in collaboration with their ERAS or perioperative medicine teams (ERAS Cardiac Society 2025; Navas-Blanco et al. 2024).

11.3.3 Evidence from Reviews and Meta-Analyses

It has been evidenced from systematic reviews and narrative reviews that the ERACS pathway is safe and also results in shorter mechanical ventilation days, ICU stay, and hospital stay, and even lesser complications at times, although the effects on mortality are not as pronounced (Hoogma et al. 2025; Navas-Blanco et al. 2024). In a systematic review carried out by Zhang et al., it was revealed that the use of the ERACS pathway led to shorter ICU stay and ventilation period without causing more reintubations or re-admissions (Zhang et al. 2022).

A study by Navas-Blanco and others carried out in 2024 found that there was evidence to show that ERACS contributes to improved postoperative outcomes based on the measurement of several parameters, although the authors noted that more high quality randomized trials were needed (Navas-Blanco et al. 2024). In another study by Hoogma et al., conducted in 2025, meta-analysis revealed that structured ER programs in cardiac surgery decreased the length of stay at hospitals without an increase in complications, when compared to the conventional fast track program (Hoogma et al. 2025).

11.4 Preoperative Phase: Patient Selection, Risk Stratification, and Optimization

11.4.1 Patient Selection and Risk Stratification for ERACS

All cardiac surgical patients may not be equal candidates for an ERACS program. Selection criteria weigh the potential advantages of early recovery against the possibility of instability or even failure (Engelman et al. 2019; Navas-Blanco et al. 2024). Patients who have low or medium risks and undergo elective CABG or single valve surgeries are usually ideal candidates for such a process, whereas those who suffer from extreme ventricular dysfunction or undergo complex surgeries, or even have high pulmonary hypertension, might need adjustments (Ender et al. 2008; Grant et al. 2024).

Risk stratification scores like EuroSCORE II and STS risk models are used to determine baseline mortality and morbidity rates that may guide ERACS preparation (Nashef et al. 2012; O'Brien et al. 2009). Preoperative spirometry, physical fitness, frailty scoring, and nutritional assessment further improve risk predictions and target prehabilitation programs (Hill et al. 2018; Navas-Blanco et al. 2024). Even patients not suitable for ultra-fast-track extubation will gain from ERACS elements like education, early mobilization, and nutrition optimization (Engelman et al. 2019). Preoperative risk stratification, prehabilitation, and carbohydrate loading, intraoperative fast-track anesthesia and hemodynamic optimization, and postoperative early extubation, mobilization, and nutritional achievement are illustrated in Fig. 11.1.

11.4.2 Preoperative Education and Patient Engagement

ERACS is characterized by patient-centered approaches, which include patient education prior to surgery and decision-making (Engelman et al. 2019). This involves counseling sessions that focus on teaching patients about the surgery process, post-operative pathway, pain management options, mobility and breathing techniques, and nutritional advice (ERAS Cardiac Society 2025; Wainwright et al. 2019). This helps increase patient satisfaction and compliance with early mobilization and feeding recommendations (Ljungqvist et al. 2017).

Patient and caregiver involvement in the process of recovery is encouraged through active participation, such as performing incentive spirometry, walking, monitoring dietary intake, and reporting symptoms early on (Navas-Blanco et al. 2024). Education before surgery serves as an ideal opportunity for setting expectations around fast-track extubation and transfer from the ICU, making it less stressful when the care pathway differs from that of prolonged ICU stay (Engelman et al. 2019).

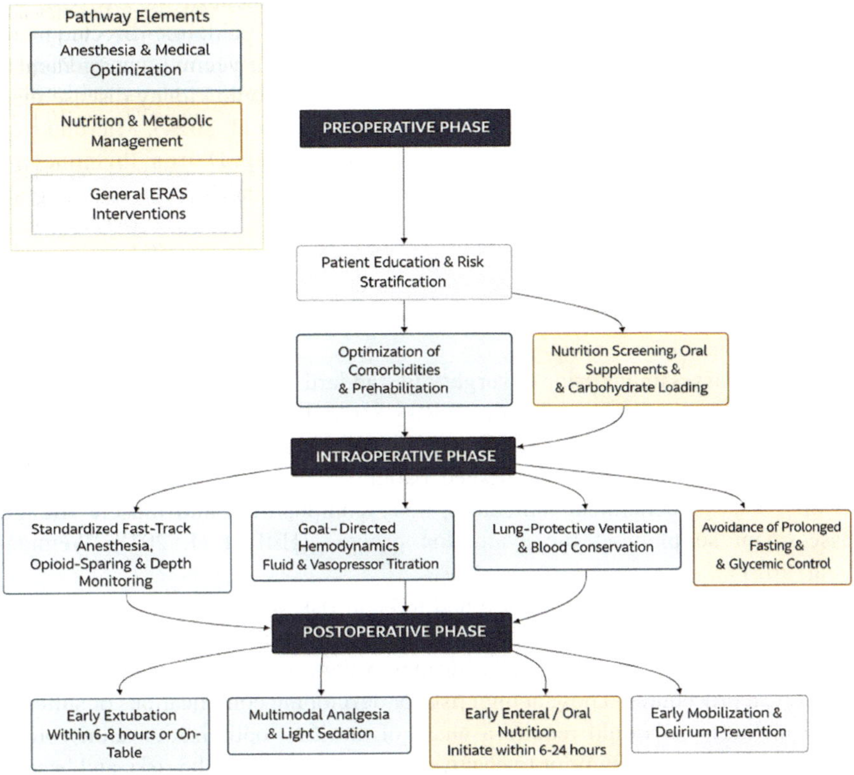

Fig. 11.1 Schematic of an ERACS pathway highlighting key anesthesia and nutrition elements across the preoperative, intraoperative, and postoperative phases. (The image has been created by using Mermaid.com)

11.4.3 Prehabilitation and Optimization of Comorbidities

There is emerging evidence supporting prehabilitation programs that integrate aerobic exercise, resistance training, respiratory physiotherapy, optimal nutrition, and psychological counseling to increase functional status before cardiac surgery and improve postsurgical outcomes (Navas-Blanco et al. 2024). Although there is limited research in cardiac surgery compared to cancer or orthopedic procedures, some preliminary results indicate an improvement in maximal oxygen uptake, muscle strength, and overall well-being (Steinmetz et al. 2026; McIsaac et al. 2022).

Comorbidities optimization is an important component of the ERACS. The tight regulation of heart failure (maximal utilization of guideline-directed medical therapy), the optimization of arrhythmia, anemia, glycemic management in diabetic patients, cessation of smoking, as well as chronic kidney disease management are suggested (Engelman et al. 2019; Grant et al. 2024). Micronutrient deficiency detection and correction (for example, vitamin D, iron, thiamine) and sarcopenia via dietitian-based intervention will help enhance metabolic resilience (Hill et al. 2018; Stoppe et al. 2017).

11.4.4 Preoperative Nutritional Assessment and Interventions

Nutritional assessment prior to surgery is standard practice in ERACS systems. Standardized tools such as Nutritional Risk Screening (NRS-2002), Malnutrition Universal Screening Tool (MUST), and Subjective Global Assessment (SGA) aid in the detection of malnourished patients (Kondrup et al. 2003; Stratton et al. 2004). Biochemical indicators, body composition, and muscle strength assessment supplement the evaluation process (Hill et al. 2018; Weimann et al. 2021).

Those patients who have been found to be at risk would also require interventions such as the use of oral nutritional supplements containing proteins and energy, treating deficiency conditions, and educating patients on caloric consumption prior to surgical procedures. Those at high risk for developing complications or suffering from malnutrition would require a phase of nutrition optimization either orally, enterally, or parenterally prior to elective surgeries, weighing the risks and benefits (Hill et al. 2018; Stoppe et al. 2017).

Insulin resistance is minimized by carbohydrate loading with carbohydrate-based drinks within 2 hours prior to anesthetization and also decreases the length of hospital stay in cases of heart surgery, just like in non-heart surgeries (Gustafsson et al. 2016; Tran et al. 2013). Carbohydrate loading is included in ERACS protocols for those not at risk of aspiration, in addition to minimizing the period of fasting (i.e., drinking clear liquids up to 2 hours and eating solids up to 6 hours prior to surgery) (Engelman et al. 2019) (Table 11.1).

Table 11.1 Core ERAS/ERACS elements in cardiac surgery with emphasis on anesthesia and nutrition

Perioperative phase	Anesthesia-focused elements	Nutrition-focused elements
Preoperative	Risk stratification, optimization of comorbidities, patient education, planning for fast-track extubation (Engelman et al. 2019; Mertes et al. 2022)	Nutrition screening, correction of deficiencies, oral supplements, carbohydrate loading, counseling (Hill et al. 2018; Stoppe et al. 2017)
Intraoperative	Standardized balanced anesthesia, depth monitoring, lung-protective ventilation, goal-directed hemodynamics, blood conservation, temperature control (Engelman et al. 2019; Grant et al. 2024)	Avoidance of unnecessary fasting, limitation of glucose-containing fluids, planning for early postoperative feeding (Engelman et al. 2019; Weimann et al. 2021)
Postoperative ICU	Fast-track extubation protocols, multimodal analgesia, light sedation, delirium prevention (Cheng et al. 1996; Ender et al. 2008)	Early enteral nutrition, progressive advancement to targets, monitoring tolerance and metabolic control (Hill et al. 2018; Reignier et al. 2018)
Ward and discharge	Analgesia optimization, mobilization, sleep, and delirium management (Navas-Blanco et al. 2024)	Ongoing nutrition counseling, adequacy of intake, preparation for home nutrition plan (Weimann et al. 2021)

11.5 Intraoperative Anesthesia Management in ERACS

11.5.1 Principles of Fast-Track and Ultra-Fast-Track Cardiac Anesthesia

Fast-track cardiac anesthesia involves techniques that will allow tracheal extubation of the patient within 6–8 hours following surgery, whereas ultra-fast-track anesthesia involves extubation within the operating theater or up to 1–3 hours after surgery (Ender et al. 2008). Fast-track anesthesia relies on balanced anesthesia using reduced amounts of long-acting opioids, fine-tuned hypnotics, tight hemodynamic control, as well as temperature and fluid management (Cheng et al. 1996; Grant et al. 2024).

According to the Cochrane systematic review and various meta-analyses conducted on fast-track heart surgeries in adults, there was no significant difference in mortality rate, incidence of myocardial infarction, stroke, or re-intubation, but shorter durations in ICU and hospital were observed in many studies conducted (Hamilton et al. 2011; Hoogma et al. 2025). Various reviews conducted later have confirmed that fast-track extubation, if performed on appropriate patients, is not dangerous and helps prevent ventilation-related complications (Navas-Blanco et al. 2024).

11.5.2 Anesthetic Drug Strategies and Depth of Anesthesia

ERACS guidelines recommend a multimodal approach to pain management, with a reduction in the usage of potent opioids. Anesthesia during surgery frequently involves a combination of one of the inhalational anesthetics like sevoflurane and desflurane or one of the intravenous drugs, namely, propofol, along with low- or moderate-dose short-acting opioids like fentanyl, sufentanil, or remifentanil and regional anesthesia in conjunction with non-opioid pain relief modalities (Kietaibl et al. 2022; Grant et al. 2024). The use of monitoring for the depth of anesthesia can prevent over- or under-sedation (Wainwright et al. 2019).

Dexmedetomidine infusion during surgery can give anxiety relief, reduce sympathetic response, and reduce opioids; however, hypotension and bradycardia should be controlled during the procedure (Navas-Blanco et al. 2024; Shehabi et al. 2019). The blockade can be reversed immediately, while body temperature is normalized before extubation (Engelman et al. 2019).

11.5.3 Hemodynamic, Fluid, and Temperature Management

Goal-directed hemodynamics is essential for effective ERACS anesthesia. This includes personalized titration of fluids, pressors, and inotropic agents using invasive and echocardiography assessments (Mertes et al. 2022). The overinfusion of fluids is minimized, with the timely application of pressor drugs such as norepinephrine and vasopressin to counter vasoplegia and inotropic agents such as dobutamine and milrinone for hypodynamic conditions (Grant et al. 2024).

CPB management should aim for minimal hemodilution (e.g., high priming hematocrit, cell salvage), maintain appropriate perfusion pressures, and minimize systemic inflammatory reactions through biocompatibility of the circuit and temperature maintenance (Gunaydin et al. 2024; Hirai 2003). Rewarming the patient and preventing postoperative shivering help to achieve extubation early. Techniques such as minimizing allogenic blood use, using restrictive transfusion criteria, point-of-care clotting tests, and protamine dosing contribute to this goal(Engelman et al. 2019; Mertes et al. 2022).

11.5.4 Airway Management, Ventilation, and Criteria for Early Extubation

Intraoperative ventilation uses lung-protective measures involving reduced tidal volumes and adequate positive end-expiratory pressure during single-lung ventilation during minimally invasive surgery and following CPB (Grant et al. 2024; Wainwright et al. 2019). Lung recruitment maneuvers are utilized appropriately. At the conclusion of the procedure, the patient's suitability for extubation is evaluated on the basis of stable hemodynamics, adequate gas exchange, normothermia, minimal bleeding, and neurologic response (Cheng et al. 1996; Ender et al. 2008).

Both retrospective and prospective analyses of early extubation protocols for cardiac surgeries have found a high percentage (>70%) of patients capable of being extubated either in the operating theater or shortly afterwards with a minimal risk of reintubation (Ender et al. 2008; Plümer et al. 1998). Predictors of successful extubation in the operating theater include low pre-operative risk scoring, good lung function, low CPB time, and no need for inotropic or vasopressor medications (O'Brien et al. 2009).

11.5.5 Interaction of Anesthesia with Perioperative Nutrition

Anesthetics and vasoactive medications can affect gut perfusion, motility, and permeability, impacting enteral feeding's timing and tolerance (Hill et al. 2018; Reignier et al. 2018). Propofol and inhalation anesthetics can cause delayed gastric emptying, whereas opioids slow down gut motility, leading to ileus (Reignier et al. 2018). Consequently, opioid-sparing approaches and minimizing anesthesia become key principles of ERACS guidelines, with the objective of transitioning to light sedation (e.g., dexmedetomidine or low-dose propofol) to enable early feeding (Navas-Blanco et al. 2024; Weimann et al. 2021).

Hemodynamic management is aligned with nutrition strategies where hemodynamically unstable patients may require withholding enteral feeding initially or using trophic feeds cautiously to prevent any potential ischemia in the intestines (Reignier et al. 2018). On the contrary, hemodynamically stable patients may reap the benefits of early enteral feeding within 6–24 hours of surgical procedures by taking advantage of their intact gastrointestinal functions (Hill et al. 2018; Stoppe et al. 2017).

11.6 Postoperative Analgesia, Sedation, and Delirium Prevention

11.6.1 Multimodal, Opioid-Sparing Analgesia

Pain relief following thoracotomy/sternotomy procedures must be optimal for adequate coughing, ventilation, mobility, and rest, and hence has direct influence on respiratory adverse effects and recovery (Engelman et al. 2019). Multimodal analgesia using regular administration of paracetamol/acetaminophen, NSAIDS when the kidney function allows it, gabapentinoids in select cases, and regional anesthesia techniques with opioids used sparingly or for moderate-to-severe pain, is recommended by ERACS (Kietaibl et al. 2022; Wainwright et al. 2019).

The regional anesthesia techniques available are paravertebral blocks, erector spinae plane blocks, pecto-intercostal fascial plane blocks, and continuous wound infiltration catheters, with all these techniques showing a reduction in opioid use and better pain scores among individuals undergoing cardiac surgery (Kietaibl et al. 2022; Macaire et al. 2019). The epidural anesthesia technique has an analgesic advantage but has the risk of developing epidural hematomas, particularly in patients on anticoagulants (Wainwright et al. 2019).

11.6.2 Sedation Strategies to Enable Early Extubation

Postoperative sedation seeks to preserve both comfort and safety while enabling neurological evaluation and ventilatory efforts. Light sedation using dexmedetomidine or propofol is recommended, whereas deep sedation utilizing benzodiazepines is discouraged (Wainwright et al. 2019). Although dexmedetomidine has analgesia-sparing properties and reduced likelihood of delirium, it can cause bradycardia and hypotension (Shehabi et al. 2019).

Sedation practices also entail regular assessment by validated instruments such as the Richmond Agitation-Sedation Scale and daily sedation breaks or spontaneous awakening tests in patients on mechanical ventilation (Wainwright et al. 2019; Grant et al. 2024). When combined with fast-track extubation programs, these allow for appropriate planning of sedation regimens relative to planned extubation dates and assessments of readiness (Cheng et al. 1996; Hamilton et al. 2011).

11.6.3 Delirium Prevention and Sleep Optimization

Delirium postoperatively is prevalent following heart surgery and linked to extended hospital stays, prolonged cognitive dysfunction, and death. The ERACS bundles have non-pharmacological measures for delirium prevention, such as orientation, early ambulation, promotion of sleep (controlling noise and lights, clustering care), visual and auditory support devices, and avoiding the use of benzodiazepines wherever possible (Wainwright et al. 2019; Grant et al. 2024).

Furthermore, proper management of pain, use of a minimal number of drugs, ensuring normoxia and normocapnia, and treatment of any infection or metabolic disturbance helps to prevent delirium (Wainwright et al. 2019). Nutrition and delirium have a relationship through glucose metabolism, nutrient deficiency such as thiamine, etc. (Hill et al. 2018; Stoppe et al. 2017).

11.7 Perioperative Nutritional Management in ERACS

11.7.1 Burden and Impact of Malnutrition in Cardiac Surgery

Many reports have noted a high prevalence of malnutrition and nutritional risks in adults who are to undergo heart surgeries, ranging from 20% to 50% (Weimann et al. 2021). The presence of malnutrition predisposes a patient to developing infections, mechanical ventilation times, ICU stay, re-hospitalization, and ultimately, higher mortality rates (Stoppe et al. 2017). Sarcopenia and frailty contribute additional risk by lowering the respiratory muscle reserve (Stoppe et al. 2017; Hill et al. 2018).

As noted by Hill et al., nutritional support in cardiac surgery patients has the potential to enhance metabolic processes, prevent catabolism, preserve gastrointestinal integrity, and minimize postoperative complications; however, randomized controlled trials are sparse (Hill et al. 2018). In the consensus statement, Stoppe et al. stressed the importance of nutritional support as an essential treatment modality for critically ill cardiac surgery patients, even in the absence of specific guidelines (Stoppe et al. 2017).

11.7.2 Preoperative Nutrition Screening and Carbohydrate Loading

Nutritional assessment before surgery using specific screening forms is suggested for ERACS patients, to be able to detect malnourished patients and refer to the dietitian (Kondrup et al. 2003). Patients showing substantial weight loss, low BMI, poor nutritional intake, and inflammatory disease require further evaluation (Hill et al. 2018; Weimann et al. 2021).

Preoperative ingestion of iso-osmotic clear fluids (e.g., 50–100 g of carbohydrates the night prior to and 2–3 hours prior to surgery) has been demonstrated in heart surgery cohorts to decrease insulin resistance, increase cardiac function indexes, and decrease hospital stay in some studies, without increased instances of aspiration if used appropriately (Tran et al. 2013). This modality should be avoided in individuals with gastroparesis, severely obese patients with reflux, or extremely high risks for aspiration (Engelman et al. 2019).

11.7.3 Early Postoperative Enteral Nutrition

Post-operative early enteral nutrition (EEN) is one of the major tenets of nutrition care pathways in ERACS. Early EEN initiation within 6–24 hours after ICU admission is feasible and linked with better patient outcomes than delayed or exclusive parenteral nutrition based on observational and experimental research evidence (Hill et al. 2018; Reignier et al. 2018). Evidence from randomized controlled trials and well-defined nutritional feeding guidelines indicates that early EEN is beneficial in improving calorie intake, growth parameters, ventilator extubation, and ICU mortality in pediatric congenital cardiac surgeries (Sahu et al. 2016; Lisanti et al. 2021).

According to international guidelines on nutrition for critically ill patients, in hemodynamically stable patients who are dependent on low-dose vasopressors, low-dose enteral feeding may be commenced after 24 hours, advancing cautiously as per tolerance (Reignier et al. 2018). Such guidelines apply to cardiology ICUs where a lot of patients are able to receive their feeds within 3–5 days, starting from low volumes (Hill et al. 2018; Weimann et al. 2021) (Table 11.2).

11.7.4 Macronutrient Targets and Route of Nutrition

While there is ongoing research on optimal macronutrient formulas for cardiac surgery patients as adults, most of the recommendations suggest a goal caloric intake between approximately 20 and 25 kcal/kg/day during the acute phase, while an increase to 25–30 kcal/kg/day can be achieved during the progressive stage, alongside sufficient protein intake amounting to at least 1.2–1.5 g/kg/day for lean mass retention (Hill et al. 2018; Stoppe et al. 2017). The proportions of carbohydrates and lipids will depend on glycaemia, lipid metabolism, and organ function (Weimann et al. 2021).

Table 11.2 Evidence examples for early enteral nutrition after cardiac surgery

Study	Population	Intervention	Main findings
Sahu et al. (2016)	Infants younger than 6 months undergoing congenital cardiac repair surgery	Early enteral nutrition initiated within the first 24 hours postoperatively using fortified breast milk or formula feeds	Early enteral nutrition was feasible and safe, improved caloric intake, reduced duration of mechanical ventilation and ICU stay, and was associated with better postoperative nutritional recovery without increasing gastrointestinal complications
Lisanti et al. (2021)	Infants with congenital heart disease requiring surgery or intensive inpatient management	Standardized feeding pathway including early nutritional assessment, defined caloric goals, feeding advancement protocols, and multidisciplinary nutrition monitoring	The standardized feeding approach reduced postoperative weight loss, improved growth trends, increased caloric intake consistency, and helped mitigate malnutrition risk during hospitalization
Hill et al. (2018)	Adult cardiac surgery (review)	Various EEN protocols	EEN feasible, may reduce infections and length of stay
Reignier et al. (2018)	Mixed critically ill with shock	Early vs. delayed EN in shock	Early low-dose EN did not increase ischemic events; supports cautious EN

Enteral nutritional support should be prioritized where possible due to maintaining gut physiology, supporting the intestinal microflora, and showing fewer rates of infection in comparison to parenteral nutrition. Parenteral nutrition becomes a choice only in situations when enteral nutrition becomes impossible within 48–72 hours despite optimization or a presence of severe malnutrition before surgery and inability to receive all nutrients enterally (Hill et al. 2018; Stoppe et al. 2017).

11.7.5 Micronutrients, Pharmaconutrition, and Special Substrates

Micronutrient deficiencies such as thiamine, vitamin D, iron, zinc, and selenium are prevalent among patients undergoing cardiac surgery, especially those suffering from heart failure, renal disease, and diuretics (Hill et al. 2018; Stoppe et al. 2017). Although there are no good clinical trials to prove their importance, their correction is logical and may help in maintaining mitochondrial health, adequate immunity, and wound healing (Weimann et al. 2021).

Pharmaconutrition products like arginine, omega-3 fatty acid preparations, glutamine, and antioxidant-enhanced formulas have been investigated in both surgical and intensive care settings, yet again yielding inconsistent results, and there are insufficient data on these supplements in cardiac surgery (Stoppe et al. 2017). The current ERACS guidelines focus on meeting essential energy and protein requirements using regular polymeric products, while specialized substrates are left for research only (Hill et al. 2018; Weimann et al. 2021).

11.7.6 Nutrition in High-Risk Subgroups

High-risk groups consist of frail elderly, obese or sarcopenic obese patients, those with diabetes, chronic renal disease, or severe heart failure, and patients on prolonged mechanical circulatory support (Hill et al. 2018). For such patients, careful assessment and customized nutritional interventions are mandatory.

For instance, when dealing with obese patients, energy prescription using actual body weight takes into consideration high protein requirements and prevention of overfeeding. In addition, the target protein requirement will be based on anabolism versus catabolism and the development of azotemia. The early intervention through physiotherapy and adequate protein will be integrated for frail patients to ensure muscle mass retention (Weimann et al. 2021). Figure 11.2 gives a simplified timeline between day 0 and day 3 for extubation, getting out of bed, walking, and enteral feeding targets.

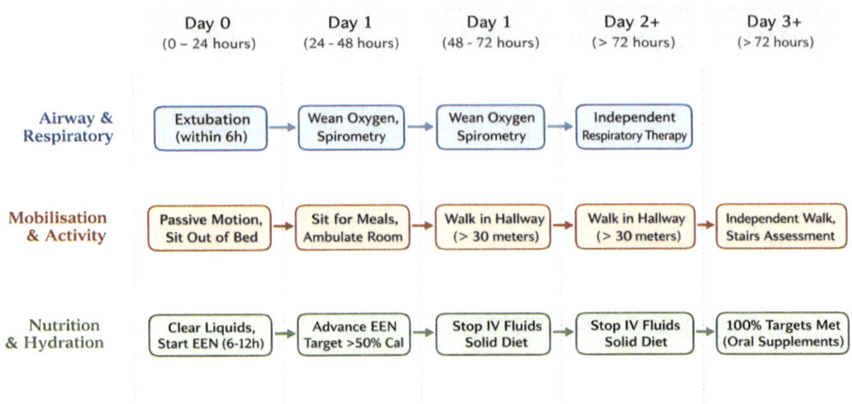

Fig. 11.2 Proposed timeline of extubation, mobilization, and nutrition milestones in an adult ERACS protocol. (The image has been created by using Mermaid.com). Abbreviations: ERACS Enhanced Recovery After Cardiac Surgery, EEN early enteral nutrition, IV intravenous, O_2 oxygen, ICU intensive care unit

11.8 Integration of Anesthesia and Nutrition Within ERACS Pathways

11.8.1 Coordinating Extubation and Feeding Milestones

In integrated ERACS approaches, schedules for extubation, early mobility, and nutrition are planned ahead and synchronized. One example may include extubation within 6 hours (or during surgery if ultra-fast-track patients are concerned), commencement of feeding at low volumes via enteral route or orally between 6 and 12 hours, sitting out of bed by days 0 to 1, and ambulation on days 1 to 2 (Navas-Blanco et al. 2024; Mertes et al. 2022).

Anesthesiologists, intensivists, and dieticians work together to make sure that sedation and vasoactive protocols permit a patient to swallow or tolerate gastric feeding and feed advancement aligns with respiratory and hemodynamic parameters (Hill et al. 2018; Weimann et al. 2021). Guidelines establish contraindications for feeding (e.g., unstable shock, high dose vasoactive agents, severe lactic acidosis, active bleeding) and indications for restarting or withdrawing feeding (Reignier et al. 2018).

11.8.2 Multidisciplinary Teamwork and Communication

For ERACS to be successfully implemented, interdisciplinary teamwork among surgeons, anesthesiologists, intensivists, cardiologists, dietitians, physiotherapists, nurses, pharmacists, and quality-improvement experts is required (Hoogma et al.

2025). Interdisciplinary rounds, development of care pathways, and employment of checklists or order sets help promote adherence to ERACS protocols and allow for the identification of discrepancies (ERAS Cardiac Society 2025; Grant et al. 2024).

Nutritionists are essential for transforming general nutritional guidance provided by ERACS into tailored diets, evaluating tolerance, and making adjustments based on laboratory and clinical assessments (Hill et al. 2018; Stoppe et al. 2017). It is necessary to coordinate work between anesthesia and intensive care staff and nutritionists to make sure that patients' hemodynamic, sedation, and analgesic state allows them to be fed according to these recommendations (Engelman et al. 2019; Navas-Blanco et al. 2024).

11.8.3 Quality Metrics, Audit, and Feedback

The measures adopted under ERACS programs are quantifiable and include process and outcome indicators, such as extubation time, percentage of extubation within specific periods, time for initial enteral feeding, achievement of nutritional goals, mobility indicators, complications, reintubation rates, duration in the ICU and the hospital as well as readmission rate (ERAS Cardiac Society 2025; Hoogma et al. 2025; Navas-Blanco et al. 2024).

Ongoing audit and feedback using dashboards and multidisciplinary conferences facilitate improvements (Grant et al. 2024). Cross-institution benchmarking based on ERAS registries adds to the motivation and is a source of data for research purposes (ERAS Society 2021; ERAS Cardiac Society 2025). Patient-reported measures (such as quality of recovery, satisfaction levels, fatigue, and appetite) form part of the assessment of ERACS effectiveness (Hoogma et al. 2025; Wainwright et al. 2019).

11.9 Clinical Outcomes of ERACS: Evidence Synthesis

11.9.1 Mechanical Ventilation and Respiratory Outcomes

Several ERACS protocols and fast-track extubation programs have demonstrated marked decreases in the duration of mechanical ventilation and associated problems. Research on rapid and ultra-rapid extubation in the operating theatre reveals that 60–80% of selected patients could be safely extubated, with lower rates of reintubation and pulmonary complications compared to traditional methods (Cheng et al. 1996; Ender et al. 2008).

According to a Cochrane review and later meta-analyses on fast-track techniques, fast-tracking is associated with decreased ICU stay, ventilator-associated events, and cost savings, with no impact on safety, especially if used on proper candidates and through a well-designed protocol (Hamilton et al. 2011; Hoogma et al. 2025). Evidence is also accumulating to show that ultra-fast extubation might benefit hemodynamic stability and ICU burden, although more randomized clinical trials are needed (Navas-Blanco et al. 2024; Zhang et al. 2022).

11.9.2 ICU and Hospital Length of Stay

Adoption of ERACS was shown to be correlated with shortened lengths of ICU and hospital stay in observational research and controlled trials (Hoogma et al. 2025). The effects of adopting ERACS included shorter ICU stay for 0.5–1.5 days and shorter hospital stay for 1–3 days due to earlier extubation, decreased complication rates, and faster mobilization (Ender et al. 2008; Gunaydin et al. 2024).

According to a systematic review, ERACS protocols were proven to lead to shortened lengths of ICU stay without increasing rates of readmission (Zhang et al. 2022). Nevertheless, not all the studies demonstrate such impressive results, as the overall healthcare system context plays an important role in lengths of stay (Navas-Blanco et al. 2024). It is vital to keep in mind that ERACS should be regarded as just one element of the perioperative care process improvement strategy.

11.9.3 Complications and Mortality

However, the effect of ERACS on complication rates and mortality is somewhat controversial, likely because of inconsistencies in protocols and patient characteristics (Hoogma et al. 2025; Zhang et al. 2022). Several ERACS programs have demonstrated decreased risks of pulmonary complications, atrial fibrillation, acute renal injury, and infections; however, there is no statistical difference (Gunaydin et al. 2024). The systematic review usually suggests that ERACS program is as effective and safe as standard treatment and has some benefits concerning selected outcomes without any signs of possible harm (Zhang et al. 2022).

To the best of my knowledge, no randomized clinical trials compare ERACS program comprehensively with standard treatment. There are many randomized clinical trials that compare one component of the ERACS with the standard approach (fast-track anesthesia, early mobility, early nutrition) (Hamilton et al. 2011; Tran et al. 2013). For that reason, it is hard to differentiate the impact of each component. However, all research data confirm the effectiveness of ERACS programs (Hoogma et al. 2025).

11.9.4 Nutritional Outcomes and Functional Recovery

Nutrition-specific components of ERACS have demonstrated beneficial effects on calorie and protein intake, faster attainment of nutritional goals, decreased negative energy balance, and preservation of lean body mass (Hill et al. 2018; Weimann et al.

Table 11.3 Comparison of conventional care versus ERACS in cardiac surgery (conceptual summary)

Outcome	Conventional care	ERACS-oriented care
Ventilation duration	Often >12–24 h, routine overnight ventilation	Targeted extubation within 6 h or on-table in selected patients (Cheng et al. 1996; Ender et al. 2008)
ICU length of stay	2–4 days typical	Reduction of 0.5–1.5 days in many programs (Hoogma et al. 2025; Zhang et al. 2022)
Nutrition	Prolonged fasting, delayed feeding, limited dietitian input	Early EN within 6–24 h, dietitian-led prescriptions, monitoring of protein/energy targets (Hill et al. 2018; Stoppe et al. 2017)
Mobilization	Bedrest for first day or longer	Sit out of bed day 0–1, ambulation day 1–2 (Engelman et al. 2019; Steinmetz et al. 2026)
Complications	Higher risk of pulmonary complications and delirium	Lower or similar complication rates, no increase in reintubation (Hoogma et al. 2025; Zhang et al. 2022)

2021). The use of early enteral nutrition was related to early recovery of bowel movements, decreased risk of infections, faster wound healing, and lower length of hospitalization among adults and children undergoing cardiac surgery (Sahu et al. 2016; Lisanti et al. 2021).

Indicators of functional recovery, including the time required to achieve ambulation independence, distance covered, and quality of recovery from the patient's perspective, were found to be positively affected by ERACS despite scarce evidence (Hoogma et al. 2025; Navas-Blanco et al. 2024). Considering the robust mechanism underpinning the role of proper nutrition in physical functioning, more research in this field is needed (Steinmetz et al. 2026; Hill et al. 2018) (Table 11.3).

11.10 Implementation Challenges and Strategies

11.10.1 Organizational and Cultural Barriers

Obstacles to ERACS implementation consist of traditional working methods (e.g., overnight ventilator usage), safety fears regarding early extubation and feeding, isolated working processes, poor staffing resources, and lack of organizational commitment (Gunaydin et al. 2024). Overcoming these obstacles demands leaders' involvement, ERACS promoters identification, and incentivization for quality and efficiency (ERAS Cardiac Society 2025; Wainwright et al. 2019).

Interprofessional training, simulation, and change management techniques may help overcome fears and create an improvement-oriented environment (ERAS Cardiac Society 2025; Grant et al. 2024). Staff participation in protocol customization is useful to achieve greater commitment and responsibility, especially concerning anesthesia and nutrition aspects that necessitate daily decisions (Engelman et al. 2019; Mertes et al. 2022).

11.10.2 Resource Constraints and Variability in Infrastructure

Resource constraints, such as ICU bed availability, the number of dietitians, physiotherapists, and advanced monitoring systems, might affect ERACS program adoption, particularly in developing countries (Gunaydin et al. 2024; Navas-Blanco et al. 2024). Adapting ERACS programs according to the local setting is crucial, for instance, by focusing on affordable yet impactful interventions such as patient education, early mobility, nutrition assessment, and fast-track extubation strategies (Hoogma et al. 2025).

Telemedicine platforms may be useful in delivering preoperative education, nutrition counseling, and post-discharge patient follow-up when face-to-face contact is restricted (Hoogma et al. 2025; Wainwright et al. 2019). Collaboration with hospital management and emphasizing the financial benefits of implementing ERACS, including shorter hospital stays and lower complication rates, might secure resources for recruiting ERAS coordinators and multidisciplinary teams (ERAS Cardiac Society 2025; Grant et al. 2024).

11.10.3 Data, Monitoring, and Iterative Refinement

Sound data infrastructures are required for monitoring ERACS compliance and performance. Health information systems, automated reporting tools, and consistent data definitions aid in accurate monitoring (Grant et al. 2024). Enrollment into ERAS or cardiac quality databases helps to compare performance and detect outliers (ERAS Society 2021; ERAS Cardiac Society 2025).

Review of collected data in multi-disciplinary meetings contributes to continuous improvement and recognition of areas requiring improvement, including delayed extubation or unresolved nutrition issues, which can be addressed with specific actions (Grant et al. 2024). Involvement of the anesthesia and nutrition specialists in the process assures the proper attention to their areas (Engelman et al. 2019; Navas-Blanco et al. 2024).

11.11 Future Directions and Research Priorities

11.11.1 Personalized and Precision ERACS

ERACS in the future will probably trend toward personalized pathways based on enhanced risk stratification that would include genomics, metabolomics, frailty scores, and comprehensive body composition analysis (Gunaydin et al. 2024). Machine learning algorithms might be able to predict which patients would most likely respond favorably to ultra-fast extubation and aggressive nutrition regimens rather than more moderate treatments (Hoogma et al. 2025; Weimann et al. 2021).

Remote monitoring using wearables might extend the use of ERACS even after discharge, with activities, sleep cycles, heart rates, and nutritional intake being monitored to determine individualized post-discharge care programs (Weimann et al. 2021). Such innovations would require seamless integration into electronic health records and patient portals (Wainwright et al. 2019).

11.11.2 High-Quality Trials on Nutrition Interventions

It is essential to conduct well-powered randomized clinical trials to assess specific nutritional interventions in cardiac surgery, like early versus delayed EN, higher protein goals, high-protein versus standard EN, and micronutrient/pharmaco-nutritional approaches (Stoppe et al. 2017). The studies should consider functional assessments, quality of life, and post-recovery markers, along with established end-points in the ICU and hospitals (Steinmetz et al. 2026; Hoogma et al. 2025).

The use of advanced imaging techniques and metabolic evaluations can provide insights into how nutrition impacts the cardiac physiology, immune system, and postoperative organ recovery following CPB (Hill et al. 2018; Weimann et al. 2021).

11.11.3 Innovations in Anesthesia and Analgesia

New approaches for anesthetic and analgesia, such as new regional blocks, non-opioid analgesia, and improved DOA monitoring, can be implemented, allowing optimization of fast-track care paths without causing delirium and chronic pain (Kietaibl et al. 2022; Macaire et al. 2019). Investigation of the concept of ultra-low or opioid-free anesthesia in cardiac surgery under the umbrella of ERACS programs is ongoing (Navas-Blanco et al. 2024; Shehabi et al. 2019).

Potential research directions within the ERACS program include patient-centered outcomes, namely cognitive, psychological, and functional outcomes, which depend on the approaches utilized during anesthesia and perioperative nutrition strategies (Steinmetz et al. 2026; Wainwright et al. 2019).

11.12 Conclusions

ERACS stands out as a revolutionary change in post-operative care, adapting the principles of ERAS into the specific setting of heart surgery. Fast-track anesthesia and enteral nutrition are critical components in ERACS, as these two play important roles in facilitating faster recovery and better results when used on carefully selected patients.

According to guideline-based literature review, systematic studies, and experiences of various institutions, ERACS has been proven as a viable and relatively risk-free method of recovery, providing reductions in mechanical ventilation time and ICU admission periods, as well as potential improvements in complications and functional restoration. Nevertheless, differences in protocol design and lack of clinical trials make further investigation necessary.

From a clinician's perspective, the key message is to integrate structured anesthetic and nutritional regimens into comprehensive ERACS protocols that can be customized according to patient risk profiles and hospital resources, with regular auditing and optimization. There is great potential for success in this area.

References

Cheng DC, Karski J, Peniston C, Asokumar B, Raveendran G, Carroll J, Nierenberg H, Roger S, Mickle D, Tong J, Zelovitsky J, David T, Sandler A. Morbidity outcome in early versus conventional tracheal extubation after coronary artery bypass grafting: a prospective randomized controlled trial. J Thorac Cardiovasc Surg. 1996;112(3):755–64. https://doi.org/10.1016/S0022-5223(96)70062-4.

Ender J, Borger MA, Scholz M, Funkat AK, Anwar N, Sommer M, Mohr FW, Fassl J. Cardiac surgery fast-track treatment in a postanesthetic care unit: six-month results of the Leipzig fast-track concept. Anesthesiology. 2008;109(1):61–6. https://doi.org/10.1097/ALN.0b013e31817881b3.

Engelman DT, Ben Ali W, Williams JB, Perrault LP, Reddy VS, Arora RC, et al. Guidelines for perioperative care in cardiac surgery: Enhanced Recovery After Surgery Society recommendations. JAMA Surg. 2019;154(8):755–66. https://doi.org/10.1001/jamasurg.2019.1153.

ERAS Cardiac Society. ERAS® Cardiac implementation and quality improvement resources. 2025. Retrieved April 18, 2026, from https://www.erascardiac.org.

ERAS Society. ERAS® Society guidelines and implementation resources. 2021. Retrieved April 18, 2026, from https://erassociety.org/guidelines.

Grant MC, Crisafi C, Alvarez A, Arora RC, Brindle ME, Chatterjee S, Ender J, Fletcher N, Gregory AJ, Gunaydin S, Jahangiri M, Ljungqvist O, Lobdell KW, Morton V, Reddy VS, Salenger R, Sander M, Zarbock A, Engelman DT. Perioperative care in cardiac surgery: a joint consensus statement by the Enhanced Recovery After Surgery (ERAS) Cardiac Society, ERAS International Society, and the Society of Thoracic Surgeons (STS). Ann Thorac Surg. 2024;117(4):669–89. https://doi.org/10.1016/j.athoracsur.2023.12.006.

Gunaydin S, Simsek E, Engelman D. Enhanced recovery after cardiac surgery and developments in perioperative care: a comprehensive review. Turk gogus kalp damar cerrahisi dergisi. 2024;33(1):121–31. https://doi.org/10.5606/tgkdc.dergisi.2024.26770.

Gustafsson UO, Oppelstrup H, Thorell A, Nygren J, Ljungqvist O. Adherence to the ERAS protocol is associated with 5-year survival after colorectal cancer surgery: a retrospective cohort study. World J Surg. 2016;40(7):1741–7. https://doi.org/10.1007/s00268-016-3460-y.

Hamilton MA, Cecconi M, Rhodes A. A systematic review and meta-analysis on the use of preemptive hemodynamic intervention to improve postoperative outcomes in moderate and high-risk surgical patients. In: Database of abstracts of reviews of effects (DARE): quality-assessed reviews [Internet]. Centre for Reviews and Dissemination (UK); 2011. Retrieved April 18, 2026, from https://www.ncbi.nlm.nih.gov/books/NBK81622/.

Hill A, Nesterova E, Lomivorotov V, Efremov S, Goetzenich A, Benstoem C, Zamyatin M, Chourdakis M, Heyland D, Stoppe C. Current evidence about nutrition support in cardiac surgery patients-what do we know? Nutrients. 2018;10(5):597. https://doi.org/10.3390/nu10050597.

Hirai S. Systemic inflammatory response syndrome after cardiac surgery under cardiopulmonary bypass. Ann Thorac Cardiovasc Surg. 2003;9(6):365–70. Systemic inflammatory response syndrome after cardiac surgery under cardiopulmonary bypass - PubMed

Hoogma DF, Van den Berg A, Van den Berg M, Van der Linden N. Efficacy of enhanced recovery programmes for cardiac surgery: a systematic review and meta-analysis. Br J Anaesth. 2025;135(1):31–9. https://doi.org/10.1016/j.bja.2025.03.019.

Kehlet H. Multimodal approach to control postoperative pathophysiology and rehabilitation. Br J Anaesth. 1997;78(5):606–17. https://doi.org/10.1093/bja/78.5.606.

Kietaibl S, Ferrandis R, Godier A, Llau J, Lobo C, Macfarlane AJ, Schlimp CJ, Vandermeulen E, Volk T, von Heymann C, Wolmarans M, Afshari A. Regional anaesthesia in patients on antithrombotic drugs: joint ESAIC/ESRA guidelines. Eur J Anaesthesiol. 2022;39(2):100–32. https://doi.org/10.1097/EJA.0000000000001600.

Kondrup J, Allison SP, Elia M, Vellas B, Plauth M. ESPEN guidelines for nutrition screening 2002. Clin Nutr. 2003;22(4):415–21. https://doi.org/10.1016/S0261-5614(03)00098-0.

Lisanti AJ, Savoca M, Gaynor JW, Mascarenhas MR, Ravishankar C, Sullivan E, Pieciak K, Costarino A, Chen J, Kennedy A, Olsen R, Min J, Mondal A, Huang J, Irving SY. Standardized feeding approach mitigates weight loss in infants with congenital heart disease. J Pediatr. 2021;231:124–130.e1. https://doi.org/10.1016/j.jpeds.2020.12.047.

Ljungqvist O, Scott M, Fearon KC. Enhanced recovery after surgery: a review. JAMA Surg. 2017;152(3):292–8. https://doi.org/10.1001/jamasurg.2016.4952.

Macaire P, Ho N, Nguyen T, Nguyen B, Vu V, Quach C, Roques V, Capdevila X. Ultrasound-guided continuous thoracic erector spinae plane block within an enhanced recovery program is associated with decreased opioid consumption and improved patient postoperative rehabilitation after open cardiac surgery: a patient-matched, controlled before-and-after study. J Cardiothorac Vasc Anesth. 2019;33(6):1659–67. https://doi.org/10.1053/j.jvca.2018.11.021.

McIsaac DI, Gill M, Boland L, Hutton B, Branje K, Shaw J, Grudzinski AL, Barone N, Gillis C, Prehabilitation Knowledge Network. Prehabilitation in adult patients undergoing surgery: an umbrella review of systematic reviews. Br J Anaesth. 2022;128(2):244–57. https://doi.org/10.1016/j.bja.2021.11.014.

Mertes P-M, Kindo M, Amour J, Baufreton C, Camilleri L, Caus T, Chatel D, Cholley B, Curtil A, Grimaud J-P, Houel R, Kattou F, Fellahi J-L, Guidon C, Guinot P-G, Lebreton G, Marguerite S, Ouattara A, Provenchère Fruithiot S, et al. Guidelines on enhanced recovery after cardiac surgery under cardiopulmonary bypass or off-pump. Anaesth Crit Care Pain Med. 2022;41(3):101059. https://doi.org/10.1016/j.accpm.2022.101059.

Nashef SAM, Roques F, Sharples LD, Nilsson J, Smith C, Goldstone AR, Lockowandt U. EuroSCORE II. Eur J Cardiothorac Surg. 2012;41(4):734–44. https://doi.org/10.1093/ejcts/ezs043.

Navas-Blanco JR, Kantola A, Whitton M, Johnson A, Shakibai N, Soto R, Muhammad S. Enhanced recovery after cardiac surgery: a literature review. Saudi J Anaesth. 2024;18(2):257–64. https://doi.org/10.4103/sja.sja_62_24.

O'Brien SM, Shahian DM, Filardo G, Ferraris VA, Haan CK, Rich JB, Normand SL, DeLong ER, Shewan CM, Dokholyan RS, Peterson ED, Edwards FH, Anderson RP, Society of Thoracic Surgeons Quality Measurement Task Force. The Society of Thoracic Surgeons 2008 cardiac surgery risk models: part 2—isolated valve surgery. Ann Thorac Surg. 2009;88(1 Suppl):S23–42. https://doi.org/10.1016/j.athoracsur.2009.05.056.

Plümer H, Markewitz A, Marohl K, Bernutz C, Weinhold C. Early extubation after cardiac surgery: a prospective clinical trial including patients at risk. Thorac Cardiovasc Surg. 1998;46(5):275–80. https://doi.org/10.1055/s-2007-1010238.

Reignier J, Boisramé-Helms J, Brisard L, Lascarrou J-B, Ait Hssain A, Anguel N, Garrouste-Orgeas M, Botoc V, Bretagnol A, Boulain T, Maxime V, Klouche K, Argaud L, Jamali S, Evrard B, Quenot J-P, Seguin P, Gibot S, Roger C, et al. Enteral versus parenteral early nutrition in ventilated adults with shock: a randomised, controlled, multicentre, open-label, parallel-group study. Lancet. 2018;391(10116):133–43. https://doi.org/10.1016/S0140-6736(17)32146-3.

Sahu MK, Singal A, Menon R, Singh SP, Mohan A, Manral M, Singh D, Devagouru V, Talwar S, Choudhary SK. Early enteral nutrition therapy in congenital cardiac repair postoperatively: a randomized, controlled pilot study. Ann Card Anaesth. 2016;19(4):653–61. https://doi.org/10.4103/0971-9784.191550.

Shehabi Y, Howe BD, Bellomo R, Arabi YM, Bailey M, Bass FE, Bin Kadiman S, McArthur C, Murray L, Reade MC, Seppelt IM, Takala J, Wise MP, Webb SA, SPICE III Investigators. Early sedation with dexmedetomidine in critically ill patients. N Engl J Med. 2019;380(26):2506–17. https://doi.org/10.1056/NEJMoa1904710.

Steinmetz C, Tran PT, Heinemann S, Arroyo-Ariza D, Jurayj J, Katz NB, Hartog J, Schmidt T, Scheenstra B, Amonoo HL, Madva EN, Qu JZ, Akeju O, Huffman JC, Kutschka I, Herrmann-Lingen C, Silver JK, von Arnim CAF, Lee A, Röver C, …, Cardiac Prehabilitation Network. Prehabilitation in patients undergoing cardiac procedures: a systematic review and meta-analysis. JACC Adv. 2026;5(3):102587. https://doi.org/10.1016/j.jacadv.2026.102587.

Stoppe C, Goetzenich A, Whitman G, et al. Role of nutrition support in adult cardiac surgery: a consensus statement from an International Multidisciplinary Expert Group on Nutrition in Cardiac Surgery. Crit Care. 2017;21:131. https://doi.org/10.1186/s13054-017-1690-5.

Stratton RJ, Hackston A, Longmore D, Dixon R, Price S, Stroud M, King C, Elia M, Stubbs R. Malnutrition in hospital outpatients and inpatients: prevalence, concurrent validity and ease of use of the 'malnutrition universal screening tool' ('MUST') for adults. Br J Nutr. 2004;92(5):799–808. https://doi.org/10.1079/BJN20041258.

Tran S, Wolever TM, Errett LE, Ahn H, Mazer CD, Keith M. Preoperative carbohydrate loading in patients undergoing coronary artery bypass or spinal surgery. Anesth Analg. 2013;117(2):305–13. https://doi.org/10.1213/ANE.0b013e318295e8d1.

Wainwright TW, Immins T, Antonis JHA, Hartley R, Middleton RG. Enhanced recovery after surgery: concepts and application to Total shoulder replacement. Orthop Nurs. 2019;38(6):375–80. https://doi.org/10.1097/NOR.0000000000000609.

Weimann A, Braga M, Carli F, Higashiguchi T, Hübner M, Klek S, Laviano A, Ljungqvist O, Lobo DN, Martindale RG, Waitzberg D, Bischoff SC, Singer P. ESPEN practical guideline: clinical nutrition in surgery. Clin Nutr. 2021;40(7):4745–61. https://doi.org/10.1016/j.clnu.2021.03.031.

Zhang Y, Chong JH, Harky A. Enhanced recovery after cardiac surgery and its impact on outcomes: a systematic review. Perfusion. 2022;37(2):162–74. https://doi.org/10.1177/0267659121988957.

12 Enhanced Recovery After Orthopedic Surgery: Integrated Strategies Addressing Anesthesia and Nutrition

Sourabh Jakhar and Nilanjan Dutta

Abstract

Enhanced Recovery After Surgery (ERAS) protocols have revolutionized the perioperative care of orthopedic surgical patients by using various evidence-based measures to reduce the surgical stress response, perioperative complications, hospital stay, and promote faster recovery from orthopedic surgeries such as total hip arthroplasty (THA), total knee arthroplasty (TKA), spinal surgeries, and fragility hip fractures.

This chapter discusses the pathophysiological basis of ERAS protocols in orthopedic surgeries and critically reviews the evidence regarding integrated anesthetic and nutritional management strategies. Special emphasis is given to the selection of neuraxial versus general anesthesia techniques, the development of multimodal analgesic regimens with motor-sparing effects, the management of postoperative nausea and vomiting, preoperative nutritional screening, and the implementation of oral nutritional support, immunonutrition, vitamin repletion, carbohydrate loading, and early enteral feeding.

Two tables are provided to discuss the essential components of ERAS protocols and the tools used in preoperative nutritional screening. Two figure placeholders are also provided to discuss the integrated anesthetic/analgesic pathway and the perioperative nutrition algorithm.

S. Jakhar
Department of Anesthesiology, Pt NRS Govt Medical College, Kolkata, West Bengal, India

N. Dutta (✉)
Department of Anesthesia & Operation Theater Technology, School of Health Sciences & Technology, Medhavi Skills University, Singtam, India

P. K. Bhattacharyya et al. (eds.), *Integrated Anesthesia and Nutrition Approaches to Enhanced Recovery after Surgery*,
https://doi.org/10.1007/978-981-92-3294-9_12

Keywords

Enhanced Recovery After Surgery (ERAS) · Orthopedic surgery · Multimodal analgesia · Perioperative nutrition · Surgical stress response

12.1 Introduction

12.1.1 Evolution of ERAS and Its Adoption in Orthopedics

The concept of ERAS was originally developed by Kehlet, who advocated the use of a multimodal approach to the management of postoperative pathophysiology and rehabilitation by optimizing the techniques of anesthesia, analgesia, fluid management, and mobilization (Kehlet 1997, 2009). It was originally applied to colorectal and abdominal surgeries but has now spread to other surgical specialities worldwide (Wainwright et al. 2020; Weimann et al. 2021).

Orthopedic surgery was one of the first surgical specialities to adopt the ERAS concept due to the high volume of surgeries involving the lower limbs and the predictable postoperative course of arthroplasty procedures, with the outcomes heavily dependent on the rehabilitation and mobilization of the patient (Zhou et al. 2024; Zhu et al. 2017). Systematic reviews and meta-analyses have consistently proven the benefit of ERAS protocols in the management of patients undergoing THA and TKA by reducing the length of stay by 1 to 3 days and the total complications compared to conventional management protocols, with no increase in the rate of readmission within 30 days of discharge (Chung et al. 2021; Changjun et al. 2023; Zhou et al. 2024). These benefits have also been seen in the management of geriatric patients with hip fractures, where the ERAS protocols reduce the length of stay and the total complications and delirium (Fox et al. 2025; Kristensen and Kehlet 2012).

12.1.2 Rationale for Focusing on Anesthesia and Nutrition

Major orthopedic surgery elicits a marked neuroendocrine and inflammatory response with concomitant hyperglycemia, insulin resistance, proteolysis, and immune suppression, as evidenced by increased catecholamines, cortisol, glucagon, and cytokine release (Kehlet 1997). These effects are particularly adverse in the elderly, frail, and multimorbid patient population with underlying sarcopenia and undiagnosed malnutrition, as noted by Gregori et al. (2023) and Weimann et al. (2021).

Anesthetic and analgesic techniques modulate the degree of surgical stress response, as they influence the degree of pain, sympathetic response, hemodynamics, and immune response, as discussed by Cusack & Buggy (2020). In parallel, the nutritional state of the patient is a key modulator of the wound healing response, immune response, and recovery of muscle mass, as discussed by Weimann et al. (2017). Observational studies have shown that preoperative malnutrition is associated with increased risk of surgical site infections, periprosthetic joint infections, wound-related complications, nonunion, readmissions, and mortality, as noted by Bohl et al. (2016), Chen and Chen (2024), De Mauro et al. (2024), and Veizi et al. (2025).

Therefore, the current recommendations of the ERAS Society for Orthopedic Surgery emphasize the importance of anesthetic technique, analgesia, and nutrition care as the cornerstones of optimization, as discussed by Wainwright et al. (2020) and Changjun et al. (2023).

12.2 Pathophysiological Basis for ERAS in Orthopedic Surgery

12.2.1 Surgical Stress, Catabolism, and Musculoskeletal Recovery

Significant orthopedic surgeries, such as THA, TKA, and spine surgery, stimulate the hypothalamic-pituitary-adrenal axis and sympathetic nervous system, resulting in increased catecholamines and glucocorticoids, which stimulate gluconeogenesis, lipolysis, and muscle protein degradation (Kehlet 2009; Weimann et al. 2021). This, combined with the effects of bed rest, results in negative nitrogen balance, hyperglycemia, and loss of lean body mass, particularly in the elderly (Weimann et al. 2021).

In addition, in arthroplasty and fracture patients, bed rest for extended periods results in increased muscle atrophy, delaying recovery milestones such as transfers, walking, and stairs (Keogh et al. 2025). Frailty and pre-existing malnutrition are associated with increased risk of complications, such as wound problems, cardiopulmonary complications, delirium, and institutionalization (Chiavarini et al. 2024; Helminen et al. 2017; Liu et al. 2022).

12.2.2 Modulation of Surgical Stress Via Anesthesia and Nutrition

Neuraxial and regional anesthesia, with short-acting general anesthetic agents and systemic analgesic agents, decrease the nociceptive and sympathetic responses and may reduce endocrine-metabolic stress (Andersen et al. 2008, 2010). Opioid-sparing regimens decrease postoperative nausea and vomiting, ileus, urinary retention, cognitive dysfunction, and respiratory depression, thereby facilitating early mobilization and oral intake (Abdelhameed et al. 2025; Grevstad et al. 2015; Cusack & Buggy 2020).

Concurrently, there is an increasing interest in optimizing perioperative nutritional care. Nutritional interventions are designed to identify and correct malnutrition, reduce fasting times, and provide early postoperative substrates that support wound healing and rehabilitation (Weimann et al. 2017, 2021). Nutritional interventions such as high-protein oral supplements, immunonutrition, micronutrient supplementation, carbohydrate loading, and early feeding have been linked with positive outcomes in surgical and orthopedic populations (He et al. 2022; Gregori et al. 2023; Deng et al. 2022).

12.3 Core ERAS Elements in Orthopedic Surgery

12.3.1 ERAS Recommendations for Hip and Knee Arthroplasty

The ERAS Society Consensus Statement for THA and TKA lists 17 key elements across preoperative, intraoperative, and postoperative phases, including patient education, optimization of comorbidities, anesthetic and analgesic modalities, surgical technique, thromboprophylaxis, fluid management, nutrition, and mobilization (Wainwright et al. 2020). These elements are supported by evidence from review articles and meta-analyses, such as multimodal analgesia, neuraxial or short-acting general anesthesia, early mobilization, and early oral nutrition (Chung et al. 2021; Changjun et al. 2023; Zhu et al. 2017). Table 12.1 highlights the major ERAS elements of THA/TKA with a focus on anesthesia and nutrition.

Table 12.1 Principal ERAS elements for total hip and knee arthroplasty with emphasis on anesthesia and nutrition

Perioperative phase	Key ERAS element	Anesthesia/nutrition focus	Evidence highlights
Preoperative	Patient education and expectation management	Explanation of anesthetic options, analgesia plan, mobilization targets, and nutrition goals	Preoperative education reduces anxiety, improves satisfaction, and may enhance adherence to early mobilization and feeding (Wainwright et al. 2020)
Preoperative	Optimization of anemia, diabetes, smoking, and nutrition	Prehabilitation, including dietitian referral; correction of anemia, vitamin D deficiency, and malnutrition	Preoperative anemia and malnutrition increase infection, transfusion, and LOS; targeted optimization improves outcomes (Bohl et al. 2016; Viola et al. 2015)
Preoperative	Fasting and carbohydrate loading	Clear fluids until 2 h pre-induction; carbohydrate drinks up to 2–3 h before anesthesia	Carbohydrate loading attenuates insulin resistance and improves comfort without raising aspiration risk in suitable patients (He et al. 2022; Weimann et al. 2021)
Intraoperative	Standardized anesthetic protocol	Neuraxial or short-acting general anesthesia; hemodynamic stability; avoidance of excessive depth	Standardized anesthetic care supports rapid emergence, fewer complications, and shorter LOS (Wainwright et al. 2020)

(Continued)

Table 12.1 (Continued)

Perioperative phase	Key ERAS element	Anesthesia/nutrition focus	Evidence highlights
Intraoperative	Multimodal, opioid-sparing analgesia	LIA, regional nerve blocks, scheduled non-opioid analgesics, minimal IV opioids	Multimodal regimens reduce pain, opioid use, and PONV, enabling early mobilization (Cusack & Buggy 2020; Wang et al. 2017)
Intraoperative	Goal-directed fluid therapy	Restriction of salt/water overload; maintenance of euvolemia	Goal-directed strategies reduce cardiopulmonary complications and LOS (Weimann et al. 2021)
Postoperative	Early oral intake and nutrition	Oral fluids and diet within hours of surgery; high-protein supplements for at-risk patients	Early feeding is safe and associated with reduced infection and preserved lean mass (Deng et al. 2022)
Postoperative	Early mobilization	Analgesia and hemodynamic stability permitting standing and ambulation on days 0–1	Early mobilization predicts shorter LOS and better functional outcomes (Keogh et al. 2025; Zhu et al. 2017)

As shown in Table 12.1, several perioperative phases offer clear opportunities to integrate anesthetic and nutritional interventions within a coherent pathway.

12.3.2 Outcomes Associated with Orthopedic ERAS Pathways

Systematic reviews and meta-analyses in THA and TKA have demonstrated that the implementation of ERAS programs in these surgical procedures has reduced the LOS in the hospital and complications without affecting the 30-day readmission rate (Chung et al. 2021; Zhou et al. 2024; Zhu et al. 2017). Patients undergoing ERAS programs in these surgical procedures have demonstrated reduced pain scores, less opioid consumption, fewer opioid-related complications, and achievement of functional milestones (Wainwright et al. 2020; Changjun et al. 2023).

Adherence to the entire ERAS bundle, including anesthetic and nutritional components, has demonstrated reduced complications and LOS, indicating the significance of the entire ERAS bundle rather than isolated components (Wainwright et al. 2020).

12.4 Anesthetic Strategies Within Orthopedic ERAS Pathways

12.4.1 Neuraxial Versus General Anesthesia

For elective THA and TKA, the ERAS Society recommendations for anesthesia are either neuraxial (spinal) anesthesia or modern short-acting general anesthesia, as long as these are used in an opioid-sparing, standardized manner (Wainwright et al.

2020). Data collected in the past indicated that, in comparison with traditional general anesthesia, the use of spinal anesthesia has been associated with reduced blood loss, transfusion, thromboembolic events, and mortality, although these differences are minimized with modern techniques of general anesthesia (Andersen et al. 2010; Kehlet 1997).

Spinal anesthesia with low-dose local anesthetics, often combined with intrathecal opioids and light sedation, remains popular for ERAS in arthroplasty because it offers profound analgesia, minimizes perioperative stress, and offers optimal immediate postoperative pain control (Wainwright et al. 2020). When neuraxial anesthesia is contraindicated or declined, a short-acting general anesthetic technique, such as that involving propofol, desflurane or sevoflurane, and remifentanil, combined with regional anesthesia techniques and systemic analgesics, has been shown to result in similar profiles for early recovery (Zhu et al. 2017).

12.4.2 Intraoperative Anesthetic Management

The important intraoperative anesthetic care practices in orthopedic ERAS are: The use of short-acting hypnotics and opioids during anesthesia care allows for rapid recovery from anesthesia and neurological assessment of the patient (Kehlet 2009; Wainwright et al. 2020). In addition, intraoperative normothermia is essential during orthopedic surgery. This is done using a forced-air warming system and intravenous fluid warming (Wainwright et al. 2020). Moreover, it is important to avoid deep anesthesia and prolonged neuromuscular blocking. These factors are linked with poor outcomes such as hypotension, postoperative delirium, and delayed mobilization (Liu et al. 2022). In addition, goal-directed fluid management is essential in the prevention of hypovolemia and fluid overload during orthopedic surgery (Weimann et al. 2021).

The use of regional anesthesia, such as spinal anesthesia, epidural analgesia (less common in primary arthroplasty), peripheral nerve blocks, and local infiltration analgesia, is important in providing afferent blocks and reducing systemic opioid use (Andersen et al. 2008; Cusack & Buggy 2020).

12.4.3 Multimodal, Opioid-Sparing Analgesia

Multimodal analgesia is key in the management of pain in the ERAS for orthopedic surgeries, aiming for optimal pain control with the least possible exposure to opioids and their associated adverse effects (Cusack & Buggy 2020). This includes:

Multimodal analgesia is recommended for optimal pain control, reducing the need for opioids. The scheduled use of paracetamol and NSAIDs or COX-2 inhibitors is recommended as the background analgesic regimen, except in those with contraindications (Wainwright et al. 2020). Gabapentinoids can be used as adjunct analgesics, but caution is recommended in their use because of variable evidence for their effectiveness and potential for sedation and dizziness (Cusack & Buggy 2020).

Periarticular local infiltration analgesia with long-acting local anesthetics, as well as adjuvants such as epinephrine and ketorolac, is commonly used, especially in total knee arthroplasty (TKA) (Andersen et al. 2013; McCartney and McLeod 2011). Regional anesthetic techniques, such as single-shot or continuous nerve blocks, e.g., adductor canal blocks in TKA or fascia iliaca blocks/pericapsular nerve group blocks in total hip arthroplasty (THA), also provide effective postoperative analgesia (Grevstad et al. 2015; Wang et al. 2017). Systemic opioids should be limited to rescue analgesia, using short-acting oral agents whenever possible, with a reduction in the use of long-acting agents and infusions to minimize opioid-related side effects (Wainwright et al. 2020).

Multimodal analgesic techniques are supported by various studies that prove that multimodal analgesia is associated with reduced pain scores, opioid consumption, postoperative nausea and vomiting, length of stay, and earlier ambulation (Cusack & Buggy 2020; Wang et al. 2017).

12.4.4 Motor-Sparing Regional Techniques

To achieve the ERAS protocol objectives of early mobilization, there has been a trend toward motor-sparing regional techniques. ACB has largely replaced femoral nerve blocks in the perioperative period for TKA, as it has been shown to provide analgesia as effective as femoral blocks while reducing the risk of falls (Grevstad et al. 2015; Wang et al. 2017). Combination ACB/LIA has been associated with high patient satisfaction, low opioid usage, and early ambulation (Andersen et al. 2013).

In the perioperative period for THA, LIA, in combination with fascia iliaca or pericapsular nerve group blocks, has been used as an adjunct to neuraxial anesthesia, although the evidence base is not as strong as for TKA (Wang et al. 2017). The choice and dose of regional anesthesia techniques should be tailored according to the dual objectives of analgesia and motor function.

12.4.5 Corticosteroids and PONV Prophylaxis

Single-dose dexamethasone, e.g., 4–8 mg IV, is commonly included in ERAS algorithms due to its analgesic-sparing and antiemetic properties (Abdelhameed et al. 2025; Xu et al. 2025). Clinical trials of dexamethasone in orthopedic surgery have demonstrated pain, opioid, and PONV reduction without increasing the risk of infection in immunocompetent patients; however, blood glucose levels should be monitored in diabetic patients.

Risk-stratified, multimodal PONV prophylaxis, commonly with dexamethasone, a 5-HT_3 antagonist, and additional agents in high-risk patients, is essential in facilitating early oral intake and mobilization of patients (Cusack & Buggy 2020). Opioid minimization is itself an effective antiemetic strategy.

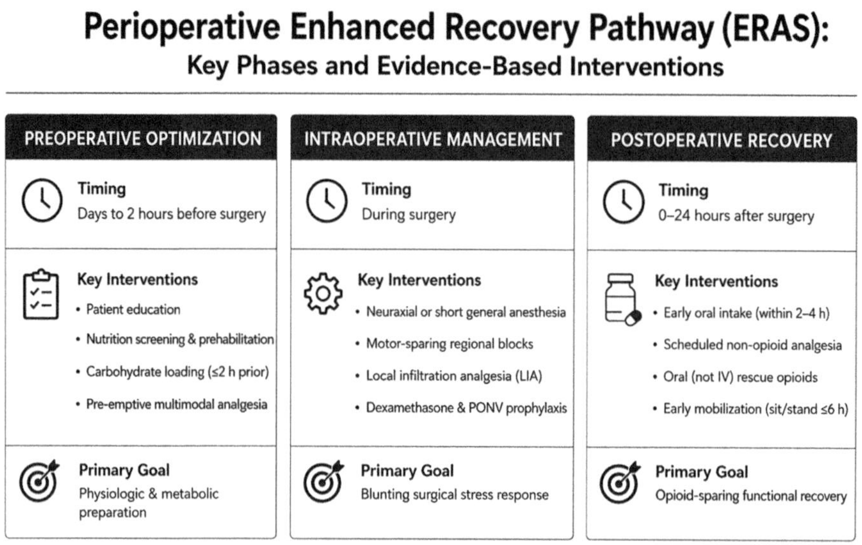

Fig. 12.1 Schematic ERAS anesthetic and analgesic pathway for total hip and knee arthroplasty. (Created by author using MS Word 2021)

12.4.6 Postoperative Analgesia and Mobilization

After surgery, ERAS programs promote continued use of non-opioid pain medication as planned, early transition to oral medication, and avoidance of continuous IV opioid infusions (Wainwright et al. 2020). When nerve blocks and/or liposomal local anesthetics are used, they help prolong pain relief. However, these must be used carefully so as not to impair movement or delay mobilization (Grevstad et al. 2015).

By integrating all these features, patients can be sitting up and standing in 6 hours or so after their operation, start mobilizing on their feet on postoperative day 0 or 1, and be discharged home within 1–3 days for uncomplicated joint replacement procedures (Keogh et al. 2025; Wainwright et al. 2020). Figure 12.1 shows a schematic of the ERAS anesthetic and analgesic pathway.

12.5 Nutritional Optimization in Orthopedic ERAS

12.5.1 Prevalence and Impact of Malnutrition

This issue of malnutrition in orthopedic patients tends to go unnoticed despite the fact that malnutrition in such patients is quite prevalent (Gregori et al. 2023). Narrative review articles indicate that as many as 8.5–50% of total joint arthroplasty patients may have at least one preoperative malnutrition criterion based on the tools used (Weimann et al. 2017, 2021). In total, as many as two-thirds of patients undergoing major surgeries may suffer from malnutrition, which may often go untreated.

In patients undergoing orthopedic surgeries, preoperative malnutrition, as indicated by low albumin, low body mass index, and controlling nutritional status, may be related to an increased risk of infections, periprosthetic infections, wound dehiscence, nonunion, readmission, and mortality (Bohl et al. 2016; Chen and Chen 2024; De Mauro et al. 2024; Veizi et al. 2025). In patients undergoing knee replacement surgeries, a controlling nutritional status of 2 or more may indicate a significantly higher rate of infections and longer hospital stays (Veizi et al. 2025). In elderly patients with femoral neck fractures undergoing arthroplasty, nutritional status may foresee more complications, lower mobility, and lower functional status (Helminen et al. 2017).

Nutritional gaps between different groups contribute to unequal access to total joint arthroplasty (TJA) as well as different outcomes following the procedure, emphasizing the significance of early screening and intervention in this regard (Chen and Chen 2024).

12.5.2 Nutritional Risk Screening Tools

It has been recommended that nutritional screening be carried out as a routine measure for all candidates undergoing orthopedic surgery, preferably weeks before the intended surgical procedure (Weimann et al. 2021). Some of the tools that are commonly used in the screening process include:

- Mini Nutritional Assessment Short Form (MNA-SF), especially in older populations, in which scores of 11 or less indicate malnutrition risk (Kaiser et al. 2009).
- Nutritional Risk Screening (NRS-2002), in which the screening tool considers the severity of the illness, body mass index, weight loss, and decreased food intake, in which scores of 3 or higher indicate malnutrition risk (Almeida et al. 2012; Sun et al. 2015).
- Perioperative Nutrition Screen (PONS), in which the tool consists of four simple questions regarding unintended weight loss, food intake less than 50% of the usual amount, body mass index, and hypoalbuminemia, in which the presence of any of these or an albumin level less than 3.0 g/dL indicates malnutrition risk (Williams et al. 2022; Zhang et al. 2021).
- Laboratory-based tools, including the CONUT score, which includes the measurement of albumin, total lymphocyte count, and cholesterol in the determination of malnutrition risk in patients undergoing total joint arthroplasty and in the orthopedic population (Veizi et al. 2025).

In addition, validation studies have confirmed that positive results for the PONS screen and abnormal nutritional biomarkers predict longer hospital stays, increased infections, and readmission rates for all surgical groups (Williams et al. 2022). Table 12.2 outlines some of the key tools and indices used for orthopedic ERAS.

Table 12.2 Selected nutritional screening tools and indices relevant to orthopedic ERAS

Tool/index	Core components	Typical cutoffs	Evidence in orthopedic/perioperative settings
MNA-SF	Weight loss, appetite, mobility, psychological stress, neurocognitive status, BMI	≤11 indicates risk of malnutrition	Widely used in geriatric hip fracture and arthroplasty cohorts; low scores predict complications and mortality (Helminen et al. 2017; Kaiser et al. 2009)
NRS-2002	BMI, recent weight loss, reduced intake, disease severity	≥3 indicates nutritional risk	Validated in mixed surgical populations; higher scores correlate with infections and LOS (Almeida et al. 2012; Sun et al. 2015)
PONS	Weight loss, intake <50% of normal, BMI thresholds, albumin <3.0 g/dL	Any positive item or albumin <3.0 g/dL defines risk	Predicts prolonged LOS and readmissions; easily implemented in preoperative clinics (Williams et al. 2022; Zhang et al. 2021)
CONUT score	Albumin, total lymphocyte count, and cholesterol	≥2 indicates malnutrition risk	Higher scores associated with infection and LOS in TKA and other orthopedic cohorts (Veizi et al. 2025)

As indicated in Table 12.2, combining simple bedside screens with laboratory indices is usually necessary to capture the full spectrum of nutritional risk (Weimann et al. 2021).

12.5.3 Preoperative Nutrition Interventions

Ideally, evidence-based nutritional optimization should start 2–4 weeks prior to elective surgery, especially in patients identified as being at risk (Weimann et al. 2021). The main aspects include:

Optimization of energy and protein: The recommendation is 1.2–2.0 g/kg/day protein, with up to 3.0 g/kg/day in highly catabolic states, with sufficient energy to prevent further weight loss (Weimann et al. 2021).

High-protein oral nutritional supplements: In THA/TKA patients, 400–600 kcal/day with 20–30 g protein, given 7–14 days prior to surgery and continued after, has been shown to improve nitrogen balance, serum albumin/prealbumin, and possibly reduce postoperative complications (Weimann et al. 2017).

Immunonutrition: Supplementation with arginine, omega-3 fatty acids, and nucleotides given 5–7 days pre- and post-surgery has been shown to reduce postoperative infectious complications and length of stay, with more studies supporting this in orthopedic patients (Gregori et al. 2023).

Micronutrient repletion: It entails correcting vitamin D deficiency, iron-deficiency anemia, as well as other nutritional deficiencies such as zinc and vitamin C. These nutritional deficiencies improve bone health, enhance immunity, and facilitate wound healing, as highlighted in recent reviews and studies (Chiavarini et al. 2024; Greenky et al. 2012; Viola et al. 2015).

Carbohydrate loading: Their loading entails taking carbohydrate-rich drinks 2–3 hours prior to undergoing anesthesia. Carbohydrate loading has been shown to reduce insulin resistance, quench thirst, as well as relieve preoperative anxiety without risking aspiration when fasting guidelines are followed (He et al. 2022; Deng et al. 2022).

Orthopedic literature on preoperative preparation suggests that all these strategies should be incorporated into preoperative preparation under a structured preoperative preparation program led by a dietician with close collaboration with orthopedic surgeons and anesthesiologists (Keogh et al. 2025; Zhang et al. 2025).

12.5.4 Intraoperative and Early Postoperative Nutrition

Long fasting before surgery and delayed feeding of patients after surgery are not in line with the objectives of ERAS. The ESPEN guidelines recommend the intake of clear fluids by patients even up to 2 hours before the administration of anesthesia and to encourage patients to resume oral intake as soon as possible after surgery when the airway is secure and the blood pressure and circulation are stable (Weimann et al. 2021).

In joint replacement surgeries, resumption of oral fluids as soon as possible, even as early as 2–4 hours after surgery, and gradual progression to a light meal have been shown to be safe and well tolerated as long as nausea and vomiting are controlled. Early feeding of patients after surgery reduces the chance of infections, preserves lean body mass, and reduces hospital stays when patients are nil by mouth as opposed to the traditional approach (Deng et al. 2022; Wainwright et al. 2020). High-protein oral nutrition supplements and immunonutrition may be continued for 1–4 weeks after surgery in patients at risk to promote healing and rehabilitation (Gregori et al. 2023). Figure 12.2 presents a step-by-step approach to the care of patients undergoing an orthopedic ERAS pathway.

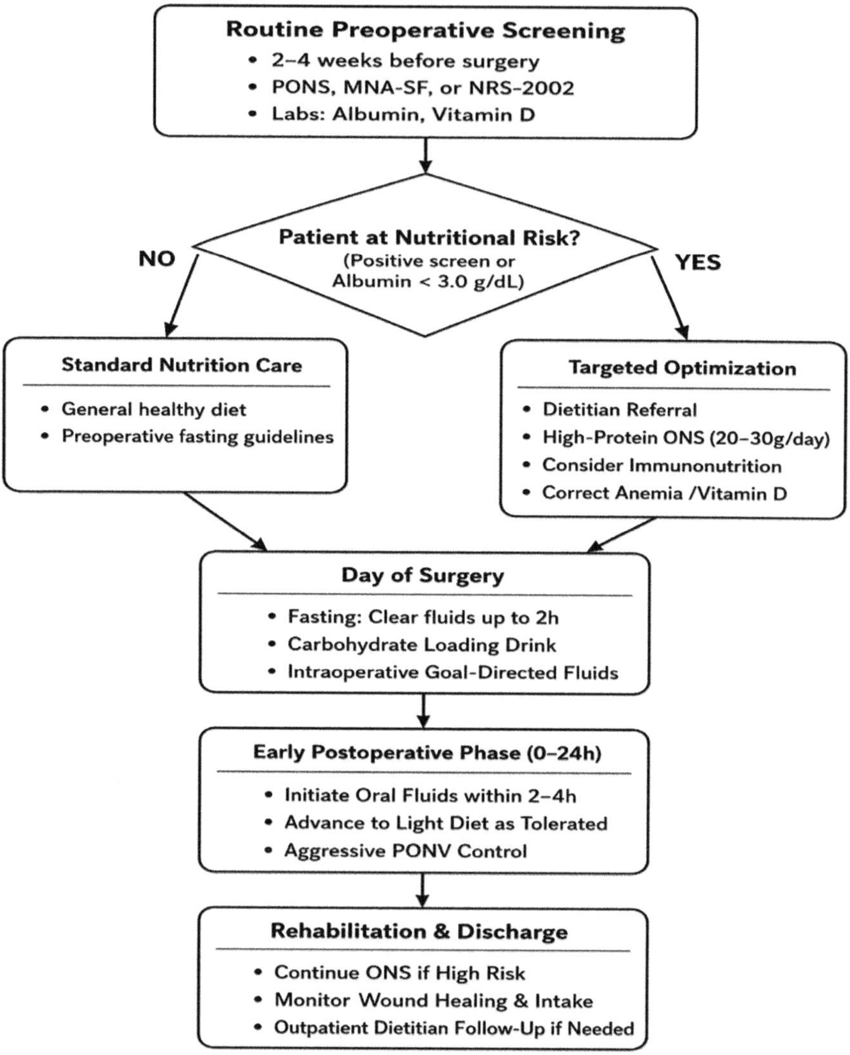

Fig. 12.2 Algorithm for perioperative nutrition optimization in elective orthopedic surgery. (Created by author using MS Word 2021)

12.6 Integrating Anesthesia and Nutrition Within ERAS Bundles

12.6.1 Interdependence of Analgesia, PONV Control, and Early Feeding

Anesthetic and analgesic care is an essential prerequisite for early feeding. Excessive systemic opioids, deep and prolonged anesthesia, and uncontrollable PONV are the main factors that impede early oral feeding in orthopedic surgery (Cusack & Buggy 2020; Xu et al. 2025). Conversely, opioid-sparing neuraxial and regional anesthesia, systemic analgesic care, and management of PONV provide an optimal environment for early oral feeding (Abdelhameed et al. 2025).

Early feeding is essential in facilitating the tolerance of physiotherapy. This is because early feeding provides the substrate required for muscle contraction and repair, maintains glycemic stability, and optimizes the general well-being of the patient (Weimann et al. 2021). Therefore, there is a two-way relationship between anesthesia and nutrition. Adequate analgesic and prophylactic care allow early feeding and physiotherapy, and early feeding optimizes the recovery and minimizes the risk of complications (Gregori et al. 2023; Wainwright et al. 2020).

12.7 An Integrated ERAS Pathway for Elective THA/TKA

A pragmatic integrated pathway for THA/TKA might encompass the following elements:

12.7.1 Preoperative (2–4 Weeks Before Surgery)

In terms of preoperative preparation, the ERAS protocols focus on patient education and optimization of the patient's health status (Wainwright et al. 2020). This is achieved by educating the patient on various aspects of the surgical recovery process, such as anesthesia, pain, early mobilization, discharge, and perioperative nutrition, through various multidisciplinary ERAS education programs. In addition, optimization of comorbid diseases, such as anemia, diabetes, cardiovascular diseases, and smoking, is carried out in consultation with the patient's primary care team and perioperative medicine specialists (Greenky et al. 2012; Viola et al. 2015).

Similarly, nutritional assessment is another crucial step in preoperative optimization (Weimann et al. 2021). This is done by using various screening tools such as the Perioperative Nutrition Screen (PONS), Mini Nutritional Assessment Short Form (MNA-SF), or Nutritional Risk Screening (NRS-2002) in addition to various biochemical tests such as albumin, vitamin D, and iron levels (Williams et al. 2022). According to these results, oral nutritional supplements with a high protein content can be started, and in certain cases, immunonutrition and vitamin supplementation can be recommended (Gregori et al. 2023). Along with this, physical prehabilitation and lifestyle modifications such as exercise, smoking cessation, and restriction of alcohol are recommended for better surgical outcomes (Keogh et al. 2025; Zhang et al. 2025).

12.7.2 Day of Surgery

On the day of surgery, patients should be given pre-specified fasting and carbohydrate-loading instructions for metabolic stability (He et al. 2022). For preemptive analgesia, oral paracetamol and NSAIDs or COX-2 inhibitors with or without gabapentinoids should be considered based on specific clinical and patient-related factors (Wainwright et al. 2020). Furthermore, it should be confirmed pre-surgery that the standardized anesthetic technique will be used, including spinal or general anesthesia, as well as regional analgesic methods such as adductor canal block (ACB), fascia iliaca or pericapsular blocks, and local infiltration analgesia (LIA) (Grevstad et al. 2015; Wang et al. 2017).

12.7.3 Intraoperative

During the intraoperative phase, anesthesia can be achieved through the use of neuraxial techniques or short-acting general anesthesia, with careful control of hemodynamic stability and normothermia to minimize perioperative complications (Wainwright et al. 2020). The motor-sparing regional analgesia techniques, in association with local infiltration analgesia (LIA), are used for effective pain relief while maintaining motor functions and promoting early mobilization (Andersen et al. 2013). It has been recommended that a single dose of dexamethasone should be given, along with prophylaxis for PONV, as well as crystalloid fluids for optimal fluid balance (Abdelhameed et al. 2025; Weimann et al. 2021; Xu et al. 2025).

12.7.4 Early Postoperative (0–24 Hours)

In the postoperative period, the resumption of oral intake is strongly encouraged as part of the enhanced recovery protocol. Patients are advised to take clear fluids within 2–4 hours post-surgery, progressing to a light diet as tolerated to promote recovery and metabolic stability (Deng et al. 2022). Pain management in the postoperative period involves the scheduled administration of paracetamol and NSAIDs or COX-2 inhibitors, with systemic opioids reserved as rescue analgesia in preference to short-acting oral opioids (Cusack & Buggy 2020).

Early mobilization is also an essential part of postoperative care, with patients encouraged to sit out of bed and stand within approximately 6 hours post-surgery, progressing to ambulation on the day of surgery or the first postoperative day (Keogh et al. 2025). Furthermore, nutritional support is continued in the postoperative recovery period, including the administration of oral nutritional supplements and immunonutrition in patients deemed at nutritional risk (Gregori et al. 2023).

12.7.5 Discharge and Follow-Up

Discharge is appropriate when pain is well controlled with oral medication, mobility and self-care are satisfactory, and oral intake is sufficient, usually after 1–3 days in uncomplicated cases (Zhu et al. 2017). An early review in the outpatient department, 1–2 weeks after surgery, should monitor pain control, nutritional status, wound healing, and functional progress with continued dietary and rehabilitation support as necessary (Wainwright et al. 2020).

12.8 Extensions to Spine Surgery and Fragility Hip Fractures

The principles of Enhanced Recovery After Surgery (ERAS) are increasingly being applied to major spine surgeries. ERAS is based on the concept of multimodal opioid-sparing analgesia, mobilization of the patient as soon as possible, fluid management, and the importance of the patient's nutritional status, especially in cases of deformity correction and fusion surgeries (Bansal et al. 2022; Tong et al. 2020).

The ERAS protocol in hip fracture patients has been shown to reduce complications by promoting prompt evaluation and management by a team, early start of surgical procedures within 1–2 days, regional anesthesia, prevention of nausea, vomiting, and delirium, early patient mobilization, and optimal nutritional support from admission through rehabilitation (Fox et al. 2025; Kristensen and Kehlet 2012). As patients with hip fractures are mostly admitted with compromised nutritional status and cognitive dysfunction, nutritional screening and prompt nutritional support are critical in this patient group (Chiavarini et al. 2024; Helminen et al. 2017).

References

Abdelhameed MA, Khalifa AA, Mahran MA, Kameel DN, Bakr HM, Abdelnasser MK. A single preoperative low dose of dexamethasone is efficacious in improving early postoperative pain, function, nausea, and vomiting after primary total knee arthroplasty: a randomized, double-blind, placebo-controlled trial. J Arthroplast. 2025;40(7):1719–25. https://doi.org/10.1016/j.arth.2024.11.061.

Almeida AI, Correia M, Camilo M, Ravasco P. Nutritional risk screening in surgery: valid, feasible, easy! Clin Nutr. 2012;31(2):206–11. https://doi.org/10.1016/j.clnu.2011.10.003.

Andersen LØ, Husted H, Otte KS, Kristensen BB, Kehlet H. High-volume infiltration analgesia in total knee arthroplasty: a randomized, double-blind, placebo-controlled trial. Acta Anaesthesiol Scand. 2008;52(10):1331–5. https://doi.org/10.1111/j.1399-6576.2008.01777.x.

Andersen KV, Bak M, Christensen BV, Harazuk J, Pedersen NA, Søballe K. A randomized, controlled trial comparing local infiltration analgesia with epidural infusion for total knee arthroplasty. Acta Orthop. 2010;81(5):606–10. https://doi.org/10.3109/17453674.2010.519165.

Andersen KV, Pfeiffer-Jensen M, Haraldsted V, Søballe K. Local infiltration analgesia for total knee arthroplasty: should ketorolac be added? Br J Anaesth. 2013;111(2):242–8. https://doi.org/10.1093/bja/aet030.

Bansal T, Sharan AD, Garg B. Enhanced recovery after surgery (ERAS) protocol in spine surgery. J Clin Orthop Trauma. 2022;31:101944. https://doi.org/10.1016/j.jcot.2022.101944.

Betül GYV, Şahan G, Cem D, Yasin E, Enejd V, Ahmet F. The role of preoperative nutritional status in predicting surgical outcomes after total knee arthroplasty: A CONUT-based analysis Joint Diseases and Related Surgery 2025;36(3):604-611. https://doi.org/10.52312/jdrs.2025.2412.

Bohl DD, Shen MR, Kayupov E, Della Valle CJ. Hypoalbuminemia independently predicts surgical site infection, pneumonia, length of stay, and readmission after total joint arthroplasty. J Arthroplast. 2016;31(1):15–21. https://doi.org/10.1016/j.arth.2015.08.028.

Changjun C, Xin Z, Yue L, Liyile C, Pengde K. Key elements of enhanced recovery after total joint arthroplasty: a reanalysis of the enhanced recovery after surgery guidelines. Orthop Surg. 2023;15(3):671–8. https://doi.org/10.1111/os.13623.

Chen Y, Chen W. Association between malnutrition status and total joint arthroplasty periprosthetic joint infection and surgical site infection: a systematic review meta-analysis. J Orthop Surg Res. 2024;19(1):660. https://doi.org/10.1186/s13018-024-05165-1.

Chiavarini M, Ricciotti GM, Genga A, Faggi MI, Rinaldi A, Toscano OD, D'Errico MM, Barbadoro P. Malnutrition-related health outcomes in older adults with hip fractures: a systematic review and meta-analysis. Nutrients. 2024;16(7):1069. https://doi.org/10.3390/nu16071069.

Chung MMT, Ng JKF, Ng FY, Chan PK, Chiu KY. Effects of enhanced recovery after surgery practices on postoperative recovery and length of stay after unilateral primary total hip or knee arthroplasty in a private hospital. Hong Kong Med J. 2021;27(6):437–43. https://doi.org/10.12809/hkmj208587.

Cusack B, Buggy DJ. Anaesthesia analgesia and the surgical stress response BJA Education 2020;20(9):321-328. https://doi.org/10.1016/j.bjae.2020.04.006.

De Mauro D, Bizzoca D, Nappi V, et al. Malnutrition affects infection rates and quality of life in patients undergoing total joint arthroplasty. J Orthop Surg Res. 2024;21:145. https://doi.org/10.5194/jbji-11-139-2026.

Deng H, Li B, Qin X. Early versus delay oral feeding for patients after upper gastrointestinal surgery: a systematic review and meta-analysis of randomized controlled trials. Cancer Cell Int. 2022;22(1):167. https://doi.org/10.1186/s12935-022-02586-y.

Fox C, Hammond SP, Shepstone L, Poland F, Henderson C, Backhouse T, et al. Enhanced recovery pathway for older people with hip fracture and cognitive impairment in acute hospitals: the PERFECTED research programme including an RCT. Programme Grants Appl Res. 2025;13(1) https://doi.org/10.3310/mdtt6530.

Greenky M, Gandhi K, Pulido L, Restrepo C, Parvizi J. Preoperative anemia in total joint arthroplasty: is it associated with periprosthetic joint infection? Clin Orthop Relat Res. 2012;470(10):2695–701. https://doi.org/10.1007/s11999-012-2435-z.

Gregori P, Franceschetti E, Basciani S, Impieri L, Zampogna B, Matano A, Manzi C, Carbone L, Marano L, Papalia R. Immunonutrition in orthopedic and traumatic patients. Nutrients. 2023;15(3):537. https://doi.org/10.3390/nu15030537.

Grevstad U, Mathiesen O, Valentiner LS, Jaeger P, Hilsted KL, Dahl JB. Effect of adductor canal block versus femoral nerve block on quadriceps strength, mobilization, and pain after total knee arthroplasty: a randomized, blinded study. Reg Anesth Pain Med. 2015;40(1):3–10. https://doi.org/10.1097/AAP.0000000000000169.

Helminen H, Luukkaala T, Saarnio J, Nuotio M. Comparison of the Mini-Nutritional Assessment short and long form and serum albumin as prognostic indicators of hip fracture outcomes. Injury. 2017;48(4):903–8. https://doi.org/10.1016/j.injury.2017.02.007.

Kaiser MJ, Bauer JM, Ramsch C, Uter W, Guigoz Y, Cederholm T, Thomas DR, Anthony P, Charlton KE, Maggio M, Tsai AC, Grathwohl D, Vellas B, Sieber CC, MNA-International Group. Validation of the Mini Nutritional Assessment short-form (MNA-SF): a practical tool for identification of nutritional status. J Nutr Health Aging. 2009;13(9):782–8. https://doi.org/10.1007/s12603-009-0214-7.

Kehlet H. Multimodal approach to control postoperative pathophysiology and rehabilitation. Br J Anaesth. 1997;78(5):606–17. https://doi.org/10.1093/bja/78.5.606.

Kehlet H. Multimodal approach to postoperative recovery. Curr Opin Crit Care. 2009;15(4):355–8. https://doi.org/10.1097/MCC.0b013e32832fbbe7.

Keogh JAJ, Keng I, Dhillon DS, Bourgeault-Gagnon Y, Simunovic N, Ayeni OR. The effects of structured prehabilitation on postoperative outcomes following total hip and total knee arthroplasty: an overview of systematic reviews and meta-analyses of randomized controlled trials. J Orthop Sports Phys Ther. 2025;55(5):344–65. https://doi.org/10.2519/jospt.2025.13075.

Kristensen MT, Kehlet H. Most patients regain prefracture basic mobility after hip fracture surgery in a fast-track programme. Dan Med J. 2012;59(6):A4447. Most patients regain prefracture basic mobility after hip fracture surgery in a fast-track programme - PubMed

Liu H, Liu H, Zhang X, Chen H, Yang L, Wang Y, Li N. Nutritional status according to the short-form Mini Nutritional Assessment and clinical outcomes in older inpatients. Front Nutr. 2022;9:815578. https://www.frontiersin.org/articles/10.3389/fnut.2022.815578

McCartney CJ, McLeod GA. Local infiltration analgesia for total knee arthroplasty. Br J Anaesth. 2011;107(4):487–9. https://doi.org/10.1093/bja/aer255.

Sun Z, Kong XJ, Jing X, Deng RJ, Tian ZB. Nutritional risk screening 2002 as a predictor of postoperative outcomes in patients undergoing abdominal surgery: a systematic review and meta-analysis of prospective cohort studies. PLoS One. 2015;10(7):e0132857. https://doi.org/10.1371/journal.pone.0132857.

Tong Y, Fernandez L, Bendo JA, Spivak JM. Enhanced recovery after surgery trends in adult spine surgery: a systematic review. Int J Spine Surg. 2020;14(4):623–40. https://doi.org/10.14444/7083.

Viola J, Gomez MM, Restrepo C, Maltenfort MG, Parvizi J. Preoperative anemia increases postoperative complications and mortality following total joint arthroplast. J Arthroplast. 2015;30(5):846–8. https://doi.org/10.1016/j.arth.2014.12.026.

Wainwright TW, Gill M, McDonald DA, Middleton RG, Reed M, Sahota O, Yates P, Ljungqvist O. Consensus statement for perioperative care in total hip replacement and total knee replacement surgery: Enhanced Recovery After Surgery (ERAS®) Society recommendations. Acta Orthop. 2020;91(1):3–19. https://doi.org/10.1080/17453674.2019.1683790.

Wang D, Yang Y, Li Q, Tang SL, Zeng WN, Xu J, Xie TH, Pei FX, Yang L, Li LL, Zhou ZK. Adductor canal block versus femoral nerve block for total knee arthroplasty: a meta-analysis of randomized controlled trials. Sci Rep. 2017;7:40721. https://doi.org/10.1038/srep40721.

Weimann A, Braga M, Carli F, Higashiguchi T, Hübner M, Klek S, Laviano A, Ljungqvist O, Lobo DN, Martindale R, Waitzberg DL, Bischoff SC, Singer P. ESPEN guideline: clinical nutrition in surgery. Clin Nutr. 2017;36(3):623–50. https://doi.org/10.1016/j.clnu.2017.02.013.

Weimann A, Braga M, Carli F, Higashiguchi T, Hübner M, Klek S, Laviano A, Ljungqvist O, Lobo DN, Martindale RG, Waitzberg D, Bischoff SC, Singer P. ESPEN practical guideline: clinical nutrition in surgery. Clin Nutr. 2021;40(7):4745–61. https://doi.org/10.1016/j.clnu.2021.03.031.

Williams DGA, Aronson S, Murray S, et al. Validation of the perioperative nutrition screen for prediction of postoperative outcomes. J Parenter Enter Nutr. 2022;46:1307–15. https://doi.org/10.1002/jpen.2310.

Xu C, Wang X, Wang M, Wang D, Kong S, Zhou Q, Lu J, Wang A. Implication of preoperative intravenous dexamethasone on pain and nausea in late-stage elderly total knee arthroplasty patients: a randomized double-blind trial. J Arthroplast. 2025;40(12):3176–85. https://doi.org/10.1016/j.arth.2025.05.065.

Yuying H, Rongrong W, Fei W, Lili C, Tingting S, Luya Z. The clinical effect and safety of new preoperative fasting time guidelines for elective surgery: a systematic review and meta-analysis Gland Surgery. 2022;11(3):563-575. https://doi.org/10.21037/gs-22-49.

Zhang F, He ST, Zhang Y, Mu DL, Wang DX. Comparison of two malnutrition assessment scales in predicting postoperative complications in elderly patients undergoing noncardiac surgery. Front Public Health. 2021;9:694368. https://doi.org/10.3389/fpubh.2021.694368.

Zhang W, Lu X, Yang N, Zhu X, Hu H. Prehabilitation is effective in relieving pain after knee arthroplasty, but has little effect on length of stay and knee function: a meta-analysis of randomized controlled trials. Front Med. 2025;12:1457407. https://doi.org/10.3389/fmed.2025.1457407.

Zhou W, Chu S, Zhou Y, Huang Y. Enhanced recovery after surgery for hip and knee arthroplasty: a systematic review and meta-analysis on randomized control trials. Geriatr Nurs. 2024;60:249–57. https://doi.org/10.1016/j.gerinurse.2024.08.002.

Zhu S, Qian W, Jiang C, Ye C, Chen X. Enhanced recovery after surgery for hip and knee arthroplasty: a systematic review and meta-analysis. Postgrad Med J. 2017;93(1106):736–42. https://doi.org/10.1136/postgradmedj-2017-134991.

Postoperative Pain Management and Early Mobilization: Pillars of Enhanced Recovery After Surgery

13

Sujata N. Walode and Pradnya Shripad Joshi

Abstract

Postsurgery pain remains a huge challenge for recovery, often standing in the way of patients' mobilization and extending the hospital stay period. This chapter explores the mechanisms involved in postsurgery pain and its management using multiple techniques, and the importance of mobilizing patients immediately after postsurgery. Enhanced Recovery After Surgery (ERAS) pathways. These approaches combine comprehensive strategies of pain relief and mobilization of patients to prevent complications, limit the use of opioids, and improve long-duration outcomes following all types of surgery. There is a latest research and meta-analyses demonstrate decrease pain, fewer hospitalizations, and better quality of life. The chapter also addresses the challenges in implementing these concepts, such as involving all health-care professionals and tackling resource constraints, and new technologies, such as AI monitoring. Ultimately, the collaboration between pain management and early mobilization is the foundation of contemporary practice around surgery and helps in getting patients up and about sooner and keeping them healthier for longer.

S. N. Walode (✉)
Assistant Professor Department of Anesthesia & Operation Theatre Technology, MGM School of Biomedical Sciences, Chhatrapati Sambhajinagar Constituent Unit of MGM Institute of Health Sciences, Navi Mumbai, Maharashtra, India

P. S. Joshi
Professor Department of Anesthesiology, MGM Medical College & Hospital, Chhatrapati Sambhajinagar, Maharashtra, India

P. K. Bhattacharyya et al. (eds.), *Integrated Anesthesia and Nutrition Approaches to Enhanced Recovery after Surgery*,
https://doi.org/10.1007/978-981-92-3294-9_13

Keywords

Postoperative pain management · Early mobilization · Multimodal analgesia · Opioid-sparing · Perioperative care · Enhanced Recovery After Surgery (ERAS)

13.1 Introduction

Postsurgical pain is one of the common and significant challenges in surgery. As new pharmacology has evolved over the past few years, pain surveys have consistently reported that between 50% and 80% of surgical patients experience moderate to severe pain during the postoperative period, and that under-managed pain is still common in both well-resourced and hard-pressed health care settings. In addition to discomfort, untreated postoperative pain is causally linked with reduced mobility, além, complications like respiratory complications (atelectasis, pneumonia, hypoxemia, and pulmonary failure, etc.), thromboembolic complications, increased length of stay, and sometimes the development of chronic pain lasting for years has been associated with poorly managed postoperative pain.

The last couple of decades have witnessed a classic shift in perioperative care, crystallized in the form of Enhanced Recovery After Surgery (ERAS) protocols. It's a strategy originally designed and conceptualized by the Danish surgeon Henrik Kehlet in the late 1990s Golder and Papalois 2012). ERAS represents an empirical, multimodal, and multidisciplinary approach to surgical care that targets each and every phase of the Before surgery stages: preoperative, during the surgery, and postoperative—with the goal of reducing physiological stress, improving recovery, and optimizing patient care (Kehlet 1997; Ljungqvist et al. 2017). Within this framework, pain management and early mobilization occupy a position of cardinal importance, as their integration unlocks the full potential of ERAS pathways.

Patients can actively engage in physical rehabilitation if effective analgesia is achieved postsurgery, particularly through multimodal and opioid-sparing strategies. This early mobilization mitigates the hazards of prolonged bed rest as it leads to conditions which include muscle atrophy, insulin resistance, pulmonary atelectasis, deep vein thrombosis, and deconditioning while it simultaneously helps promote gastrointestinal recovery, psychological well-being, and immune function (Wainwright et al. 2020; Brower 2009). So, the reciprocal interaction between ERAS efficacy.

This chapter provides a comprehensive, evidence-based discussion in the two areas of post-operative pain physiology and the array of pain relief techniques available in the peri-operative environment, on one hand, and the framework and protocol that governs the early mobilization of patients in a setting of ERAS, on the other. There is a particular emphasis on issues in the implementation of the system, interdisciplinary coordination needs, evidence of outcomes, and future directions in the use of technology in the care of patients undergoing surgery. Through the explanation of these interconnected and interrelated principles, the chapter will help medical practitioners, nurses, physiotherapists, and health care systems to facilitate patient-centered, coordinated, and effective recovery after surgery.

13.2 Physiology of Postoperative Pain

13.2.1 Nociception and the Pain Cascade

Postoperative pain is fundamentally a consequence of surgical tissue injury, which gets activated due to a complex cascade of nociceptive, inflammatory, and neuroplastic processes. When the incision is taken, at the site of incision or due to organ manipulation, tissue damage fundamentally triggers the release of pro-inflammatory mediators, including prostaglandins, bradykinin, histamine, substance P, and cytokines such as interleukin-1β (IL-1β), interleukin-6 (IL-6), and tumor necrosis factor-alpha (TNF-α) (Woolf and Salter 2000; Brennan 2011; Sherwood 2012). These mediators activate the peripheral nociceptors, i.e., primarily A-delta and C-fiber that results in primary hyperalgesia, this is a state where the pain threshold at the wound site is markedly reduced.

Nociceptive signals are sent from peripheral tissues to the dorsal horn of the spinal cord via afferent nerve fibers. At this synaptic junction, glutamate, substance P, and calcitonin gene-related peptide (CGRP) are released, activating N-methyl-D-aspartate (NMDA) receptors, alpha-amino-3-hydroxy-5-methyl-4-isoxazolepropionic acid (AMPA) receptors, and neurokinin-1 (NK-1) receptors on postsynaptic neurons. This activation triggers wind-up, a process in which dorsal horn neurons gradually amplify pain signals in response to repeated nociceptive input (Dickenson and Sullivan 1987). The persistent stimulation of NMDA receptors is critical in the development of central sensitization, which is a state of higher excitation of the central nervous system (CNS) that causes secondary hyperalgesia (pain beyond the injury's site), allodynia (pain from generally non-painful stimuli), and time summation.

13.2.2 Central Sensitization and Chronic Pain Development

Though often overlooked, central sensitization plays a key role in clinical relevance, as it represents the neurophysiological substrate underlying poorly managed acute postoperative pain to the development of chronic postsurgical pain (CPSP). This CPSP affects approximately 10–50% of patients after commonly done procedures such as thoracotomy, mastectomy, inguinal herniorrhaphy, and total knee arthroplasty, with the incidence depending significantly on the type of procedure, intensity of the acute pain, and individual patient factors (Kehlet et al. 2006). Psychological distress before the surgery, exaggeration, and genetic polymorphisms in pain-processing genes have been detected as a major predisposing factor, highlighting the biopsychosocial dimensions of postoperative pain (VanDenKerkhof et al. 2012).

The descending modulation system, which compromises signal from the periaqueductal gray (PAG), rostral ventromedial medulla (RVM), and locus coeruleus, can cause bidirectional influences on spinal nociception, capable of both inhibiting and boosting pain transmission. As surgical stress disrupts this descending inhibitory control, it eventually contributes to the elevated pain sensitivity observed in the postoperative period (Ossipov et al. 2010). Understanding these mechanisms facilitates a compelling ground for multimodal analgesia for better efficacy: by targeting the multiple sites in the pain cascade altogether, it is possible to achieve a superior analgesic effect while reducing the doses and therefore eventually reducing the adverse effects of individual agents.

13.2.3 Impact of Pain on Surgical Recovery

Inadequately managed postoperative pain triggers multiple physiological disruptions that collectively hinder the surgical recovery. Among all complications, respiratory complications are among the most consequential, as pain restricts chest wall expansion and the cough reflex, making patients susceptible to splinting, atelectasis, hypoxemia, and pneumonia. These are the risks that are particularly occurring after thoracic and upper abdominal surgery (Ballantyne et al. 1998). For example, cardiac events include sympathetic activation mediated by pain, causing tachycardia, hypertension, and increased oxygen consumption by the heart muscle, which can again lead to cardiac events in predisposed patients (Kehlet and Dahl 2003).

There is also a neuro-endocrine response to surgical pain, which involves the surge in levels of cortisol, catecholamines, glucagon, and growth hormone, while suppressing insulin, which leads to hyperglycemia, catabolism, immunosuppression, and delayed wound healing. Pain (including opioids) also causes a reduced gastrointestinal motility, which results in prolonged postoperative ileus and restores the ability for oral feeding. Psychologically, inadequate pain management is associated with anxiety, depression, sleep deprivation, and decreased patient satisfaction, resulting in the physiological toll of recovery. These multisystem effects highlight the need for active, diverse, and patient-specific approaches to pain management in an ERAS.

13.3 Multimodal Analgesia in the ERAS Framework

13.3.1 Principles of Multimodal Analgesia

Multimodal analgesia (MMA) refers to the simultaneous administration of multiple analgesic agents or techniques with different mechanisms of action, which is administered at different points alongside the pain pathway, with an intention of achieving additive or combined analgesic effects while reducing the adverse effects of any single agent (Kehlet and Dahl 1993). This major concept has now become the fundamental approach in pain management guidelines established by several anesthesia societies nationally and internationally, including the American Society of Anesthesiologists (ASA), the European Society of Anaesthesiology (ESA), and ERAS Society policies (Chou et al. 2016; Gustafsson et al. 2019).

The rationale behind MMA is grounded in receptor pharmacology and scientific evidence. Since postoperative pain involves more than one type of receptor system, i.e., opioid receptors, NMDA receptors, cyclooxygenase (COX) enzymes, sodium channels, and adrenergic receptors, combining these mechanisms would be superior to high-dose single-agent therapy. Numerous randomized controlled trials and systematic reviews consistently prove that MMA reduces opioid consumption by 20–60%, lowers pain scores by 20–40%, and diminishes opioid-related side effects, including nausea, vomiting, drowsiness, ileus, and breathing problems. Opioid-related side effects include nausea, vomiting, drowsiness, ileus, and breathing problems. Opioid-related side effects include nausea, vomiting, drowsiness, ileus, and breathing problems (Manion and Brennan 2011; Memtsoudis et al. 2018). Thus, integration of opioid-sparing MMA into ERAS pathways is both clinically advantageous and consistent with the current emphasis on responsible opioid stewardship.

13.3.2 Pharmacological Analgesic Agents

Paracetamol (acetaminophen) is chosen as the analgesic backbone in the context of ERAS protocols due to its favorable safety profile, central and peripheral analgesic action, and efficacy in opioid-sparing properties. Intravenous paracetamol is mostly preferred in the immediate postoperative period for consistent bioavailability. Evidence from systematic reviews indicates that morphine-sparing effects of approximately 9 mg over 24 hours when paracetamol is administered as a scheduled agent (Remy et al. 2005). Non-steroidal anti-inflammatory drugs (NSAIDs), including ketorolac, ibuprofen, celecoxib, and diclofenac, act via inhibiting cyclooxygenase enzymes with consequent reduction in peripheral prostaglandin synthesis and attenuating inflammatory hyperalgesia. The benefit associated with the use of COX-2 selective inhibitors (coxibs) offers limited gastrointestinal and antiplatelet adverse effects compared to non-selective NSAIDs, making them preferable in many perioperative settings (White 2005).

Gabapentinoids, namely gabapentin and pregabalin, act on voltage-gated calcium channels in dorsal horn neurons, helping to control central sensitization and reducing wind-up. The results of meta-analyses demonstrate that postoperative opioid consumption is reduced by 20–35% and pain scores are also decreased at rest and during movement when gabapentinoids are incorporated into multimodal regimens (Tiippana et al. 2007). However, concerns related to dose-dependent sedation, dizziness, and the emerging possibility of respiratory depression in opioid-naive patients should be considered for cautious use of gabapentinoids, especially in elderly and obese patients (Hah et al. 2017; Laskowski et al. 2011). Dexmedetomidine, a selective alpha-2 adrenergic agonist, decreases sympathetic responses, offers anxiolysis and sedation without minimal respiratory depression, and has opioid-sparing properties based on spinal and supraspinal mechanisms (Blaudszun et al. 2012).

13.3.3 Regional Anesthetic Techniques

Regional anesthesia is the strongest component of multimodal analgesia, with segmental blocking of afferent nociceptive transmission and providing effective opioid-sparing. Administration of epidural analgesia via a catheter positioned in the epidural space delivers local anesthetics and/or opioids in proximity to spinal nociceptive pathways, achieving optimal analgesia, particularly for thoracic, abdominal, and lower limb procedures. Multiple meta-analyses confirmed that in high-risk surgery, thoracic epidural analgesia significantly improves pain scores, decreases the neuroendocrine stress response, increases pulmonary function, and reduces postoperative morbidity compared to systemic opioid analgesia. (Block et al. 2003; Popping et al. 2014).

The advent of ultrasound-guided peripheral nerve blocks has expanded the list of regional analgesia considerably, providing procedure-specific, opioid-free analgesia for an encompassing range of surgical procedures. The Transversus Abdominis Plane (TAP) block, quadratus lumborum (QL) block, erector spinae plane (ESP) block, pectoral nerve (PECS) blocks, and adductor canal block stand out as milestones in the field of regional anesthesia that have been seamlessly incorporated into ERAS pathways across surgical specialties (Abdallah and Brull 2013; El-Boghdadly et al. 2017). Liposomal bupivacaine formulations have extended the duration of local infiltration analgesia up to 72 hours, eliminating the need for catheterization, thus making ambulatory procedures possible (Bramlett et al. 2012). Intrathecal administration of opioids, as a component of spinal anesthesia, provides up to 12–24 hours of superior postoperative analgesia, particularly for orthopedic and obstetric procedures, with long-acting formulations further extending this duration.

13.3.4 Pre-emptive and Preventive Analgesia

Pre-emptive analgesia—the administration of an analgesic before the nociceptive impulses are generated as a result of surgical stimuli is conceptually designed to prevent or eliminate central sensitization by ensuring adequate CNS analgesic conditions before the barrage of nociceptive input occurs. While clinical evidence for strict pre-emptive analgesia (defined as treatment before versus after incision) has not been supported, the broader idea of preventive analgesia that attempts to minimize afferent nociceptive signaling throughout the entire perioperative period has been proven beneficial (Ong et al. 2005). The current ERAS protocols now incorporate preoperative analgesic loading with drugs, i.e., celecoxib, gabapentin, paracetamol, as a standard element of premedication. This pre-emptive approach, combined with intraoperative maintenance of analgesia and structured postoperative analgesia, results in a temporal integration of analgesia with minimal sensitization at every phase of the perioperative journey (Chou et al. 2016).

The analgesic agents employed within ERAS-based multimodal pain management protocols vary considerably in their efficacy profiles, adverse effect burdens, and clinical applicability. Table 13.1 provides a structured comparison of the principal analgesic classes currently utilized in perioperative settings, outlining their relative effectiveness, associated risks, representative drug examples, specific roles within ERAS pathways, and key clinical limitations. This comparative overview is intended to guide clinicians in selecting and combining agents to achieve optimal opioid-sparing analgesia while minimizing postoperative complications.

The rationale underlying multimodal analgesia in ERAS lies in the simultaneous targeting of distinct neuroanatomical pain processing pathways, thereby reducing dependence on any single analgesic agent. As illustrated in Fig. 13.1, analgesic agents within ERAS protocols act at three hierarchical levels of the nociceptive pathway—peripheral sensitization, spinal modulation, and supraspinal processing—each addressed by pharmacologically distinct drug classes. At the peripheral level, NSAIDs exert their effect through COX enzyme inhibition alongside local anesthetics, while ketamine (NMDA antagonist), gabapentinoids, and epidural analgesia modulate pain transmission at the spinal cord. Opioids and dexmedetomidine act centrally at the supraspinal level to further attenuate pain perception. This layered, mechanism-based approach reflects the core ERAS principle of achieving synergistic painkiller while limiting the dose-specific side effects related to opioid monotherapy.

Table 13.1 Comparison of analgesic agents used in ERAS-based multimodal pain management

Analgesic class	Efficacy	Adverse effects	Examples	Clinical role in ERAS	Limitations
Opioids	High	Respiratory depression, constipation, nausea, dependence	Morphine, fentanyl, oxycodone	Widely used; WHO analgesic ladder	High risk PONV, tolerance
NSAIDs	Moderate-high	Renal impairment, GI bleeding, platelet dysfunction	Ketorolac, ibuprofen, diclofenac	Effective opioid-sparing; anti-inflammatory	Contraindicated in renal disease
Paracetamol	Mild-moderate	Hepatotoxicity (overdose)	IV/PO paracetamol	Safe, widely available, baseline analgesic	Ceiling effect
Gabapentinoids	Moderate	Sedation, dizziness, respiratory depression	Gabapentin, pregabalin	Reduce opioid consumption by 20–30%	CNS depression risk
Regional Anesthesia	High	Hematoma, nerve injury, local toxicity	Epidural, TAP block, nerve block	Gold standard for procedure-specific pain	Requires skill, equipment
Ketamine (sub-anesthetic)	Moderate-high	Dysphoria, hallucinations at high doses	IV ketamine infusion	NMDA antagonist; prevents central sensitization	Psychomimetic side effects
Dexmedetomidine	Moderate	Bradycardia, hypotension	IV infusion	Alpha-2 agonist; reduces opioid need and anxiety	Hemodynamic monitoring needed
Local infiltration	Moderate	Local toxicity, infection	Bupivacaine, ropivacaine	Wound infiltration; simple administration	Short duration

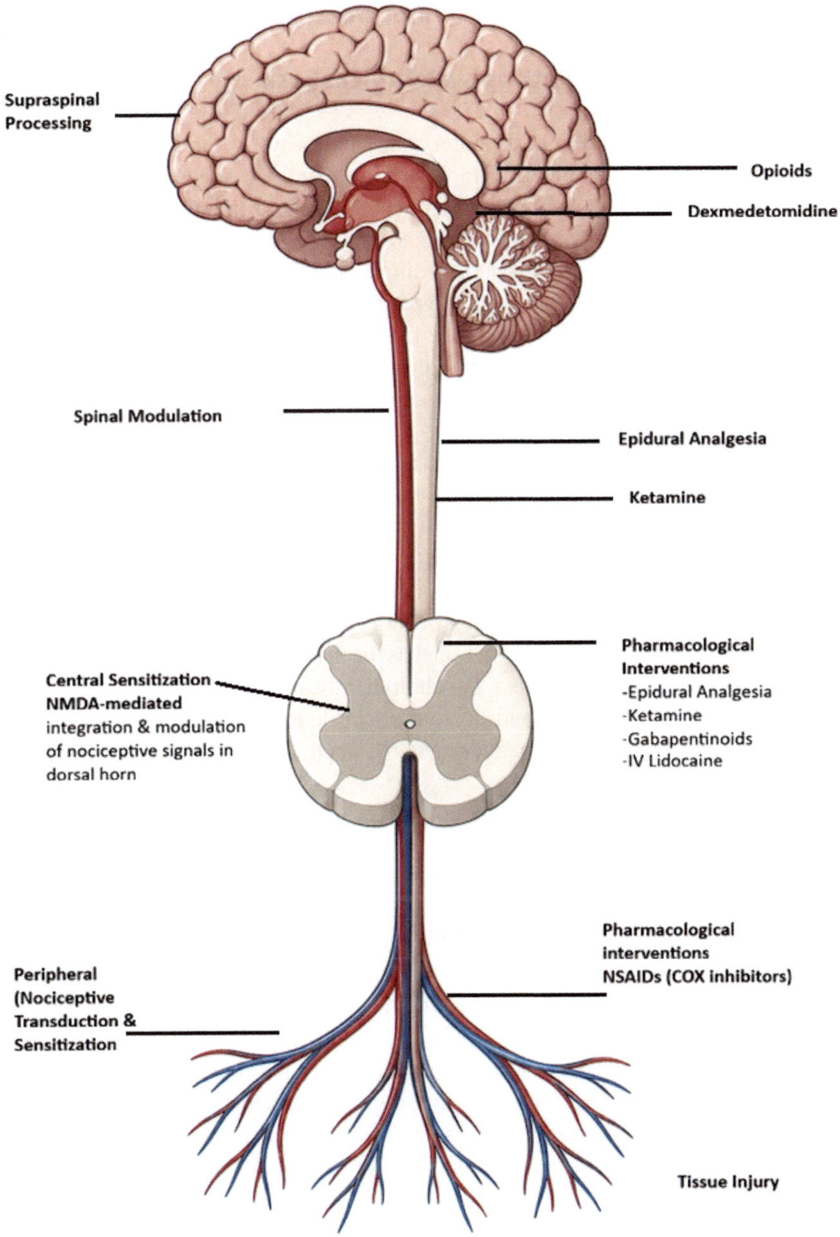

Fig. 13.1 Multimodal analgesic pathways in ERAS. (Created by author using MS Word 2021)

13.4 Early Mobilization as a Pillar of ERAS

13.4.1 Rationale and Pathophysiological Basis

Physiological risks of immobility enter many pathways in many steps, which are becoming increasingly defined. Immobilization results in skeletal muscle wasting within 24 hours due to selective protein degradation via the ubiquitin-proteasome pathway and decreased formation of anabolic proteins such as FaK. Prolonged recumbency results in insulin resistance, similar to the type 2 diabetes mellitus metabolic state and can cause postsurgery hyperglycemia. Immobility can be damaging to the lungs, as it can lead to a decrease in the functional residual capacity (FRC), clearance of mucus, atelectasis, ventilation-perfusion mismatch, and the risk of pneumonia, especially in aged and obese patients, and patients undergoing thoracotomy and abdominal surgery.

The stasis of blood because of decreased muscle pump in the lower-most part of the body, because of immobility, and the hypercoagulation effect following the surgery make one susceptible to postoperative complications such as deep vein thrombosis (DVT) and pulmonary embolism (PE), which are cited as the number one cause of death following surgery. Intestinal motility, which is decreased by the use of opioid analgesics and manipulation during surgery, is also further decreased by immobility; however, early ambulation has been demonstrated to recover bowel motility more rapidly than bedrest. Psychologically, immobility is a source of anxiety, depression, helplessness, and decreased self-learning efficacy, which all contribute to poor motivation for recovery and the need for long-term compliance with rehabilitation.

13.4.2 Definition and Timing of Early Mobilization

Early mobilization (EM) within ERAS is defined as structured, progressive, and goal-directed physical activity initiated by medical professionals within 6–24 hours postsurgery, when patients demonstrate both physiological stability and adequate analgesia (Wainwright et al. 2020). The mobilization continuum includes various activities that start with passive repositioning and active leg exercises in bed and progress through bedside sitting and standing, until patients can walk freely in the corridor, with their advancement depending on their ability to tolerate activities and their current physical state and specific medical requirements.

According to ERAS Society guidelines in colorectal surgery, among the most evidence-based guidelines, the patient must be awake for a minimum of 2 hours during surgery and reach mobilization of at least 6 hours on the first-day postsurgery (Gustafsson et al. 2019). In orthopedics, the ERAS guidelines for total hip and knee replacement aim to mobilize patients 4–6 hours after surgery, which is a paradigm shift from the previous notion of prolonged bed rest after arthroplasty surgery (Wainwright et al. 2020). In thoracic surgery involving video-assisted thoracoscopic surgery (VATS), the mobilization of the patient hours after surgery has become the standard of care in most centers. The common principle across all specialties is that earlier mobilization, safely initiated, consistently yields superior outcomes to delayed ambulation.

13.4.3 Evidence Base for Early Mobilization

Early mobilization has ample support in multiple surgical specialties, patient populations, and healthcare systems. A landmark systematic review and meta-analysis conducted by Willner et al. (2023) examining gastrointestinal and orthopedic surgery revealed that early mobilization reduces hospital length of stay (LOS) by a mean of 1.5–2.5 days, lowers pulmonary complication rates by 40–50%, and significantly reduces DVT incidence compared to standard care. On the other hand, in colorectal surgery, application of early mobilization procedures in the Enhanced Recovery After Surgery pathways leads to decreased prevalence of postoperative ileus by 30–50% and reduction in LOS by 2–4 days (Greco et al. 2014).

In cardiac surgeries, a randomized controlled trial conducted by Stiller and Phillips (2003) found that structured physiotherapy with early mobilization had significantly fewer cases of atelectasis and pneumonia than the unstructured care. In orthopedics, studies on ERAS have shown that immediate mobilization after Total Knee and Total Hip Arthroplasty surgeries significantly decreases the rate of re-admissions (by 20–35%), enhances functional recovery scores at 6 weeks postsurgery, and lowers the incidence of adverse events related to joint replacement surgery (Wainwright et al. 2020). It is important to note that early mobilization does not actually cause the increased rates of surgical complication, wound dehiscence, or pain scores when done alongside adequate multimodal analgesia, an observation which highlights their synergism within the ERAS framework (Kehlet and Wilmore 2008).

13.4.4 Structured Mobilization Protocols

To achieve optimal postoperative mobilization, it is important to adopt structured protocols as part of the ERAS protocol, together with interprofessional collaboration. Prior to surgery, through proper education about the importance of early mobilization, prehabilitation aiming to improve the initial function of the body, and psychological support to avoid fear-avoidant behaviors. During surgery, the type of anesthesia is selected using short-acting drugs to abolish any residual neuromuscular blockade and regional anesthesia.

Postoperatively, the early mobility starts once the patient is medically stable; there is a structured program that defines the exercise program for patients within hours or days after the surgery. Nurses are trained in assisting patients to mobilize, fall prevention, and motivation for mobilization. Physiotherapists formally assess and provide plans for progressive exercise sessions based on the patient's progress and procedure. Electronic medical record documentation of mobilization data supports protocol compliance and outcome audits. Patient-reported time logs and pedometers are now also being used to supplement formal assessments, to increase ambulation data, achieving personalized progression.

Early mobilization is a key component of ERAS protocols, with its timing and structure differing widely across varied surgical fields. Table 13.2 offers a comparison of specialty-specific early mobilization guidelines, including the suggested timing for initial mobilization, activity progression steps, clinical outcomes, and common barriers to implementation. This overview is designed to help clinicians and ERAS teams benchmark and standardize mobilization practices across various surgical populations.

Table 13.2 Early mobilization protocols across surgical specialties: timing, strategies, and outcomes

Surgical procedure	Timing of first mobilization	Recommended mobilization protocol	Outcomes	Barriers
Cardiac surgery	Hours 6–12 postextubation	Supervised passive-to-active mobilization, respiratory physiotherapy	Reduced ICU stay by 1–2 days, lower pulmonary complications	Hemodynamic instability, drains, invasive lines
Colorectal surgery	POD 1 (target: 2 h out of bed)	Ambulation, progressive sitting and standing, core exercises	LOS reduced by 2–3 days; lower ileus rates, reduced DVT	Pain, fatigue, nasogastric tubes
Orthopedic (TKR/THR)	POD 0 within 4–6 h	Full weight-bearing as tolerated; structured physiotherapy	Faster functional return; reduced readmission by ~30%	Quadriceps weakness, fear of falling, prosthetic concerns
Thoracic surgery	POD 0-1 post-VATS	Sit-to-stand, corridor ambulation, inspiratory muscle training	Reduced atelectasis, pneumonia; shorter chest drain duration	Chest tubes, pain, limited mobility
Gynecologic oncology	POD 0-1	Early ambulation, pelvic floor exercises, graded activity	Reduced VTE, earlier return to function; shorter LOS	Fatigue, abdominal wound discomfort
Abdominal/ HPB surgery	POD 1	Ambulation 3–6 times/day with physiotherapy support	Improved GI function recovery, lower pneumonia rates	Abdominal distension, drain management
Bariatric surgery	POD 0 within 6 h	Early ambulation; breathing exercises; progressive ambulation	Reduced respiratory complications; shorter LOS by 1–2 days	Obesity-related mobility challenges, wound care

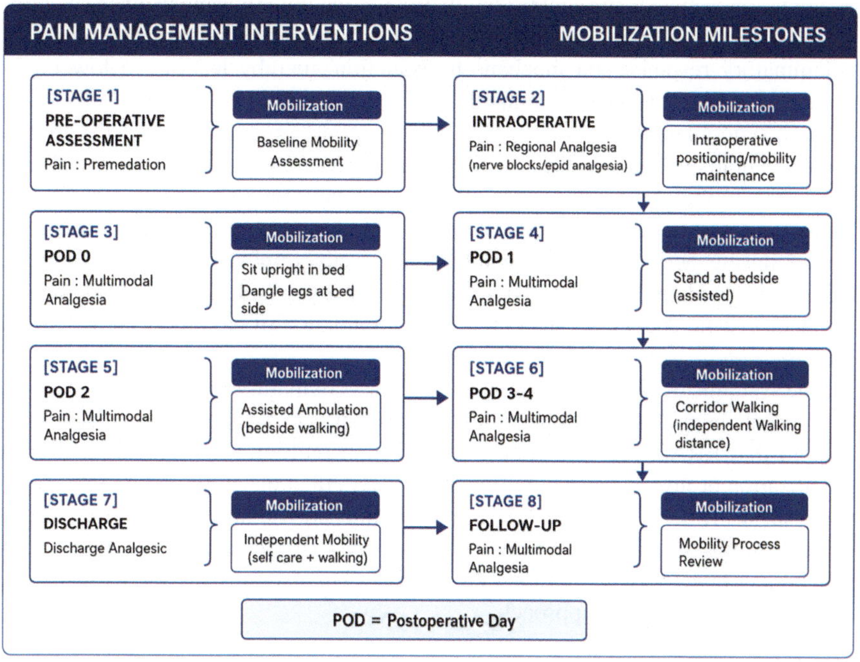

Fig. 13.2 ERAS continuum: integration of pain management and early mobilization. (Created by author using MS PowerPoint 2021)

The eight-stage Enhanced Recovery After Surgery (ERAS) pathway, spanning from preoperative assessment through postoperative follow-up is a part of Integrating Pain Management and Early Mobilization, where each stage pairs pain management strategies—primarily multimodal analgesia targeting a Visual Analog Scale (VAS) score below 4/10—with corresponding mobilization milestones, ranging from baseline mobility assessment and sitting upright in bed (POD 0) to independent corridor walking (POD 3–4) and self-care at discharge. The bidirectional arrows between paired stages reflect the mutually reinforcing relationship between adequate pain control and progressive early mobilization, a core principle of ERAS protocols aimed at reducing postoperative complications and accelerating recovery, as shown in Fig. 13.2.

13.5 The Synergistic Relationship Between Pain Management and Early Mobilization

Pain control and early rehabilitation have a profound inter-relationship and synergy. Pain management is essential to optimal mobilization: pain-induced limitations in movement, fear of re-injury, and balances in non-pain/distracter effects of analgesia all limit the initiation and intensity of exercise programs. Similarly, effective early mobilization mitigates the centralization of pain that underlies persistent postoperative pain, increases endogenous opioid and endocannabinoid release, and blunts the inflammatory response via mechano-transduction, thereby leading to lower pain scores and reduced analgesic demand.

Such synergism is reflected in the "dose–response" relationship for ERAS outcomes: patients with the highest quality of analgesic care scores mobilize first, and those who mobilize first have the lowest subsequent pain scores and opioid use. Underlying mechanisms for this synergy include improved oxygenation of the wound during activity (faster healing), increased lymphatic drainage (reducing inflammatory edema), preservation of muscle glycogen and mitochondrial activity, and neuroplastic changes in the descending modulation of pain induced by aerobic exercise.

The systemic evidence for synergism includes comparative effectiveness studies. In a recent meta-analysis of 16 studies across surgery types, Greco et al. (2014) showed that ERAS strategies that included both multimodal analgesia and early mobilization protocols had a significantly greater effect on complication rates (relative risk: 0.71, 95% CI: 0.60–0.83), and readmissions than protocols that implemented only one of these "pillars." This provides strong empirical evidence that pain and early activity are not only concomitant but also intricately interdependent components of an ERAS approach.

13.6 Challenges in Implementing ERAS Pain and Mobilization Protocols

13.6.1 Interdisciplinary and Organizational Barriers

Optimal ERAS pathways require a level of interdisciplinary collaboration that extends beyond traditional "command and control" approaches to surgery. The surgeon, anesthetist, nurse, physiotherapist, dietician, pharmacist, and psychologist should function as a cohesive team with common goals, clear roles, and effective communication. Pragmatically, the way departments are organized, differences in hierarchies and approaches to practice can make protocol adherence difficult. A systematic review identified inter-professional disharmony, lack of effective leadership, and poor documentation levels as the most common organizational barriers.

Analgesic prescribing practice is a common problem. While evidence favors a multimodal opioid-sparing approach to pain management, the standard practice in many surgical settings is for pain to be managed principally by opioids, due to prescriber habit, patient expectations, the fear of being judged for under-treating pain, and limited time for execution of regional anesthesia techniques. Cultural views on pain and pain management (both provider and patient) also play a role in the uptake of non-opioid-based pain management. Opioid-sparing educational programs for all members of the surgical team, combined with prescriber order sets inputted into the electronic health record to guide protocol-driven prescribing, have been successful in shifting and improving prescribing habits.

13.6.2 Patient-Related Barriers

Individual factors significantly impact early mobilization. Elderly, obese, and cancer patients, who are at high risk of deconditioning before surgery, have lower physiological reserves and are at higher risk of falls, dizziness, and heart disease during early mobilization attempts. Pain anticipation, catastrophizing thoughts, and low perceived self-efficacy are strong predictors of dysfunctional avoidance of mobilization and subsequent functional recovery, highlighting the need for pre-treatment psychological screening and education to reduce fear of pain and increase self-efficacy in ERAS.

Complications such as peripheral sensory loss, severe osteoarthritis, heart failure, and chronic obstructive pulmonary disease (COPD) require tailored mobility programs that consider physiological constraints while still working towards planned activity schedules. Postoperative nausea and vomiting (PONV), a frequent adverse effect of opioids and general anesthesia, substantially impairs early mobilization by inducing debilitating nausea, limiting oral fluid intake, and reinforcing bed-bound behavior. ERAS-aligned PONV prophylaxis using combination antiemetics like ondansetron, dexamethasone, and scopolamine dramatically reduces this barrier and is considered an integral component of opioid-sparing multimodal protocols (Gan et al. 2020).

13.6.3 Resource and System-Level Constraints

One of the problems associated with ERAS is that of resource constraints in the middle- and lower-income health care context. The use of regional anesthesia in terms of ultrasonography and peripheral nerve blocks, as well as epidural analgesia, demands special equipment, time allocation, skilled personnel, and monitoring facilities. However, due to the absence or limited availability of the above elements in resource-constrained environments, ERAS can be implemented only partially, including pharmacological means of pain relief only (Kehlet and Wilmore 2008). In addition, the ratio between staff and patients admitted into the recovery wards may prevent frequent mobilization sessions, especially after work hours (Kehlet and Wilmore 2008).

The financial mechanisms through which health care systems are reimbursed also impact ERAS uptake: Fee-for-service may not appropriately align incentives with the initial investment required to establish an infrastructure to sustain the ERAS protocol, teamwork, and patient education, given the long-term cost-benefit of reducing LOS and complications. Fees for services and bundled payment systems more closely "pay for the protocol." Global ERAS implementation networks, which includes ERAS Society's implementation initiatives and the Global ERAS Initiative, offer standardized audit and monitoring tools, mentoring, and evidence-based tools for implementing ERAS that have been shown to be effective in improving adherence and outcomes across multiple settings.

13.7 Outcomes and Quality Metrics in ERAS

13.7.1 Clinical Outcomes

The clinical outcome data for integrated ERAS protocols, including multimodal analgesia and early mobilization, are the most reliable in surgery. In the year 2014, Nicholson et al., meta-analysis of 13 RCT's in colorectal surgery showed a weighted mean LOS reduction of 2.5 days (95% CI: 1.8–3.2) in ERAS compared to standard care, which showed no significant differences in readmission or death. The incidence of postoperative complications was 30–40% lower, with benefits for pulmonary events, ileus, wound infection, and thromboembolism. In orthopedics, the adoption of ERAS for total knee and hip arthroplasty has led to reductions in LOS from a mean of 5–7 days previously to 1–3 days in many orthopedic units, with improvements in patient-reported outcome measures (PROMs) at 6 weeks and 3 months, decreased transfusion rates, and readmissions. Opioid consumption figures consistently report a 30–60% reduction in morphine equivalent dose (MED) at 24- and 48-hours after surgery in ERAS patients compared to historical controls, a result which has important implications for opioid-related side effects, potential risks for chronic opioid use, and financial implications Memtsoudis et al. (2018). Critically, the reductions in opioid consumption do not come at the expense of diminished quality of pain relief, with non-inferior or improved pain scores on a variety of validated scales such as the Numerical Rating Scale (NRS) and Visual Analog Scale (VAS).

13.7.2 Patient-Reported Outcomes and Quality of Life

Using ERAS protocols results in better patient-reported outcomes than conventional care beyond the immediate recovery period. Health-related quality of life (HRQoL) measures using validated questionnaires such as the EuroQol 5-Dimension Questionnaire (EQ-5D), which is a standardized instrument to measure health-related quality of life (HRQoL), the Short Form (36) Health Survey (SF-36), which is a comprehensive quality-of-life questionnaire, and procedure-specific Patient Reported Outcome Measures (PROMs) consistently indicate such benefits for ERAS patients at 4–12 weeks postsurgery, in dimensions of physical function, pain, fatigue, emotional well-being, and social participation. ERAS patients also report higher rates of patient satisfaction due to improved pain, nausea, patient participation and empowerment, and shorter recovery periods, enabling a quicker return to home and normal activities.

Health-Related Quality of Life (HRQoL) is considerably enhanced by Enhanced Recovery After Surgery (ERAS) protocols, especially after major cancer surgeries, where there is significant functional decline and physiological deterioration following surgery. In contrast to standard perioperative care, which frequently results in prolonged bed rest, impaired nutritional recovery, and prolonged hospital stays, which accelerate sarcopenia and disability, ERAS involves a multimodal evidence-driven strategy that encompasses superior pain management, early enteral feeding, and mobility to expedite functional recovery.

This, in turn, allows for an earlier start to adjuvant treatment such as chemotherapy and radiotherapy, which are essential for cancer control since starting them too late is associated with tumor progression and reduced survival. Meanwhile, ERAS protocols also improve psychological well-being, a critical factor for HRQoL, through early mobilization, which increases self-confidence, lowers anxiety and depression, and restores circadian disruption through improved sleep quality and architecture, and this is supported by decreased opioid use and shorter lengths of stay. Finally, longer-term follow-up studies in colorectal cancer show enhanced survival at 3–5 years in ERAS patients, likely reflecting mitigation of the stress response to surgery, which leads to neuroendocrine and inflammatory processes that downregulate immune response, including natural killer cells that play a key role in surveillance against tumor presence. Absent suppression of immunology during the perioperative period, with early resumption of cancer treatments, ERAS ensures optimal recovery, not only in the short term but also in terms of chronic function and survival, stressing the unequivocal contribution of ERAS in improving clinical (HRQoL and quality of life) and patient-reported outcomes of oncological diseases.

13.8 Future Innovations in Postoperative Pain Management and Mobilization

13.8.1 Artificial Intelligence and Predictive Analytics

Artificial intelligence (AI) and machine learning (ML) technologies will revolutionize pain management and early mobilization by predicting, prescribing, and monitoring. AI models applied to large perioperative data sets can identify risk factors for developing severe postoperative pain, opioid consumption, PONV, and Chronic Post-Surgical Pain (CPSP) in individual patients, allowing for risk-adapted analgesia planning. Natural language processing (NLP) software integrated into the electronic health record can monitor nursing documentation, vital signs, and patient-reported pain evaluations for inadequate pain relief in real time and prompt timely analgesic adjustments. Predictive algorithms of readiness for early mobilization that incorporate vital signs, analgesic dosing doses, and the patient's self-report pain scores can schedule individualized early mobilization programs and notify physiotherapists of the highest readiness for mobilization. Deep learning approaches in pain assessment are progressing objective pain assessment by examining physiognomy, vocal cues, kinematics, and parameters of the autonomic nervous system measured in real time via bedside cameras and body-worn sensors. Such objective pain parameters may be useful in patients with compromised verbal communication, such as elderly patients with diminished cognition, children, and patients on ventilation, in whom reliance on subjective self-reported pain measures is limited.

Artificial intelligence-based decision support systems in anesthesia information management systems (AIMS) can make real-time recommendations for analgesic dosing based on patient pharmacogenomics, co-morbidities, and intraoperatively administered medications.

13.8.2 Wearable Technology and Remote Monitoring

Wearable technology platforms (accelerometers, gyroscopes, heart rate, pulse oximeters, electrodermal activity devices embedded in smart watches, patches, and garments) allow objective continuous measurement of postoperative ambulation, vital signs, and sympathetic responses to pain in the hospital ward and home after discharge. Accelerometery-based step count, walking speed, and activity signals yield objective surrogate measures of function more sensitive and precise than intermittent physiotherapy evaluation. These data streams, integrated with hospital electronic medical record systems, allow physicians to quantify protocol compliance, early physiological responses and can be used to give patients feedback about mobilization progress against protocol standards.

Postsurgical wearable monitoring extends surveillance for ERAS beyond hospital discharge by facilitating early identification of suboptimal recovery, pain, or progressive function loss that might require early readmission. Telehealth platforms integrating wearable data with patient-reported symptom questionnaires and video consultations are increasingly demonstrating feasibility and patient acceptability, with pilot data suggesting reductions in unplanned readmission rates and emergency department visits (Hashimoto et al. 2020). As these technologies mature and become economically accessible, they are expected to fundamentally alter the temporal and geographic boundaries of perioperative care.

13.8.3 Pharmacological Innovations

Some of the new developments that are revolutionizing the delivery and management of postoperative pain management include the use of new long-acting local anesthetic agents like liposomal bupivacaine, extended-release bupivacaine microspheres, and sustained-release meloxicam, among others, which have increased the time period of action of local anesthetics to more than 8 hours, thus making single-shot nerve blocks possible. There is ongoing research into new targeted pain medication delivery using nanoparticles.

Emerging biologic approaches to postoperative pain management include monoclonal antibodies targeting growth factor (NGF), a key mediator of inflammatory and neuropathic pain, combined with anti-IL-6 receptor antibodies, and pro-resolving lipid mediators derived from omega-3 fatty acids, known as specialized pro-resolving mediators (SPMs). Nevertheless, these agents introduce novel mechanisms for pain relief and could meet the needs of patients who do not respond to traditional multimodal treatments. Moreover, the pharmacogenomic profiling, which is used to predict individual responses to analgesics, receptor sensitivity, and adverse effects based on genetic polymorphisms such as CYP2D6 and OPRM1 variants, sheds light on personalized perioperative pain management, although it is still in early development stages.

13.9 Conclusion

Postoperative pain management and early mobilization are the two pillars of Enhanced Recovery After Surgery, and their combination has driven the paradigm shift in perioperative care over the past 25 years. The complex neurophysiology of postoperative pain, including peripheral sensitization, spinal wind-up, central sensitization, and descending pain modulation, requires a pain management strategy that matches its complexity and extends through the pre-, intra-, and postoperative period. But it remains crucial to note that because the effect of immobility can affect many organ systems (respiratory, cardiovascular, metabolic, gastrointestinal, and psychological), it is critical that early mobilization be undertaken as soon as possible with the most effective pain relief measures. The body of evidence for a multimodal, integrated system is significant, consistent, and relevant across a spectrum of medical disciplines. Randomized controlled trials, systematic reviews, and large-scale registry-based trials all point to the fact that ERAS protocols involving multimodal opioid-sparing pain relief and early mobilization decrease hospital length of stay, rates of complications, opioid use, improve patient-reported outcomes, quality of life, and possibly long-term survival in cancer patients. These positive outcomes are obtainable across diverse surgical operations, patient cohorts, and health-care environments, albeit requiring protocol tailoring to accommodate local health-care system attributes and patient needs. Barriers to implementation—related to interdisciplinary communication, prescription culture, patient factors, and limited resources—are present but conquerable by ensuring leadership in organizations to develop policy and practice change, provide protocol infrastructure, educate all members of the team, engage patients, and align health system priorities. With new AI-based pain monitors, devices, extended-release analgesics, and pharmacogenomic personalization, we look towards the future of ever more targeted, responsive, and personalized perioperative pain and rehabilitation. The integrated ERAS approach must be embraced, developed, and promoted by clinicians, health care organizations, and health care systems worldwide as the future of perioperative practice. In doing so, they honor the primary tenets of medical practice to relieve suffering, expedite recovery, and restore function, which is the functional objective of surgery.

References

Abdallah FW, Brull R. Facilitatory effects of perineural dexmedetomidine on neuraxial and peripheral nerve block: a systematic review and meta-analysis. Br J Anaesth. 2013;110(6):915–25. https://doi.org/10.1093/bja/aet066.

Ballantyne JC, Carr DB, deFerranti S, Suarez T, Lau J, Chalmers TC, Angelillo IF, Mosteller F. The comparative effects of postoperative analgesic therapies on pulmonary outcome: cumulative meta-analyses of randomized, controlled trials. Anesth Analg. 1998;86(3):598–612. https://doi.org/10.1097/00000539-199803000-00032.

Blaudszun G, Lysakowski C, Elia N, Tramèr MR. Effect of perioperative systemic α2 agonists on postoperative morphine consumption and pain intensity. Anesthesiology. 2012;116(6):1312–22. https://doi.org/10.1097/ALN.0b013e31825681cb.

Block BM, Liu SS, Rowlingson AJ, Cowan AR, Cowan JA, Wu CL. Efficacy of postoperative epidural analgesia: a meta-analysis. JAMA. 2003;290(18):2455–63. https://doi.org/10.1001/jama.290.18.2455.

Bramlett K, Onel E, Viscusi ER, Jones K. A randomized, double-blind, dose-ranging study comparing wound infiltration of DepoFoam bupivacaine, an extended-release liposomal bupivacaine, to bupivacaine HCl for postsurgical analgesia in total knee arthroplasty. Knee. 2012;19(5):530–6. https://doi.org/10.1016/j.knee.2011.12.004.

Brennan TJ. Pathophysiology of postoperative pain. Pain. 2011;152(3 Suppl):S33–40. https://doi.org/10.1016/j.pain.2010.11.005. Epub 2011 Jan 12. PMID: 21232860; PMCID: PMC3073562.

Brower RG. Consequences of bed rest. Crit Care Med. 2009;37(10 Suppl):S422–8. https://doi.org/10.1097/CCM.0b013e3181b6e30a.

Chou R, Gordon DB, de Leon-Casasola OA, Rosenberg JM, Bickler S, Brennan T, Carter T, Cassidy CL, Chittenden EH, Degenhardt E, Griffith S, Manber R, Turk DC, Perkal MF, Prasad R, Sluka K, Strassels S, Thirlby R, Viscusi E, Wu CL. Management of postoperative pain: a clinical practice guideline from the American Pain Society, the American Society of Regional Anesthesia and Pain Medicine, and the American Society of Anesthesiologists' Committee on Regional Anesthesia, Executive Committee, and Administrative Council. J Pain. 2016;17(2):131–57. https://doi.org/10.1016/j.jpain.2015.12.008.

Dickenson AH, Sullivan AF. Evidence for a role of the NMDA receptor in the frequency dependent potentiation of deep rat dorsal horn nociceptive neurones following C fibre stimulation. Neuropharmacology. 1987;26(8):1235–8. https://doi.org/10.1016/0028-3908(87)90275-9.

El-Boghdadly K, Chin KJ, Chan VWS. Phrenic nerve palsy and regional anesthesia for shoulder surgery: anatomical, physiologic, and clinical considerations. Anesthesiology. 2017;127(1):173–91. https://doi.org/10.1097/ALN.0000000000001668. PMID: 28514241.

Gan TJ, Belani KG, Bergese S, Chung F, Diemunsch P, Habib AS, Jin Z, Kovac AL, Meyer TA, Urman RD, Apfel CC, Ashraf S, Hanna MN, Hedrick TL, Kranke P, Lee PK, Lipman D, Minkowitz HS, Morton J, Philip BK. Fourth consensus guidelines for the management of postoperative nausea and vomiting. Anesth Analg. 2020;131(2):411–48. https://doi.org/10.1213/ANE.0000000000004833.

Golder HJ, Papalois V. Enhanced recovery after surgery: history, key advancements and developments in transplant surgery. J Clin Med. 2012;10(8):1634. https://doi.org/10.3390/jcm10081634.

Greco M, Capretti G, Beretta L, Gemma M, Pecorelli N, Braga M. Enhanced recovery program in colorectal surgery: a meta-analysis of randomized controlled trials. World J Surg. 2014;38(6):1531–41. https://doi.org/10.1007/s00268-013-2416-8.

Gustafsson UO, Scott MJ, Hubner M, Nygren J, Demartines N, Francis N, Rockall TA, Young-Fadok TM, Hill AG, Soop M, de Boer HD, Urman RD, Chang GJ, Fichera A, Kessler H,

Grass F, Whang EE, Fawcett WJ, Carli F, Lobo DN. Guidelines for perioperative care in elective colorectal surgery: Enhanced Recovery After Surgery (ERAS) Society recommendations (2018). World J Surg. 2019;43(3):659–95. https://doi.org/10.1007/s00268-018-4844-y.

Hah JM, Bateman BT, Ratliff J, Curtin C, Sun E. Chronic opioid use after surgery: implications for perioperative management in the face of the opioid epidemic. Anesth Analg. 2017;125(5):1733–40. https://doi.org/10.1213/ANE.0000000000002458.

Hashimoto DA, Witkowski E, Gao L, Meireles O, Rosman G. Artificial intelligence in anesthesiology: current techniques, clinical applications, and limitations. Anesthesiology. 2020;132(2):379–94. https://doi.org/10.1097/ALN.0000000000002960.

Kehlet H. Multimodal approach to control postoperative pathophysiology and rehabilitation. Br J Anaesth. 1997;78(5):606–17. https://doi.org/10.1093/bja/78.5.606.

Kehlet H, Dahl JB. The value of 'multimodal' or 'balanced analgesia' in postoperative pain treatment. Anesth Analg. 1993;77(5):1048–56. https://doi.org/10.1213/00000539-199311000-00030.

Kehlet H, Dahl JB. Anaesthesia, surgery, and challenges in postoperative recovery. Lancet (London, England). 2003;362(9399):1921–8. https://doi.org/10.1016/s0140-6736(03)14966-5. PMID: 14667752.

Kehlet H, Jensen TS, Woolf CJ. Persistent postsurgical pain: risk factors and prevention. Lancet. 2006;367(9522):1618–25. https://doi.org/10.1016/S0140-6736(06)68700-X.

Kehlet H, Wilmore DW. Evidence-based surgical care and the evolution of fast-track surgery. Ann Surg. 2008:189–98. https://doi.org/10.1097/SLA.0b013e31817f2c1a. PMID: 18650627.

Laskowski K, Stirling A, McKay WP, Lim HJ. A systematic review of intravenous ketamine for postoperative analgesia. Can J Anesth. 2011;58(10):911–23. https://doi.org/10.1007/s12630-011-9560-0.

Ljungqvist O, Scott M, Fearon KC. Enhanced recovery after surgery: a review. JAMA Surg. 2017;152(3):292–8. https://doi.org/10.1001/jamasurg.2016.4952.

Manion SC, Brennan TJ. Thoracic epidural analgesia and acute pain management. Anesthesiology. 2011;115(1):181–8. https://doi.org/10.1097/ALN.0b013e318220847c.

Memtsoudis SG, Poeran J, Zubizarreta N, Cozowicz C, Mörwald EE, Mariano ER, Mazumdar M. Association of multimodal pain management strategies with perioperative outcomes and resource utilization: A population-based study. Anesthesiology, 2018;128(5):891–902. https://doi.org/10.1097/ALN.0000000000002132

Ong CK, Lirk P, Seymour RA, Jenkins BJ. The efficacy of preemptive analgesia for acute postoperative pain management: a meta-analysis. Anesth Analg. 2005;100(3):757–73. https://doi.org/10.1213/01.ANE.0000144428.98767.0E.

Ossipov MH, Dussor GO, Porreca F. Central modulation of pain. J Clin Invest. 2010;120(11):3779–87. https://doi.org/10.1172/JCI43766.

Popping DM, Elia N, Van Aken HK, Marret E, Schug SA, Kranke P, Wenk M, Tramèr MR. Impact of epidural analgesia on mortality and morbidity after surgery: systematic review and meta-analysis of randomized controlled trials. Ann Surg. 2014;259(6):1056–67. https://doi.org/10.1097/SLA.0000000000000237.

Remy C, Marret E, Bonnet F. Effects of acetaminophen on morphine side-effects and consumption after major surgery: meta-analysis of randomized controlled trials. Br J Anaesth. 2005;94(4):505–13. https://doi.org/10.1093/bja/aei085.

Sherwood L. Human Physiology: From Cells to Systems. 8th ed. Belmont, CA: Brooks/Cole, Cengage Learning; 2012. ISBN: 978-1111577438.

Stiller K, Phillips A. Safety aspects of mobilising acutely ill inpatients. Physiother Theory Pract. 2003;19(4):239–57. https://doi.org/10.1080/09593980390246751.

Tiippana EM, Hamunen K, Kontinen VK, Kalso E. Do surgical patients benefit from perioperative gabapentin/pregabalin? A systematic review of efficacy and safety. Anesth Analg. 2007;104(6):1545–56. https://doi.org/10.1213/01.ane.0000261517.27532.80.

VanDenKerkhof EG, Hopman WM, Goldstein DH, Wilson RA, Towheed TE, Lam M, Harrison MB, Reitsma ML, Johnston SL, Medd JD, Gilron I. Impact of perioperative pain intensity, pain qualities, and opioid use on chronic pain after surgery: a prospective cohort study. Reg Anesth Pain Med. 2012;37(1):19–27. https://doi.org/10.1097/AAP.0b013e318237516e.

Wainwright TW, Gill M, McDonald DA, Middleton RG, Reed M, Sahota O, Yates P, Ljungqvist O. Consensus statement for perioperative care in total hip replacement and total knee replacement surgery: Enhanced Recovery After Surgery (ERAS) Society recommendations. Acta Orthop. 2020;91(1):3–19. https://doi.org/10.1080/17453674.2019.1683790.

White PF. The changing role of non-opioid analgesic techniques in the management of postoperative pain. Anesth Analg. 2005;101(5 Suppl):S5–S22. https://doi.org/10.1213/01.ANE.0000177099.28914.A7.

Willner A, Teske C, Hackert T, Welsch T. Effects of early postoperative mobilization following gastrointestinal surgery: Systematic review and meta-analysis. BJS Open, 2023;7(5):zrad102. https://doi.org/10.1093/bjsopen/zrad102

Woolf CJ, Salter MW. Neuronal plasticity: increasing the gain in pain. Science. 2000;288(5472):1765–9. https://doi.org/10.1126/science.288.5472.1765.

Enhanced Recovery After Surgery (ERAS) Implementation Challenges: Multidisciplinary Teamwork, Logistics, and Digital Governance

14

James Raj K and K. S. Jyothsna Prabhat

Abstract

ERAS stands for a revolutionary change in perioperative medicine. There are several high-quality randomized controlled trials and meta-analyses that prove that ERAS programs decrease the rates of postoperative complications, hospital length of stay, and even re-admissions and mortality in certain cases. Nonetheless, the actual implementation of ERAS in clinical practice demonstrates high heterogeneity due to the variability in both ERAS compliance and patient outcomes between different institutions and healthcare systems. The current problem of perioperative medicine lies not in the validation of the clinical efficacy of ERAS protocols but in the efficient and consistent application of complex multidisciplinary treatment approaches.

The considerably extended chapter presents a synthesis of current research findings from both clinical practice and implementation sciences related to ERAS. The chapter analyzes the physiopathological background of stress in surgery, the physiological underpinnings of ERAS intervention elements, and the essential importance of multidisciplinary collaboration, logistics in implementing the program, digital technologies, and information management. Using the prism of evidence-based research, the chapter focuses on the reliance of successful ERAS implementation on adherence to all components, the crucial importance of

J. R. K (✉)
Department of Medical & Surgical Nursing, College of Nursing Sciences, Dayananda Sagar University (DSU), Bengaluru, Karnataka, India

K. S. Jyothsna Prabhat
Department of Anesthesiology, Dr. Chandramma Dayananda Sagar Institute of Medical Education and Research (CDSIMER), Dayananda Sagar University (DSU), Bengaluru, Karnataka, India

P. K. Bhattacharyya et al. (eds.), *Integrated Anesthesia and Nutrition Approaches to Enhanced Recovery after Surgery*,
https://doi.org/10.1007/978-981-92-3294-9_14

nursing care, dietitian interventions, anesthesia, and physiotherapy, and obstacles to effective implementation. With the help of the conceptual framework of implementation science, including the CFIR and NPT models, a strategic map of the process is created. Specific tactics to overcome the challenges related to workforce shortage, logistic limitations, and cultural obstacles are discussed. Finally, a multi-level model of the successful implementation of enhanced recovery programs is developed, which includes formal governance, clinical champions, auditing, and contextual adaptation.

Keywords

Enhanced Recovery After Surgery (ERAS) · Implementation science · Perioperative pathways · Multidisciplinary teamwork · Audit and feedback · Digital health · Data governance · Surgical stress response · Immunonutrition · Opioid-free anesthesia

14.1 Introduction and Historical Context

14.1.1 The Evolution of Enhanced Recovery

The idea of ERAS first became a reality during the 1990s when Professor Henrik Kehlet developed the "fast-track" surgery concept. According to his studies, a patient's body suffers severe physiological stress in reaction to the surgery, which is believed to be a primary factor leading to postoperative malfunctioning of internal organs, prolonged recovery period, and possible complications (Kehlet 1997). Using various methods to minimize this reaction (such as epidural anesthesia, early feeding, and obligatory mobility), he succeeded in proving that patients who had undergone major colonic surgery can safely recover and be discharged within just 2–3 days, which is drastically different from the usual 10–14 days (Kehlet and Wilmore 2008).

After these landmark findings, the ERAS Study Group was founded in 2001 and finally became an international organization, the ERAS Society. In 2005, the first set of consensus guidelines for colorectal and rectal surgery incorporated the fast-track concepts of Kehlet to form evidence-based guidelines for perioperative care (Fearon et al. 2005). The guidelines defined a seamless process of care that involved the preoperative, intraoperative, and postoperative stages with an explicit focus on addressing insulin resistance, protein catabolism, and immune dysregulation. During the last two decades, ERAS principles have become applicable beyond colorectal surgery, and evidence-based guidelines have been formulated for hepatopancreatobiliary, gynecological, urological, orthopedic, bariatric, and cardiac surgeries (Carmichael et al. 2017; Melloul et al. 2016; Nygren et al. 2013).

14.1.2 Pathophysiology of the Surgical Stress Response

It is crucial to comprehend the basic physiologic process of the stress response to gain maximum benefit from the application of ERAS in the perioperative setting. Significant surgical injuries trigger a substantial neuroendocrine and immune response. Neurologic impulses generated by the injured tissues activate the hypothalamus-pituitary-adrenal (HPA) axis and sympathetic nervous system to release several anti-insulin hormones like cortisol, glucagon, growth hormone, and catecholamines (Kehlet 1997).

This combination of hormones leads to a condition characterized by extreme catabolism and peripheral insulin resistance. Insulin resistance prevents glucose from being taken up by cells, resulting in hyperglycemia that affects leukocytes' functionality, slows down wound healing, and causes a greater likelihood of surgical site infection (Smith et al. 2014). Simultaneously, proteins in the skeletal muscles break down rapidly to provide amino acids for the production of acute-phase proteins and hepatic gluconeogenesis. The mechanisms of ERAS address the problem of such a response. Carbohydrate loading prior to surgery reduces insulin resistance, minimal invasive methods cause less damage to tissues, and anesthesia prevents sensory input to the neuroendocrine system (Kehlet and Wilmore 2008; Tong et al. 2022).

14.1.3 From Evidence to Everyday Practice

The use of meta-analysis from randomized clinical trials now yields strong evidence to support the use of ERAS in decreasing hospital LOS, morbidity, and readmissions among diverse categories of surgery (Sauro et al. 2024; Zhang et al. 2023; Limbu et al. 2023). For instance, a meta-analysis involving 74 randomized studies with more than 9000 patients has shown that the implementation of ERAS protocols leads to a reduction of 2 days in LOS and decreases mortality and complication rate with no increased risk of death (Sauro et al. 2024).

In spite of all the evidence presented above, implementation audits show that practice does not always correspond to what the guidelines state. In general, hospitals have partially implemented the guidelines, implementing the less complicated components such as minimal invasive surgery or use of particular anesthesia techniques, but skipping the more complicated ones like prehabilitation routines, strict mobilization criteria, and discharge management (Cakir et al. 2013; Gustafsson et al. 2011). It appears that the reasons for this type of implementation failure relate to the interaction of several factors (Pearsall et al. 2015; Wang et al. 2022).

14.1.4 Global Scalability and Contextual Adaptation

Starting out in tertiary care centers in well-resourced academic institutions, ERAS programs are now becoming common among community hospitals, rural institutions, and under-resourced health care facilities around the world (Norcross et al.

2019; Pearsall et al. 2015). From experience in such environments, it is clear that ERAS can be successfully implemented and result in improved LOS and recovery functionally if the program is contextualized according to local staff arrangements (Temple-Oberle et al. 2019; Pearsall et al. 2015).

One notable multicenter study carried out in China revealed some of the major structural constraints associated with the scalability of ERAS; these included the shortage of medical personnel, inadequate health policies, and the obsolescence of clinical models (Wang et al. 2022). Process-related obstacles included poor multidisciplinary teamwork and the use of conventional communication approaches between doctors and patients. All these point to the need for context-specific implementation of ERAS using the fewest yet most influential measures when limited resources cannot support the strict application of ERAS guidelines.

14.2 Core Components of the ERAS Pathway

The success of ERAS depends on the synergy created by combining small gains from several different approaches within the perioperative process.

14.2.1 Preoperative Optimization and Education

Education of the patient and counseling are essential components of the ERAS philosophy, as they ensure that the expectations of the patients are managed well, preoperative anxiety is minimized, and the patient becomes a proactive participant in their recovery process (Fearon et al. 2005). The use of prehabilitation strategies such as aerobic exercises, strength training, nutrition enhancement, and psychological preparation seeks to improve the physiological capacity of the patient before he undergoes the stress of surgery.

14.2.2 Nutritional Screening and Carbohydrate Loading

Preoperative routine fasting starting at midnight (nil per os since midnight) worsens preoperative dehydration, anxiety, and postoperative insulin resistance. According to ERAS recommendations, preoperative consumption of solid food should be allowed up to 6 h before surgery, while clear fluids can be taken up until 2 h before anesthesia induction (Gustafsson et al. 2013). In addition, preoperative carbohydrate loading (PCL), consisting of administering an 800 mL of carbohydrate-enriched drink the day before surgery and another 400 mL drink 2 h prior to surgery, was proved to effectively reduce postoperative insulin resistance, protein catabolism, and overall subjective satisfaction (Tong et al. 2022).

New meta-analyses of clinical randomized trials have demonstrated the ability of PCL to reduce hunger, thirst, and fatigue without any risks of increased pulmonary aspiration and delay in gastric emptying (Smith et al. 2014; Tong et al. 2022).

Further studies related to ERAS approach conducted on orthopedic and gastrointestinal surgery patients revealed a positive impact on length of stay and inflammation (Soffin and YaDeau 2016; Bilku et al. 2014). Nonetheless, there were many reported failures in using this technique owing to the poor communication between ward and operating room staff regarding scheduling problems (Wang et al. 2022).

14.2.3 Intraoperative Management: Anesthesia and Fluids

Intraoperative management involves reducing surgery-related stress, limiting the use of long-acting opioid drugs, ensuring normothermia, and using goal-directed fluid therapy (GDFT).

Opioid-Sparing and Opioid-Free Anesthesia (OFA) The conventional approach to anesthesia involved the use of high doses of intraoperative opioids, leading to a myriad of postoperative issues, including PONV, postoperative ileus, respiratory depression, and opioid-induced hyperalgesia (Kehlet and Wilmore 2008). The modern ERAS protocol involves the use of multimodal pain management strategies using regional blocks such as TAP blocks, ESP blocks, and thoracic epidurals alongside non-opioid systemic medications, including paracetamol, NSAIDS, ketamine, dexmedetomidine, magnesium, and intravenous lidocaine (Xu et al. 2025).

Opioid-Free Anesthesia (OFA) is a new approach in anesthesia, which seeks to eliminate opioids from being administered to patients intraoperatively. Studies conducted on bariatric and gastrointestinal surgeries indicate that OFA decreases postoperative morphine requirements, reduces PONV frequency, and hastens bowel recovery, but it needs close monitoring of the hemodynamics because it causes hypotension and bradycardia (Dagher et al. 2025; Ao et al. 2025).

Goal-Directed Fluid Therapy (GDFT) Hypovolemic state (leading to inadequate splanchnic perfusion and kidney damage) and hypervolemic state (contributing to fluid accumulation in tissues, ileus, and anastomotic dehiscence) are not beneficial for the postoperative process. The use of goal-directed fluid therapy (GDFT), based on such parameters as SVV or PPV, is recommended by the ERAS philosophy for optimization of intravascular volume and cardiac output (Thiele et al. 2015).

14.2.4 Postoperative Recovery: Feeding and Mobilization

Early Enteral Feeding The traditional teaching of surgery required postponing eating until the appearance of bowel sounds and flatus. The concept of ERAS directly contradicts this notion by showing that early feeding following gastrointestinal surgery within 24 h is safe, well tolerated, and favorable. Early feeding initiates gastrocolic reflexes, helps maintain the integrity of the mucosa, prevents translocation of bacteria, and quickens the recovery from postoperative ileus

(Reissman et al. 1995; Feo et al. 2004). However, early feeding is possible only if there is proper PONV management and no bowel dysfunction caused by opioids (Slim et al. 2020).

Early Mobilization Increased bedridden time promotes muscle wastage, leads to insulin resistance, affects pulmonary functions, and substantially increases the chances of developing venous thromboembolism and pneumonia. ERAS guidelines set strict mobilization goals, such as getting out of bed to sit for 2 h on the surgery day and 6 h later, on a daily basis. Meeting such goals necessitates adequate pain management without using opioids, early removal of physical restraints like IV catheters, urinary catheters, and surgical drainages, as well as appropriate nursing and physiotherapy assistance (Yeom and Lim 2022; Liu et al. 2025).

14.3 Implementation Science and ERAS

This ongoing mismatch between ERAS guideline publications and actual practice has sparked the use of frameworks from implementation science for understanding and addressing barriers to implementation.

14.3.1 Adherence Thresholds and Clinical Outcomes

There have been consistent studies confirming the existence of a dose-response relationship between adherence to ERAS protocol and outcomes. Significant decreases in both LOS and complication rates can only be observed after adherence rates to the pathway exceed 70–80% (Cakir et al. 2013; Norcross et al. 2019). The relationship between compliance and shorter LOS and less morbidity has been proven by Cakir et al. (2013), who stated that compliance with certain components of ERAS protocol is the strongest independent factor associated with shortened hospital stays and morbidity rate. Registry studies indicate that adherence improvements over several years lead to gradual LOS reductions, but not readmission rate increase (Norcross et al. 2019).

14.3.2 Implementation Frameworks: CFIR and NPT

The implementation of such complicated programs as ERAS can be better assessed through existing models. For example, the CFIR (Consolidated Framework for Implementation Research) divides the barriers and facilitators into five categories: intervention characteristics (such as complexity, evidence), outer setting (such as policy, incentive), inner setting (such as organizational climate, leadership engagement), individual characteristics (such as knowledge, belief), and implementation process (such as plan, engage, reflect) (May et al. 2009; Gotlib Conn et al. 2015).

The Normalization Process Theory (NPT) deals with the social organization of work by paying particular attention to the processes involved in the embedding of innovations into routine clinical practice. According to NPT, four types of work should be performed: achieving coherence (understanding the innovation, ERAS); cognitive participation (clinician support of the protocol); collective action (actual implementation of ERAS); and reflexive monitoring (evaluation of the impacts of the protocol) (May et al. 2009). Research conducted using qualitative methodology indicates that poor coherence among the healthcare professionals, who treat the ERAS protocol as a transient trend from the administration, leads to fast implementation failure (Pearsall et al. 2015; Lyon et al. 2014).

14.3.3 Audit, Feedback, and Regional Implementation

A&F is a powerful behavioral intervention that ensures adherence during all stages of the ERAS continuum (Fig. 14.1). The effectiveness of this approach was proven in a stepped-wedge, cluster-randomized study conducted among 29 Italian colorectal surgery units, which showed that the implementation of an ERAS protocol along with educational initiatives and continuous, data-driven A&F led to improved compliance and a reduction in adjusted length of stay (LOS) exceeding half a day, without affecting surgical outcomes (Pagano et al. 2024). Supplying the clinical staff

Preoperative Clinic

↓

Patient assessment, risk stratification, counselling, and prehabilitation

Anaesthesia Assessment

↓

Optimization of comorbidities, planning of regional anaesthesia and analgesia strategy

Surgery

↓

Minimally invasive techniques, fluid management, temperature control

Recovery Room (PACU)

↓

Early extubation, pain control, monitoring, initiation of recovery protocols

Ward Care

↓

Early feeding, catheter and drain removal, monitoring for complications

Physiotherapy

↓

Early mobilization, respiratory exercises, functional recovery support

Discharge Planning

↓

Criteria-based discharge, patient education, follow-up planning

Fig. 14.1 The ERAS pathway as a continuous flow of care across the perioperative continuum

with honest and unblinded feedback on their rate of adherence during all stages of patient care, from preoperative consultation to discharge planning (see Fig. 14.1), shatters the "illusion of compliance," which is the erroneous belief that clinicians are already implementing ERAS (Elias et al. 2019).

14.4 Multidisciplinary Teamwork and Clinical Roles

The implementation of the ERAS protocol is crucially dependent upon the management of the MDT that should function effectively. There should be a shift from the traditional hierarchical approach in surgical medicine toward a collaborative approach in which all medical specialties participate in achieving the goals of recovery (RAS; Elias et al. 2019).

14.4.1 Team Roles and Responsibilities

Surgeons It is the surgeons' responsibility to offer pre-operative surgical advice, perform minimally invasive surgical procedures using laparoscopy or robotics, avoid nasogastric intubation and prophylactic peritoneal drainages, and set out explicit discharge criteria (Carmichael et al. 2017).

Anesthesiologists The anesthesiologist is responsible for maintaining physiological stability during surgery. This involves using opioid-sparing or OFA approaches, performing regional anesthesia, precise goal-directed fluid therapy, stringent temperature regulation (normothermia), and multi-modal prophylaxis against PONV (Xu et al. 2025; Dagher et al. 2025).

Nurses The ward nurses are the primary coordinators of the ERAS process. They ensure daily recovery efforts, monitor the attainment of specified benchmarks, motivate early mobilization and nutritional goals, oversee the timely withdrawal of any physical constraints (catheter/ drainage), and consistently educate the patients. Dedicated ERAS nursing services have been proven to be significantly linked to better pain management, early mobilization, and high levels of patient satisfaction (Yeom and Lim 2022; Liu et al. 2025).

Dietitians Dietitians play an essential role in conducting preoperative nutrition risk assessment by using proven techniques (such as the NRS-2002 or GLIM criteria), organizing all PCL activities, administering immuno-nutritional supplementation, and formulating high-protein enteral feedings after surgery to counteract the catabolic state (August and Huhmann 2009; Sun et al. 2015).

Physiotherapists Physiotherapists create customized early mobilization protocols that they monitor closely, perform essential breathing exercises to avoid atelectasis,

Table 14.1 Roles of multidisciplinary team members in ERAS implementation

Team member	Key role	Example responsibilities
Surgeon	Operative care and pathway design	Minimally invasive surgery; early drain/catheter removal; discharge criteria
Anesthesiologist	Physiological stability and analgesia	OFA; regional blocks; GDFT; PONV prophylaxis
Nurse	Day-to-day pathway coordination	Monitoring; documentation; mobilization; catheter/drain management
Dietitian	Perioperative nutrition	NRS-2002 screening; PCL; immunonutrition; protein-targeted feeding
Physiotherapist	Functional recovery	Early ambulation; respiratory exercises; progressive mobilization
ERAS coordinator	Implementation and audit	Compliance monitoring; data abstraction; feedback; staff education

and develop personalized functional rehabilitation objectives based on the patient's preoperative mobility status and type of surgery (Soffin and YaDeau 2016).

ERAS Coordinators The ERAS coordinator, who is typically an advanced practice nurse, serves as the glue that binds together all aspects of the program. Their job involves maintaining compliance, abstracting information with a high degree of precision to the registries, producing reports for clinical feedback, training the team, and ensuring effective communication among various departments (Temple-Oberle et al. 2019; Norcross et al. 2019). These roles and their interrelationships are captured in Table 14.1.

14.4.2 Structural Barriers and Coordination Bottlenecks

Structural barriers create huge hindrances for ERAS processes. Consistently, audits have found systemic failures in the form of neglected pre-operative nutritional orders, delayed physiotherapy assessments, and delayed removal of urinary catheters despite having ERAS protocols in place (Sauro et al. 2024; Norcross et al. 2019). For hospitals that operate under high volumes and are publicly funded, severe time constraints and complex logistics pose huge challenges. If ERAS duties are imposed on already overloaded nursing routines without additional staffing, pathway adherence is bound to falter (Wang et al. 2022).

According to nursing personnel, it is difficult to balance strict documentation demands, provision of direct care, patient mobilization, and patient education. This imbalance often results in the selection of easier protocol components while leaving labor-intensive aspects, such as repeated mobilizations per day, undone (Yeom and Lim 2022).

14.4.3 Behavioral and Cultural Determinants

Cultural barriers must be addressed if structural approaches are to succeed. Qualitative studies in ERAS suggest there is significant resistance by clinicians who perceive a standardized approach to represent an encroachment on their professional autonomy. For instance, surgeons often display apprehension over the removal of drains shortly after surgery owing to their concern about anastomotic leakage, while anesthesiologists may be doubtful whether an opioid-sparing approach is sufficient to manage postoperative pain after complex surgeries (Lyon et al. 2014; Pearsall et al. 2015).

In order to address cultural barriers, it is necessary to build common mental models about recovery through frequent multidisciplinary team discussions. Open communication on both achievements and challenges fosters the belief that the protocol is safe (Herbert et al. 2017; Wang et al. 2022).

14.5 Anesthesia and Nutrition Integration in ERAS

14.5.1 The Clinical Interdependence of Anesthesia and Nutrition

There exists a fundamental connection between anesthesia and perioperative nutrition under the ERAS framework. For the success of oral feeding, the ability of the anesthetist to avoid PONV and opioid-related ileus is vital. On the other hand, appropriate fluid therapy facilitates adequate gut mucosal perfusion and the recovery of bowel motility (Kehlet and Wilmore 2008; Xu et al. 2025).

When high-dose opioids are administered during surgery, or if there is a marked volume overload resulting in bowel edema or volume depletion causing splanchnic ischemia, recovery of gut function does not occur quickly. In such cases, it is impossible to follow the guidelines for early oral feeding, resulting in nausea, vomiting, and increased chances of aspiration (Reissman et al. 1995; Slim et al. 2020). Hence, coordination is essential in terms of the time of administering antiemetics, managing pain, and advancing nutrition (Fig. 14.2).

14.5.2 Immunonutrition and Nutritional Risk Screening

Malnutrition represents an independent and strong predictor of poor surgical outcomes. It is imperative to perform preoperative nutritional risk assessment using instruments like the NRS-2002. The results from meta-analyses of large prospective cohorts show that high-risk individuals (NRS-2002) have more complications, higher LOS, and mortality rates (Sun et al. 2015; Limbu et al. 2024).

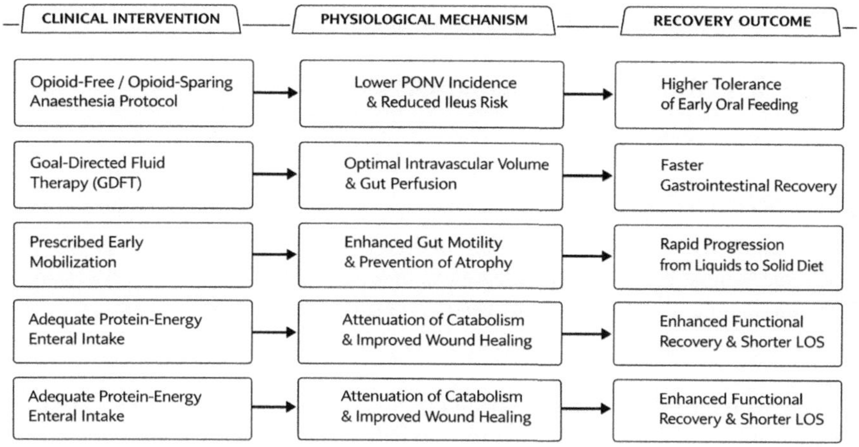

Fig. 14.2 Interaction between anesthesia, fluid therapy, and nutrition in ERAS. (The image has been created by using Mermaid.com)

Immunonutrition involves providing enteral feeding supplements with pharmacologic nutrients like arginine, omega-3 fatty acids, and nucleotides. The objective of immunonutrition therapy is to regulate the host immune system and promote microperfusion. There is considerable evidence from randomized controlled trials among elective colorectal surgeries, including the SONVI trial, which showed that incorporating immunonutrition within ERAS protocols resulted in significantly fewer cases of infections, especially surgical site infections (Moya et al. 2016; Braga et al. 1999; Cerantola et al. 2011). Nevertheless, cost constraints and absence of responsibility for perioperative nutrition services are major challenges for implementation (August and Huhmann 2009).

14.5.3 Governance and Ownership of Perioperative Nutrition

One important observation from the studies on implementing ERAS protocols is that nutrition management frequently ends up as "orphan." Whereas there are definite proponents of both surgical and anesthesia interventions, nutrition assessment, PCL planning, and protein management after surgery are not firmly assigned to either of these two professions (Yeom and Lim 2022; Liu et al. 2025). Recruiting specialized dieticians to preoperative settings and establishing explicit nutrition-related KPIs like timing of first food ingestion and target protein achievement rate are some ways to address this challenge (Freeman et al. 2019).

14.6 Organizational and Logistical Barriers

14.6.1 Logistics as a Determinant of Clinical Workflow

In numerous cases, ERAS pathway failure is due to logistics rather than clinical reasons. In many cases where patients have fulfilled all clinical requirements for recovery (such as eating solid foods, walking around unaided, and managing pain with oral medication), the reason behind their extended hospitalization is primarily logistical. Logistical issues include delays in scheduling physiotherapy assessments after surgery, delays in distributing medications from the hospital pharmacy, and the absence of pre-arranged transportation for patients (Sauro et al. 2024; Norcross et al. 2019).

Process mapping, an approach inspired by Lean Six Sigma processes, has proven to be useful in ERAS implementations to determine and reduce such non-clinical bottlenecks. The prioritization of ERAS patients who undergo frequent turnover for early surgery scheduling and matching the nursing shift pattern with peak discharges are very efficient logistic measures (Norcross et al. 2019; Temple-Oberle et al. 2019).

14.6.2 Institutional Leadership and Change Fatigue

Organizational fragmentation significantly hinders ERAS uptake. Findings from multi-center trials have shown that surgical wards without a structured ERAS implementation lead to the practice's "cherry-picking" whereby select protocol components are applied independently and inconsistently, leading to extreme disparities in compliance (Norcross et al. 2019). The primary cause of implementation resistance is typically due to conflicting objectives within the organization, inadequate backing from hospital management, and a lack of economic or career rewards to encourage departments to adopt ERAS (Wang et al. 2022; Lyon et al. 2014). A detailed list of logistical hurdles, associated patient consequences, and recommended interventions is outlined in Table 14.2.

Table 14.2 Organizational and logistical barriers and potential solutions

Domain	Barrier	Impact	Strategy
Teamwork	Siloed services; poor communication	Partial execution of ERAS elements	Regular MDT huddles; joint ERAS ward rounds
Scheduling/ discharge	Rigid OR lists; discharge delays	Discharge bottlenecks; longer LOS	Align OR slots, bed flow, physiotherapy staffing
Data systems	Incomplete/low-quality registry data	Unreliable performance monitoring	Data-quality audits; ERAS flags in the EMR
Leadership/ governance	No central ERAS ownership	Project fatigue; variable adherence	ERAS steering committee; ERAS KPIs in dashboards
Workforce	Insufficient ERAS-literate staff	Protocol attrition; nurse burnout	ERAS education; dedicated coordinators

14.7 Digital Health, Data Governance, and Performance Monitoring

14.7.1 Digital Health Tools and Telemonitoring in ERAS

ERAS pathways have undergone rapid changes due to digital health innovations. Technologies such as mHealth applications and telemonitoring devices have been used to offer patients pre-operative education and remind them of the fast and carbohydrate loading requirements. A randomized clinical trial conducted on patients undergoing oncologic surgeries found significant improvements in patients' quality of recovery scores in 2 and 6 weeks post-operation when compared to conventional care using home monitoring by smartphones (Temple-Oberle et al. 2023).

The systematic review proves that ERAS applications for smartphones positively affect patient engagement, compliance, and satisfaction without raising the risks of developing complications and re-hospitalization (Temple-Oberle et al. 2022; D'Ambrosio et al. 2026). Wearable devices with capabilities to measure physiological parameters and physical activity provide objective data on functional recovery, allowing clinicians to identify any changes in patients' clinical status (Posthuma et al. 2024; Haveman et al. 2024).

14.7.2 Electronic Medical Record Integration and Data Quality

The sustainability of ERAS is extremely reliant on continuous auditing processes that are driven by reporting standards like the RECOvER audit checklist (Elias et al. 2019). Nevertheless, the usefulness of ERAS registries and EMR-based auditing depends greatly on the quality of the data itself. Clinical quality registry auditing often reveals extremely high levels of data completeness with relatively moderate data agreement based on the primary sources (Tan et al. 2019).

Dimensions of quality of EHR data, including completeness, accuracy, concordance, plausibility, and recency, should be strictly controlled (Weiskopf and Weng 2013). Innovative informatics techniques, based on EMR order set flagging and automated case request identification, have been created to measure ERAS metrics effectively without substantial abstraction efforts (Freeman et al. 2019). Clinical decision support reminders incorporated into the EHR serve as behavioral safeguards, prompting physicians to withdraw catheters, administer multimodal pain management, and introduce an early diet (Temple-Oberle et al. 2019; Temple-Oberle et al. 2023).

14.8 ERAS in Special Populations and Complex Contexts

Whereas the basic physiological concepts underlying ERAS apply to all patients, the particular interventions employed and the timeline of the pathway need to be carefully tailored to accommodate at-risk and complicated surgical groups.

14.8.1 Geriatric and Frail Patients

However, the presence of frailty, sarcopenia, preexisting cognitive deficits, and medical comorbidities makes geriatric surgery significantly different from other procedures regarding patient risk factors. Geriatric patients with frailty are prone to postoperative complications such as delirium, deterioration of function, and adverse events. Therefore, ERAS protocols for geriatric patients should include comprehensive preoperative assessment, prehabilitation with multiple modalities, opioid-sparing pain management to avoid delirium, and gradual rehabilitation sessions (August and Huhmann 2009; Limbu et al. 2024).

14.8.2 Emergency Surgery

Use of ERAS in emergency surgery is complicated since it is not possible to optimize patients before surgery, do carbohydrate loading, or prehabilitate them. Nevertheless, systematic review results have shown that shortened ERAS pathways, which mainly emphasize GDFT during surgery, multimodal pain management, early removal of catheters, and vigorous postoperative mobilization, can effectively decrease LOS and complications following emergency surgery for colorectal and abdominal surgeries despite the unfeasibility of adhering strictly to the ERAS principles (Mac Curtain et al. 2023).

14.8.3 Subspecialty Adaptations (Pediatrics, Bariatrics, Orthopedics)

The ERAS program for newborns and pediatrics highlights aspects such as parental education, reduction in fasting time before surgery, accurate fluid resuscitation, and regional anesthesia based on neonatal physiology (Brindle et al. 2020). ERAS for bariatric surgeries concentrates heavily on patient mobilization to counteract the very high risk of developing venous thromboembolism (VTE) and pulmonary atelectasis because of the patient's extremely high body mass index, and OFA to prevent postoperative respiratory depression (Dagher et al. 2025). Elective orthopedic surgeries, specifically arthroplasty procedures, use the ERAS approach to mobilize patients very quickly after surgery, with some patients being able to walk within a few hours of having undergone surgery using local anesthetics and tranexamic acid (Soffin and YaDeau 2016).

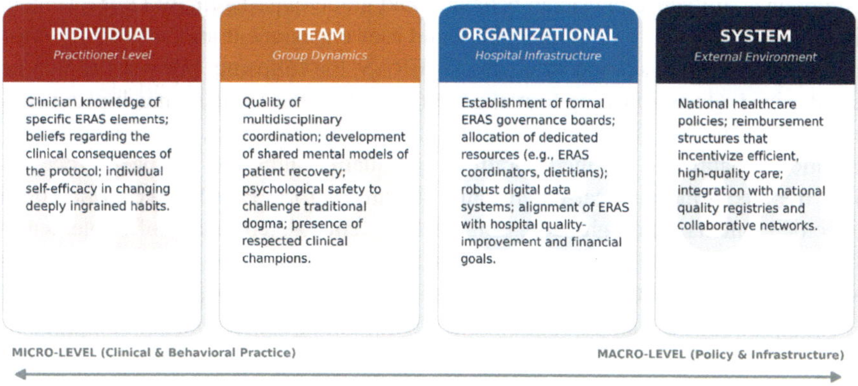

Fig. 14.3 Multi-level implementation framework for ERAS. (The image has been created by using Mermaid.com)

14.9 Implementation Framework for ERAS Integration

The successful implementation of ERAS is an intricate multi-level organizational change management strategy which requires strategic planning on individual, group, organization, and systemic levels (Fig. 14.3).

Implementation theories suggest that the process of implementation is non-linear and iterative. The most durable and effective ERAS protocols involve tactics that work at all levels of the framework, namely grassroots education and strong audit feedback at the team level, together with hospital leadership endorsement and allocated budgeting at the organizational level (May et al. 2009; Norcross et al. 2019; Pagano et al. 2024).

14.10 Conclusion

Provided there is high fidelity and compliance in the adoption of such ERAS protocols, the consistent and significant reduction in the incidence of postoperative complications, reduced LOS, and faster recovery have been demonstrated for an extensive spectrum of surgical disciplines. In the modern era of perioperative medicine, the task is not to determine the effectiveness of each component of ERAS; the challenge lies in delivering them in concert with precision.

Collaboration among various disciplines underpins the ERAS approach. The role of nurses, dietitians, physiotherapists, and even anesthesiologists is comparable to that of the operating surgeon for reaching the recovery targets. But such collaboration is often hampered by structural gaps, behavioral dogmatism, and manpower shortage. In addition, logistic factors such as scheduling of the OR, bed management, and discharge from pharmacy take precedence over readiness to discharge.

The use of digital health technologies, advanced audit processes, and effective data governance frameworks offers strong modern mechanisms to ensure protocol compliance, influence physician behavior, and guide ongoing quality improvement initiatives, as long as strict data quality and user engagement are ensured. In terms of practical implementation strategies for ERAS, the following priorities should be emphasized: (1) establishing formal governance processes with ownership and clinical champions at the institutional level; (2) investing in nursing, nutrition, and coordination capabilities; (3) incorporating high-quality audit and feedback processes into the electronic medical record; and (4) tailoring the ERAS bundles based on specific contexts. Through addressing such systemic determinants of implementation, instead of continually refining individual care practices, healthcare systems will be able to unlock their transformative power.

References

Ao Y, Ma J, Zheng X, Zeng J, Wei K. Opioid-sparing anesthesia versus opioid-free anesthesia for the prevention of postoperative nausea and vomiting after laparoscopic bariatric surgery: a systematic review and network meta-analysis. Anesth Analg. 2025;140(2):385–96. https://doi.org/10.1213/ANE.0000000000006942.

August DA, Huhmann MB, the American Society for Parenteral and Enteral Nutrition (A.S.P.E.N.) Board of Directors. A.S.P.E.N. clinical guidelines: nutrition support therapy during adult anticancer treatment and in hematopoietic cell transplantation. JPEN J Parenter Enteral Nutr. 2009;33:472–500. https://doi.org/10.1177/0148607109341804.

Bilku DK, Dennison AR, Hall TC, Metcalfe MS, Garcea G. Role of preoperative carbohydrate loading: a systematic review. Ann R Coll Surg Engl. 2014;96(1):15–22. https://doi.org/10.1308/003588414X13824511650614.

Braga M, Gianotti L, Radaelli G, Vignali A, Mari G, Gentilini O, Di Carlo V. Perioperative immunonutrition in patients undergoing cancer surgery: results of a randomized double-blind phase 3 trial. Arch Surg. 1999;134(4):428–33. https://doi.org/10.1001/archsurg.134.4.428.

Brindle ME, McDiarmid C, Short K, Miller K, MacRobie A, Lam JYK, Brockel M, Raval MV, Howlett A, Lee KS, Offringa M, Wong K, de Beer D, Wester T, Skarsgard ED, Wales PW, Fecteau A, Haliburton B, Goobie SM, Nelson G. Consensus guidelines for perioperative care in neonatal intestinal surgery: enhanced recovery after surgery (ERAS®) society recommendations. World J Surg. 2020;44(8):2482–92. https://doi.org/10.1007/s00268-020-05530-1.

Cakir H, van Stijn MF, Lopes Cardozo AM, Langenhorst BL, Schreurs WH, van der Ploeg TJ, Bemelman WA, Houdijk AP. Adherence to enhanced recovery after surgery and length of stay after colonic resection. Colorectal Dis. 2013;15(8):1019–25. https://doi.org/10.1111/codi.12200.

Carmichael JC, Keller DS, Baldini G, Bordeianou L, Weiss E, Lee L, Boutros M, McClane J, Feldman LS, Steele SR. Clinical practice guidelines for enhanced recovery after colon and rectal surgery from the American Society of Colon and Rectal Surgeons and Society of American Gastrointestinal and Endoscopic Surgeons. Dis Colon Rectum. 2017;60(8):761–84. https://doi.org/10.1097/DCR.0000000000000883.

Cerantola Y, Hübner M, Grass F, Demartines N, Schäfer M. Immunonutrition in gastrointestinal surgery. Br J Surg. 2011;98(1):37–48. https://doi.org/10.1002/bjs.7273.

D'Ambrosio PD, Passos FS, da Nobrega Oliveira REN, Alvarenga-Bezerra V, Hirayama P, Kawano AHA, Terra RM, Moretti-Marques R. Mobile applications in enhanced recovery after surgery: a systematic review of protocol adherence and outcomes. Mhealth. 2026;12:9. https://doi.org/10.21037/mhealth-25-37.

Dagher C, Mattar R, Aoun M, et al. Opioid-free anesthesia in bariatric surgery: a prospective randomized controlled trial. Eur J Med Res. 2025;30:320. https://doi.org/10.1186/s40001-025-02565-9.

Elias KM, Stone AB, McGinigle K, et al. The reporting on ERAS compliance, outcomes, and elements research (RECOvER) checklist: a joint statement by the ERAS® and ERAS® USA societies. World J Surg. 2019;43:1–8. https://doi.org/10.1007/s00268-018-4753-0.

Fearon KCH, Ljungqvist O, Von Meyenfeldt M, Revhaug A, Dejong CHC, Lassen K, Nygren J, Hausel J, Soop M, Andersen J, Kehlet H. Enhanced recovery after surgery: a consensus review of clinical care for patients undergoing colonic resection. Clin Nutr. 2005;24(3):466–77. https://doi.org/10.1016/j.clnu.2005.02.002.

Feo CV, Romanini B, Sortini D, Ragazzi R, Zamboni P, Pansini GC, Liboni A. Early oral feeding after colorectal resection: a randomized controlled study. ANZ J Surg. 2004;74(5):298–301. https://doi.org/10.1111/j.1445-1433.2004.02985.x.

Freeman NLB, McGinigle KL, Leese PJ. Using electronic medical records to identify enhanced recovery after surgery cases. EGEMS (Washington, DC). 2019;7(1):34. https://doi.org/10.5334/egems.304.

Gotlib Conn L, McKenzie M, Pearsall EA, McLeod RS. Successful implementation of an enhanced recovery after surgery programme for elective colorectal surgery: a process evaluation of champions' experiences. Implement Sci. 2015;10:99. https://doi.org/10.1186/s13012-015-0289-y.

Gustafsson UO, Hausel J, Thorell A, Ljungqvist O, Soop M, Nygren J. Adherence to the enhanced recovery after surgery protocol and outcomes after colorectal cancer surgery. Arch Surg. 2011;146(5):571–7. https://doi.org/10.1001/archsurg.2010.309.

Gustafsson UO, Scott MJ, Schwenk W, Demartines N, Roulin D, Francis N, McNaught CE, Macfie J, Liberman AS, Soop M, Hill A, Kennedy RH, Lobo DN, Fearon K, Ljungqvist O, Enhanced Recovery After Surgery (ERAS) Society, for Perioperative Care, European Society for Clinical Nutrition and Metabolism (ESPEN), International Association for Surgical Metabolism and Nutrition (IASMEN). Guidelines for perioperative care in elective colonic surgery: Enhanced Recovery After Surgery (ERAS(®)) Society recommendations. World J Surg. 2013;37(2):259–84. https://doi.org/10.1007/s00268-012-1772-0.

Haveman ME, Jonker LT, van den Heuvel B, Verhoef C, Wiggers T, de Vries J-PPM. Effectiveness of current perioperative telemonitoring on postoperative outcome in patients undergoing major abdominal surgery: a systematic review of controlled trials. J Telemed Telecare. 2024;30(2):215–29. https://doi.org/10.1177/1357633X211047710.

Herbert G, Sutton E, Burden S, Lewis S, Thomas S, Ness A, Atkinson C. Healthcare professionals' views of the enhanced recovery after surgery programme: a qualitative investigation. BMC Health Serv Res. 2017;17(1):617. https://doi.org/10.1186/s12913-017-2547-y.

Kehlet H. Multimodal approach to control postoperative pathophysiology and rehabilitation. Br J Anaesth. 1997;78(5):606–17. https://doi.org/10.1093/bja/78.5.606.

Kehlet H, Wilmore DW. Evidence-based surgical care and the evolution of fast-track surgery. Ann Surg. 2008;248(2):189–98. https://doi.org/10.1097/SLA.0b013e31817f2c1a.

Limbu Y, Raut S, Pudasaini P, Regmee S, Ghimire R, Maharjan DK, Thapa PB. Correlation of the nutritional risk screening 2002 score with post-operative complications in gastrointestinal and hepatopancreatobiliary oncosurgeries. Cureus. 2024;16(4):e58514. https://doi.org/10.7759/cureus.58514.

Lyon A, Solomon MJ, Harrison JD. A qualitative study assessing the barriers to implementation of enhanced recovery after surgery. World J Surg. 2014;38:1374–80. https://doi.org/10.1007/s00268-013-2441-7.

Mac Curtain BM, O'Mahony A, Temperley HC, Ng ZQ. Enhanced recovery after surgery protocols and emergency surgery: a systematic review and meta-analysis of randomized controlled trials. ANZ J Surg. 2023;93(10):2424–32. https://doi.org/10.1111/ans.18550.

May CR, Mair F, Finch T, et al. Development of a theory of implementation and integration: Normalization Process Theory. Implement Sci. 2009;4:29. https://doi.org/10.1186/1748-5908-4-29.

Melloul E, Hübner M, Scott M, Snowden C, Prentis J, Dejong CH, Garden OJ, Farges O, Kokudo N, Vauthey JN, Clavien PA, Demartines N. Guidelines for perioperative care for liver surgery: Enhanced Recovery After Surgery (ERAS) Society recommendations. World J Surg. 2016;40(10):2425–40. https://doi.org/10.1007/s00268-016-3700-1.

Moya P, Miranda E, Soriano-Irigaray L, et al. Perioperative immunonutrition in normo-nourished patients undergoing laparoscopic colorectal resection. Surg Endosc. 2016;30:4946–53. https://doi.org/10.1007/s00464-016-4836-7.

Norcross W, Miller TE, Huang S, et al. Implementation of a successful enhanced recovery after surgery program in a community hospital. Cureus. 2019;11(10):e6029. https://doi.org/10.7759/cureus.6029.

Nygren J, Thacker J, Carli F, et al. Guidelines for perioperative care in elective rectal/pelvic surgery: Enhanced Recovery After Surgery (ERAS®) Society recommendations. World J Surg. 2013;37:285–305. https://doi.org/10.1007/s00268-012-1787-6.

Pagano E, Pellegrino L, Robella M, Castiglione A, Brunetti F, Giacometti L, Rolfo M, Rizzo A, Palmisano S, Meineri M, Bachini I, Morino M, Allaix ME, Mellano A, Massucco P, Bellomo P, Polastri R, Ciccone G, Borghi F, ERAS-colorectal Piemonte group. Implementation of an enhanced recovery after surgery protocol for colorectal cancer in a regional hospital network supported by audit and feedback: a stepped wedge, cluster randomised trial. BMJ Qual Saf. 2024;33(6):363–74. https://doi.org/10.1136/bmjqs-2023-016594.

Pearsall EA, Meghji Z, Pitzul KB, Aarts MA, McKenzie M, McLeod RS, Okrainec A. A qualitative study to understand the barriers and enablers in implementing an enhanced recovery after surgery program. Ann Surg. 2015;261(1):92–6. https://doi.org/10.1097/SLA.0000000000000604.

Posthuma LM, Breteler MJM, Lirk PB, Nieveen van Dijkum EJ, Visscher MJ, Breel JS, Wensing CAGL, Schenk J, Vlaskamp LB, van Rossum MC, Ruurda JP, Dijkgraaf MGW, Hollmann MW, Kalkman CJ, Preckel B. Surveillance of high-risk early postsurgical patients for real-time detection of complications using wireless monitoring (SHEPHERD study): results of a randomized multicenter stepped wedge cluster trial. Front Med. 2024;10:1295499. https://doi.org/10.3389/fmed.2023.1295499.

Reissman P, Teoh TA, Cohen SM, Weiss EG, Nogueras JJ, Wexner SD. Is early oral feeding safe after elective colorectal surgery? A prospective randomized trial. Ann Surg. 1995;222(1):73–7. https://doi.org/10.1097/00000658-199507000-00012.

Sauro KM, Smith C, Ibadin S, et al. Enhanced recovery after surgery guidelines and hospital length of stay, readmission, complications, and mortality: a meta-analysis of randomized clinical trials. JAMA Netw Open. 2024;7(6):e2417310. https://doi.org/10.1001/jamanetworkopen.2024.17310.

Slim K, Reymond T, Joris J, Paul S, Pereira B, Cotte E. Intolerance to early oral feeding in enhanced recovery after colorectal surgery: an early red flag? Colorectal Dis. 2020;22(1):95–101. https://doi.org/10.1111/codi.14785.

Smith MD, McCall J, Plank L, Herbison GP, Soop M. Preoperative carbohydrate treatment for enhancing recovery after elective surgery. Cochrane Database Syst Rev. 2014;2014(8):CD009161. https://doi.org/10.1002/14651858.CD009161.pub2.

Soffin EM, YaDeau JT. Enhanced recovery after surgery for primary hip and knee arthroplasty: a review of the evidence. Br J Anaesth. 2016;117(Suppl 3):iii62–72. https://doi.org/10.1093/bja/aew362.

Sun Z, Kong XJ, Jing X, Deng RJ, Tian ZB. Nutritional risk screening 2002 as a predictor of postoperative outcomes in patients undergoing abdominal surgery: a systematic review and meta-analysis of prospective cohort studies. PLoS One. 2015;10(7):e0132857. https://doi.org/10.1371/journal.pone.0132857.

Tan AC, Armstrong E, Close J, Harris IA. Data quality audit of a clinical quality registry: a generic framework and case study of the Australian and New Zealand Hip Fracture Registry. BMJ Open Qual. 2019;8(3):e000490. https://doi.org/10.1136/bmjoq-2018-000490.

Temple-Oberle C, Yakaback S, Webb C, Assadzadeh GE, Nelson G. Mobile app post-operative home monitoring after oncologic surgery using ERAS protocols improves quality of recovery: results of a randomized controlled trial. Clin Nutr ESPEN. 2022;51:493. https://doi.org/10.1016/j.clnesp.2022.06.020.

Temple-Oberle C, Yakaback S, Webb C, Assadzadeh GE, Nelson G. Effect of smartphone app postoperative home monitoring after oncologic surgery on quality of recovery: a randomized clinical trial. JAMA Surg. 2023;158(7):693–9. https://doi.org/10.1001/jamasurg.2023.0616.

Thiele RH, Rea KM, Turrentine FE, Friel CM, Hassinger TE, McMurry TL, Goudreau BJ, Umapathi BA, Kron IL, Sawyer RG, Hedrick TL. Standardization of care: impact of an enhanced recovery protocol on length of stay, complications, and direct costs after colorectal surgery. J Am Coll Surg. 2015;220(4):430–43. https://doi.org/10.1016/j.jamcollsurg.2014.12.042.

Tong E, Chen Y, Ren Y, Zhou Y, Di C, Zhou Y, Shao S, Qiu S, Hong Y, Yang L, Tan X. Effects of preoperative carbohydrate loading on recovery after elective surgery: a systematic review and Bayesian network meta-analysis of randomized controlled trials. Front Nutr. 2022;9:951676. https://doi.org/10.3389/fnut.2022.951676.

Wang D, Liu H, Zhang Y, Li X, Zhang L, Wang H, et al. Barriers to implementation of enhanced recovery after surgery (ERAS) by a multidisciplinary team in China: a multicentre qualitative study. BMJ Open. 2022;12(3):e053687. https://doi.org/10.1136/bmjopen-2021-053687.

Weiskopf NG, Weng C. Methods and dimensions of electronic health record data quality assessment: enabling reuse for clinical research. J Am Med Inform Assoc. 2013;20(1):144–51. https://doi.org/10.1136/amiajnl-2011-000681.

Xu Y, Zhong M, Li S. Opioid-free anesthesia in enhanced recovery after surgery for gastrointestinal surgery: current status, challenges, and prospects. Front Pharmacol. 2025;16:1662818. https://doi.org/10.3389/fphar.2025.1662818.

Yeom J, Lim H-S. Effects of the enhanced recovery after surgery (ERAS) program for colorectal cancer patients undergoing laparoscopic surgery. Clin Nutr Res. 2022;11(2):75–83. https://doi.org/10.7762/cnr.2022.11.2.75.

Zhang W, Wang F, Qi S, Liu Z, Zhao S, Zhang N, Ping F. An evaluation of the effectiveness and safety of the Enhanced Recovery After Surgery (ERAS) program for patients undergoing colorectal surgery: a meta-analysis of randomized controlled trials. Wideochir Inne Tech Maloinwazyjne. 2023;18(4):565–77. https://doi.org/10.5114/wiitm.2023.131426.

Future Directions: Personalised ERAS and Emerging Technologies in Integrated Anaesthesia–Nutrition Pathways

15

Ravi Yadav and Nekita Sharma

Abstract

The advent of ERAS protocols has brought about immense changes to perioperative care, making the process much safer with fewer complications and shorter stays. Nevertheless, standard ERAS care paths depend largely on the "one size fits all" principle, which ignores genetic variability, metabolism, and even microbiome differences from one patient to another. In this chapter, the authors investigate the required shift from standardised ERAS protocols to personalised, integrated anaesthesia-nutrition care paths through precision medicine technologies. Through a "precision within protocol" strategy, the authors assess how pharmacogenomics, multi-omics, digital medicine, and artificial intelligence play crucial roles.

The precision of anaesthesia allows customised risk assessment, real-time AI-supported physiological monitoring, and personalised multimodal pain management according to patient-specific parameters, allowing the minimal use of opioids and early restoration of bowel function. Simultaneously, perioperative nutrition based on the principle of precision employs cutting-edge technologies in the field of preoperative phenotyping, including the analysis of body composition using imaging and continuous glucose monitoring, enabling personalised interventions, including immunonutrition and modulation of the microbiota based on biomarkers. Wearable devices and mobile apps, along with machine learning, provide the ability to adjust interventions based on real-time information on physiological and functional parameters of patients.

In the end, adopting the new ERAS paradigm will certainly lead to the optimisation of recovery outcomes for all patients. The successful adoption of such

R. Yadav · N. Sharma (✉)
Department of Anesthesia & Operation Theater Technology, Medhavi Skills University, School of Health Sciences & Technology, Singtam, Sikkim, India

P. K. Bhattacharyya et al. (eds.), *Integrated Anesthesia and Nutrition Approaches to Enhanced Recovery after Surgery*,
https://doi.org/10.1007/978-981-92-3294-9_15

an approach would necessitate effective data infrastructures that are interoperable, multi-disciplinary governing structures, as well as measures that would ensure access to such technologies is equal and ethical.

Keyword

Enhanced Recovery After Surgery (ERAS) · Precision medicine · Perioperative nutrition · Artificial intelligence · Multi-omics

15.1 Introduction

In essence, Enhanced Recovery after Surgery (ERAS) has revolutionised perioperative management by moving away from empirically based practices to systematic approaches based on evidence throughout the pre- to post-surgery period (Ljungqvist et al. 2017). The core of ERAS involves reduction of the body's stress response, maintaining physiological functioning, and early resumption of normal activity via an integrated approach of managing anaesthesia, pain relief, fluid, nutrition, and mobility (Altman et al. 2019; Ljungqvist 2019a, Ljungqvist 2019b). ERAS implementation in several specialities has yielded favourable outcomes such as decreased risk of complications, fewer lengths of stay in hospitals, reduced costs, and comparable or better patient satisfaction than conventional care (Engelman et al. 2019; Sauro et al. 2024).

However, the current ERAS protocols have mainly been developed as procedural checklists. The patients are mainly stratified based on the type of surgical procedures performed and their associated risks, using a standard set of interventions for a diverse population that varies biologically, medically, physiologically, and socioeconomically (Ljungqvist 2019a, Ljungqvist 2019b). On the other hand, precision medicine is focused on the customisation of disease diagnosis, prevention, and treatment based on the patient's genomic, environmental, microbiological, and behavioural profile (Zeng et al. 2024). With recent developments in genomics, omics sciences, imaging, artificial intelligence, and digital health, ERAS protocols can be personalised.

Personalised care may find great potential in anaesthesia and perioperative nutrition, as both are highly relevant to surgery-associated physiological processes. Specifically, there is a strong scientific base for both fields, as well as a significant degree of individual variability within responses to interventions, which cannot be accounted for by existing ERAS pathways (Weimann et al. 2017; Lia et al. 2024). Also, both fields are becoming increasingly data-driven and suitable for optimisation through algorithms.

This chapter delves into the potential avenues for development of "personalised ERAS" with specific emphasis on the integration of anaesthesia-nutrition pathway approaches. The chapter first provides an overview of the history and shortcomings of conventional ERAS. Secondly, the chapter evaluates the recent advancements in precision medicine technologies for anaesthesia and perioperative nutrition. Thirdly, the chapter considers digital medicine, telemedicine, and AI technologies as facilitators of adaptive ERAS pathways. Lastly, the chapter presents guidelines for implementing personalised anaesthesia-nutrition interventions for future-generation ERAS programs.

15.2 From Standardised to Personalised ERAS

15.2.1 Evolution and Impact of ERAS Pathways

The initial ERAS protocols in colorectal surgeries questioned established beliefs like preoperative fasting, bowel cleansing, abundant fluid administration, delayed ambulation, and delayed feeding (Ljungqvist et al. 2017). Using prospective protocols, minimally invasive surgical procedures, short-acting anaesthetic agents, multimodal analgesia, limited fluid administration, and early catheter and feeding were all integrated into ERAS protocols. Several clinical trials and studies confirmed that using ERAS reduced hospital stay by 30–50% without higher admission rates or mortality (Ljungqvist et al. 2017; Altman et al. 2019).

In recent years, however, these principles have also found applicability to surgeries involving the upper gastrointestinal tract, hepatopancreatobiliary system, urogenital organs, female reproductive system, orthopaedic system, and the heart (Engelman et al. 2019; Altman et al. 2019; Ljungqvist 2019a, Ljungqvist 2019b). Pre-, intra-, and post-operative guidelines for various types of surgeries, formulated by the ERAS® Society and collaborating institutions, provide comprehensive guidance for these procedures (Ljungqvist 2019a, Ljungqvist 2019b; Grant and Engelman 2025).

A more recent meta-analysis of ERAS randomised trials found that following the ERAS guidelines is related to a decrease in the number of complications, readmissions, and deaths in various surgeries (Sauro et al. 2024). Cardiac surgery and orthopaedic surgery are other areas where improvements were seen using the ERAS protocol (Engelman et al. 2019; Ljungqvist 2019a, Ljungqvist 2019b).

15.2.2 Heterogeneous Treatment Effects and the Need for Personalisation

While ERAS guidelines enhance overall outcomes, not all patients will experience positive impacts from such protocols. Even in compliant ERAS programs, there still exists heterogeneity among patients in terms of post-operative complications, recovery time, chronic pain, and quality of life (Altman et al. 2019; Li & Shuang 2024). These variations result from:

- *Baseline risk:* comorbid conditions, organ system dysfunction, frailty, sarcopenia, dementia, and psychological risks
- *Biology:* genetic polymorphisms involved in pharmacokinetics, pharmacodynamics, inflammation, and pain perception (Zeng et al. 2024; Malviya and Khanna 2024)
- *Metabolic and nutritional status:* malnutrition, obesity, obesity with sarcopenia, insulin resistance, and micronutrient deficiencies (Li & Shuang 2024; Weimann et al. 2017)
- *Microbiome composition:* dysbiosis, which results from the patient's dietary intake, antibiotic administration, or other underlying diseases that affect infections and metabolism (Keskey et al. 2022; Masi et al. 2026)

In terms of application within the clinical setting, the ERAS bundles tend to be used in quite a similar fashion among these different phenotypes. The consequence is that certain patients are given "not enough" of important elements (e.g., nutritional support, prehabilitation, and intensive monitoring), whereas other patients end up receiving "too much" (e.g., excessive feeding or early hospital discharge).

15.2.3 Precision Within Protocol: A Hybrid Model

While some clinicians have concerns about personalisation because of the potential to introduce variability, thereby negating the benefits of standardisation, which has been key to the success of ERAS, precision medicine can coexist alongside protocolisation according to thought leaders (Althans et al. 2024). In the "precision-within-protocol" approach:

ERAS fundamental principles are standard among different patients and hospitals, and include counselling before surgery, thromboprophylaxis, multimodal pain management, mobility, and early enteral nutrition. It is important to note, however, that personalisation comes through the way in which these fundamental principles are applied, especially with respect to timing, frequency, mode of delivery, and thresholds. High-quality patient information is used to personalise perioperative care in order to be congruent with each patient's physiology and risk factors (Althans et al. 2024; Zain et al. 2024).

For instance, early feeding could be an essential goal, but at different rates of progression, types of feed, and requirements of immunonutrition based on the patient's nutritional risks, glycaemic phenotype, and microbiome (Li & Shuang 2024; Weimann et al. 2017). All patients might be offered multimodal analgesia therapy, but the drugs used, dosage, techniques of regional analgesia, and extent of monitoring after surgery depend on the pharmacogenomics of patients, their pain profile, and psychotherapeutic issues (Zeng et al. 2024; Malviya and Khanna 2024).

Anaesthesia and nutrition are among the most important topics where precision might be combined with standard Enhanced Recovery After Surgery protocols at the level of individuals.

15.3 Precision Anaesthesia in ERAS

15.3.1 Personalised Risk Assessment and Perioperative Phenotyping

Previously, anaesthesiologists relied on the ASA classification of physical status along with some comorbidities for patient risk stratification. However, precision anaesthesia demands a more comprehensive analysis that includes frailty, sarcopenia, sleep apnoea, autonomic dysfunction, and cognitive status (Zeng et al. 2024). Frailty scores offer more accurate predictions regarding postoperative complications and mortality compared to just age or ASA score and could provide anaesthetic and analgesic guidance and postoperative monitoring indications (Zeng et al. 2024).

New strategies utilise information from imaging-based body composition (using preoperative CT or MRI scans) and physiologic measurements (for instance, cardiopulmonary exercise test) to develop risk prediction models. Quantification of muscle mass, muscle quality, and visceral fat automatically provides an objective assessment of physiological reserve capacity (Li & Shuang 2024). Such data will allow choosing the type and dose of anaesthesia, the necessity of regional blocks and after-care requirements.

15.3.2 Pharmacogenomics and Individualised Drug Therapy

Pharmacogenomics is an area that centres on the impact of genetics on drug metabolism and response. Genetic differences in enzymes like CYP2D6, CYP3A4, OPRM1, COMT, and others lead to differences in sensitivity to opioids, effectiveness of pain relief, and vulnerability to respiratory depression (Malviya and Khanna 2024; Zeng et al. 2024). People who are poor metabolisers for CYP2D6 cannot effectively obtain pain relief from the pro-drugs opioids like codeine and tramadol.

In a personalised ERAS pathway, targeted pharmacogenomic testing could be used to:

- Avoid certain opioids based on genetic profiles and consider other options such as morphine, hydromorphone, or non-opioid therapy.
- Individualise PCA parameters based on predicted sensitivity and the risk of developing chronic pain.
- Individually adjust antiemetics for patients genetically susceptible to postoperative nausea and vomiting.

Although data supporting routine perioperative pharmacogenetic testing are not yet available, it can be implemented at the outset in a small and selected group of patients in ERAS pre-assessment clinics (Malviya and Khanna 2024; Zeng et al. 2024).

15.3.3 AI-Based Monitoring and Closed-Loop Control

AI techniques and improved capabilities in signal processing have allowed for a better understanding of physiological signals during surgery. AI-based machine learning techniques are used to process arterial waveforms, Electrocardiograph (ECG), Electroencephalogram (EEG), and pain proxies to predict the depth of anaesthesia, nociceptive balance, and the risk of hemodynamic instability (Singam 2023; Zain et al. 2024).

Indices for predicting hypotension from the arterial pressure waveform have proven capable of accurately predicting instances of intraoperative hypotension ahead of time, enabling preventive therapy to preserve perfusion and avoid organ damage (Singam 2023). Closed-loop delivery systems for propofol or volatile agents, based on processed EEG measures, can sustain a specific level of hypnotic effect with minimised drug consumption and hemodynamic stability (Zain et al. 2024).

In a personalised ERAS context, such systems could:

- Preserve the patient's baseline blood pressure and anaesthesia level as closely as possible.
- Create "stress exposure" parameters that will guide the decision on postoperative nutrition and activity (such as cumulative hypotensive minutes or the burden of nociception).
- Cut down the inconsistency between the anaesthesia technique used by different clinicians, thus enabling us to understand the additional effect that each ERAS step creates.

It is important to note that, according to systematic reviews, many AI applications in anaesthesia are still in their early stages of development and do not have sufficient external validation and evidence of better patient-related outcomes (Bellini et al. 2022; Singam 2023).

In the course of surgery, information about the patient's physiology is gathered and analysed in real time, which is used to regulate the dosage of the anaesthesia drugs delivered to the patient, as illustrated in Fig. 15.1.

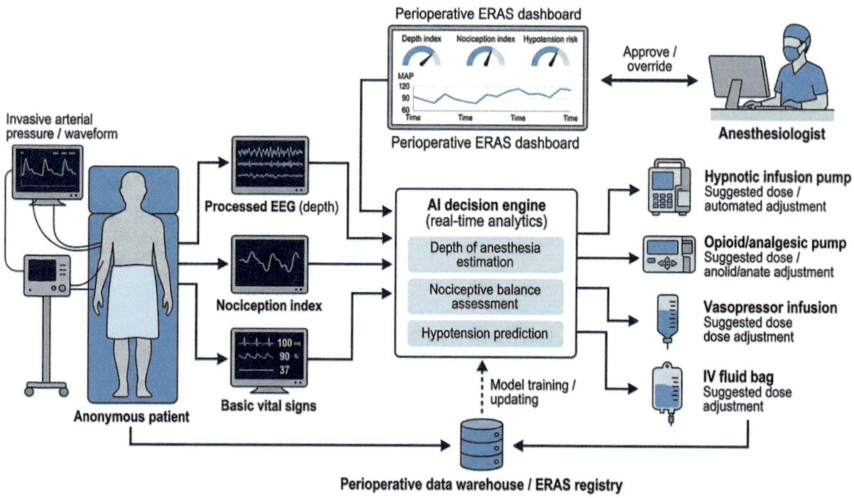

Fig. 15.1 AI-enhanced anaesthetic control loop. (Figure created by the author using draw.io (diagrams.net))

15.3.4 Precision in Multimodal and Regional Analgesia

The ERAS protocol for different medical specialisations recommends using a multimodal, opioid-sparing analgesic approach that includes regional anaesthesia, paracetamol, non-steroidal anti-inflammatory drugs, and other medications. However, the effectiveness of pain medication is highly variable. Some patients may need very high doses of opioids despite the use of multimodal therapy, whereas others can suffer side effects even from small doses.

Personalised analgesia in ERAS may involve:

- Identifying patients likely to suffer from acute severe or postoperative chronic pain using preoperative questionnaires and models that predict their occurrence (Bellini et al. 2022).
- Offering them enhanced regional anaesthesia techniques (such as continuous catheter blocks or fascial plane blocks), ketamine/lidocaine infusion, and consultation by pain specialists.
- Personalising the technique used for the regional anaesthesia and the dose of local anaesthetics based on the individual patient's body size, anatomical differences, and surgery-related characteristics.

Integration of digital devices makes it even more personalised. For instance, pain scores after surgery and opioid use collected using mobile devices can be integrated with anaesthesia and regional data to improve care and help find those requiring timely intervention for ineffective pain management (Sierra et al. 2025).

15.3.5 Anaesthetic Decisions and Early Nutrition

The selection of the anaesthetic may affect the motility of the GI tract, nausea, vomiting, and hunger. Overuse of opioids and excessive use of volatile anaesthetics are linked with POI and PONV, and the latter could lead to delayed feeding (Weimann et al. 2017). However, neuraxial and regional anaesthesia, low doses of opioids, and multimodal strategies help promote early resumption of bowel movement.

In a personalised ERAS framework, anaesthesia teams and dietitians can jointly:

- Classify patients according to their susceptibility to ileus (e.g., excessive bowel handling, high opioid needs, pre-existing motility problems) and tailor anaesthetic techniques to suit.
- Timing of antiemetic strategies must be synchronised with anticipated early nutrition targets.
- Monitor haemodynamic and stress responses during surgery to assess the rate at which oral/enteral feedings can be increased postoperatively.

15.4 Precision Perioperative Nutrition in ERAS

15.4.1 Nutritional Risk and Contemporary Guidelines

Malnutrition, obesity, and sarcopenia are prevalent conditions among the surgical patient population that significantly increase the risk of morbidity, infections, poor wound healing, and mortality (Weimann et al. 2017; Weimann et al. 2025). ESPEN Guidelines for nutrition in surgery (2017 & 2025), which are based on the ERAS approach

- Routine risk assessment for nutrition with validated scales (for instance, NRS-2002, MUST).
- Nutritional optimisation before surgery for high-risk individuals, such as oral nutritional supplementation and enteral nutrition.
- Shortening fasting time before surgery and carbohydrate loading in eligible candidates.
- Oral or enteral nutrition started early postoperatively, ideally within 24 hours, where applicable (Weimann et al. 2017; Weimann et al. 2025).

Nevertheless, audits indicate that nutrition interventions are underused compared with other aspects of the protocol (Li & Shuang 2024). Personalised nutrition is designed to solve this problem by tailoring the intensity of the intervention to patient risks and using novel sources of data to determine how, what, and when to feed patients.

15.4.2 From Generic Screening to Data-Rich Phenotyping

Conventional diagnostic tools only account for standard anthropometric measurements, weight loss, and decreased intake, while failing to identify sarcopenic obesity, malnutrition, and functional impairment (Li & Shuang 2024). Technological advancements have allowed for a better understanding of these phenotypes:

- CT imaging performed before surgery for tumour staging can be utilised to calculate skeletal muscle mass, muscle density (as a marker of myosteatosis), and abdominal fat mass.
- They are better predictors of post-surgical complications and costs than BMI and can be objectively assessed by algorithms incorporated in radiological imaging processes (Li & Shuang 2024).
- The body composition phenotype can determine nutritional intervention type and urgency, physiotherapy intensity, and even eligibility for surgery.

The paradigm shift towards personalising perioperative nutrition within ERAS pathways is reflected in Table 15.1. It presents a comparison between conventional approaches, where all patients are treated equally regardless of their metabolism

Table 15.1 From standardised to personalised perioperative nutrition in ERAS

Domain	Conventional ERAS practice	Precision-oriented evolution
Risk screening	Manual NRS-2002/ MUST, limited body composition assessment	Automated EHR algorithms combining screening tools, labs, and imaging-derived body composition (Li & Shuang 2024; Weimann et al. 2025)
Preoperative fasting and carbohydrate loading	Uniform fasting times; standard carbohydrate drink for most elective patients	Tailored regimens based on diabetes status, CGM-derived glycaemic variability, and aspiration risk (Weimann et al. 2017; Li & Shuang 2024)
Route and timing of feeding	Early oral or enteral feeding, with PN as fallback	Algorithmic selection of route and rate based on hemodynamic stability, gut perfusion, and microbiome status (Ljungqvist et al. 2017; Masi et al. 2026)
Immunonutrition	Offered by procedure (e.g., major GI, oncology)	Biomarker-guided IMN for patients with high inflammatory or immunosuppressive profiles (Weimann et al. 2017; Ho et al. 2024)
Follow-up	Weight and basic labs at set intervals	Continuous logging of intake, symptoms, and function via digital tools, with alerts for deviation from expected recovery (Wu et al. 2023; Sierra et al. 2025)

ERAS Enhanced Recovery After Surgery, *NRS-2002* Nutritional Risk Screening 2002, *MUST* Malnutrition Universal Screening Tool, *EHR* Electronic Health Records, *CGM* Continuous Glucose Monitoring, *PN* Parenteral Nutrition, *GI* Gastrointestinal, *IMN* Immunonutrition

and nutrition requirements, and contemporary techniques in which the patients' metabolic and nutritional needs are taken into account when designing treatment plans.

15.4.3 Glycaemic Phenotyping and Metabolic Flexibility

Insulin resistance in the perioperative period leads to hyperglycaemia, infection, and poor wound healing. Previously, glycaemic management has been based on glucose levels measured from intermittent blood samples and sliding scale insulin (Li & Shuang 2024). However, continuous glucose monitoring (CGM) provides detailed information on glycaemic variability and time-in-range pre- and post-operatively.

Within ERAS, CGM could help:

- Detect "metabolically fragile" patients who need intensive preparation before surgery and tight glucose management after the operation.
- Optimise carbohydrate loading and early nutrition administration for minimising fluctuations in blood glucose level.
- Consider the effect of anaesthesia and analgesia protocols on metabolic processes; therefore, connecting anaesthesia with nutrition.

15.4.4 Microbiome Readiness and Perioperative Modulation

The gut microbiota impacts immune function, barrier integrity, and metabolism. Dysbiosis caused by Western diets, antibiotic use, and other comorbid conditions could lead to a higher risk for infections and anastomotic leakage (Keskey et al. 2022). Preoperative dietary modifications like high fibre, low-fat diets, in experiments and clinical trials, have been shown to improve microbiota composition and lower postoperative risks (Keskey et al. 2022).

Omics-based studies on bariatric surgery reveal that surgery produces alterations in the microbiome and metabolome unique to surgery compared to dietary weight loss alone, which contribute to metabolic improvements (Masi et al. 2026; Gopalakrishnan et al. 2025). There may be grounds to suggest that perioperative nutrition based on the microbiome can lead to similar results in other surgeries.

15.4.5 Immunonutrition and Targeted Metabolic Therapies

Formulations of immunonutrition (IMN) that contain arginine, omega-3 fatty acids, and nucleotides have demonstrated efficacy in reducing infection and decreasing hospital stay in high-risk gastrointestinal and cancer surgeries, particularly in patients with malnutrition (Weimann et al. 2017; Ho et al. 2024). The current approach to ERAS involves using IMN according to procedure, not patient-specific risks.

Personalised ERAS could incorporate:

- IMN selection through inflammatory and immune markers such as C-reactive protein and lymphocytes.
- Multi-modal treatments involving IMN with microbiota-modulating therapies using probiotics, according to metabolic information from stool samples (Masi et al. 2026; Armetta et al. 2025).
- Technology that tracks IMN adherence and tolerability, allowing quick changes to treatment schedules (Wu et al. 2023).

15.5 Digital Health and Remote Monitoring in Personalised ERAS

15.5.1 Telemedicine in Preoperative and Postoperative Phases

Telemedicine is now considered a key element in both preoperative assessment and postoperative follow-up. The literature, which includes spine surgery, indicates that telemedicine can ensure diagnostic accuracy and patient safety equal to those of in-person consultations with high levels of satisfaction and fewer logistics (Williams et al. 2018; Shinwari et al. 2025). In ERAS, telemedicine can facilitate:

- Preoperative counselling, risk assessment, and decision-making process.
- Specialised virtual optimisation clinics (anaemia clinic, nutritional clinic, diabetes clinic), managed by anaesthesia and nutritional staff.
- Postoperative symptom screening, wound monitoring, and complication management.

Telemedicine also offers an opportunity for personalised ERAS elements on the basis of evolving needs and preferences of patients.

15.5.2 mHealth Applications for ERAS Education and Self-management

Applications on smartphones tailored to the use of ERAS principles may include educational tools, interactive checklists, drug administration, symptom logging, nutritional intake monitoring, and exercise activity monitoring. An application on a smartphone to manage nutrition and health integrated into the ERAS approach for surgery involving malignant tumours enhanced compliance, reduced complications, and decreased length of hospital stay when compared with traditional education (Wu et al. 2023). Other applications have demonstrated potential utility in monitoring postoperative pain and complications (Sierra et al. 2025; Sivachalam et al. 2024).

These interfaces offer a seamless way to make individualised recommendations and gather detailed information. For instance, dietary suggestions can be customised according to risk of nutrition deficiency, early satiety, or nausea, whereas activity goals can be adapted according to pre- and post-surgical benchmarks.

15.5.3 Wearables and Remote Automated Monitoring

Wearable technologies like smart watches, accelerometers, and wireless vital sign monitors allow for constant or frequent monitoring of heart rate, activity level, sleep, and sometimes blood oxygen level. Remote automated monitoring systems have proven effective at detecting post-operative complications and providing earlier interventions, although proving their impact on mortality rates has been difficult (McGillion et al. 2021).

Within ERAS, wearables and RAM can facilitate personalisation by:

- Ensuring that progress toward mobilisation objectives is monitored and initiating further physiotherapy or nursing interventions if mobility is not progressing as predicted.
- Detecting signs of deconditioning (such as elevated heart rate at rest, reduced activity, or poor sleep) that may indicate problems or suboptimal pain management.

Table 15.2 Digital health modalities and their role in personalised ERAS

Modality	Key ERAS functions	Personalisation opportunities
Video telemedicine	Preoperative counselling; postoperative review; complication triage	Visit frequency and content tailored to risk and recovery trajectory (Williams et al. 2018; Shinwari et al. 2025)
ERAS smartphone apps	Education; reminders; pain, nutrition, and mobility logging	Adaptive content and alerts based on engagement, symptoms, and biometric data (Wu et al. 2023; Sierra et al. 2025)
Wearable sensors	Monitoring of steps, heart rate, sleep, and sometimes oxygen saturation	Individualised mobility targets and early warnings for deterioration (Knight et al. 2021)
Remote wound monitoring	SSI detection using photos and questionnaires	Risk-stratified follow-up and early intervention (McLean et al. 2023)
Remote automated monitoring	High-acuity monitoring outside ICU	Selection of candidates based on risk models; dynamic adjustment of monitoring intensity (McGillion et al. 2021)

ERAS Enhanced Recovery After Surgery, *SSI* Surgical Site Infection, *ICU* Intensive Care Unit

- Offering quantifiable measures to determine the effects of nutritional and anaesthetic approaches on functional outcomes.

The different ways in which digital technologies play an important role in enabling personalised ERAS can be seen from the examples provided in Table 15.2. It discusses how wearable technology, telehealth, and m-health can help monitor patients' vitals and compliance with pre- and post-operative guidelines. The table shows the power of digital technology in empowering patients to modify care pathways.

15.5.4 Integration and Workflow Challenges

With the increasing availability of technology, implementation within daily operations is still difficult. Some systems work in isolation, where information cannot easily be accessed from the main EHR. Alert fatigue can occur, and there might be confusion about which person will monitor the information stream (Knight et al. 2021; Sierra et al. 2025).

Addressing these challenges requires:

- Standardisation of interoperability and funding for integration middleware.
- Establishment of roles regarding monitoring and intervention with digital information (such as ERAS nurse coordinators and virtual care teams).
- Development of interfaces together with healthcare practitioners to be relevant to their work (Sivachalam et al. 2024).

15.6 Artificial Intelligence, Machine Learning, and ERAS Optimisation

15.6.1 Risk Prediction and Stratified Care

ML techniques have been employed to create prediction models for perioperative complications, length of hospital stay, ICU admissions, and readmissions (Bellini et al. 2022). This type of model often outperforms logistic regression due to its ability to handle interaction and non-linear relationships. In the case of ERAS, ML models could be employed for:

- Classify patients based on their risk profile to assess how much optimisation, monitoring, and follow-up are needed.
- Locate patients whose rapid discharge after surgery in an ERAS program would pose risks, necessitating prolonged hospitalisation or RAM.
- Focus on higher-risk patients for co-operative anaesthesiology-nutrition prehabilitation clinics.

The authors suggested that an ERAS program is designed to be a learning system that improves risk stratification and process development based on accumulating evidence (Zain et al. 2024).

15.6.2 Dynamic, Adaptive ERAS Pathways

ERAS protocols are usually static documents, revised occasionally by committees. AI-assisted ERAS would allow dynamic ERAS pathways that change dynamically based on an individual's risk and response characteristics (Zain et al. 2024). This is exemplified through:

- Daily postoperative risk scoring using vitals, laboratory test results, and wearables will aid decision-making regarding patient discharge and frequency of telemonitoring and home visits.
- Digital reporting of symptoms and pain scores can be used to invoke predefined action steps, such as adjusting analgesics and nutritional plans.
- Longitudinal data collected from multiple patients contribute to performance dashboards used for protocol improvements.

Categorisation of the artificial intelligence-assisted tasks throughout the various stages of the ERAS pathway, such as the preoperative, intraoperative, and postoperative stages, is presented in Table 15.3. This table illustrates the potential use of machine learning algorithms and prediction models that will be able to predict the risks associated with patients, determine the appropriate dosage of anaesthetics, and identify potential complications before they arise.

Table 15.3 AI-enabled functions across the ERAS timeline

Phase	Example AI application	Impact on anaesthesia–nutrition ERAS
Preoperative	Predict complications and malnutrition using EHR and imaging	Triage to intensive prehabilitation, anaemia management, and dietitian–anaesthesiologist joint clinics (Li & Shuang 2024; Bellini et al. 2022)
Pre-assessment clinic	Intelligent chatbots for education and symptom screening	Personalise fasting instructions, smoking cessation advice, and nutrition counselling based on risk and literacy (Sivachalam et al. 2024)
Intraoperative	Closed-loop anaesthesia and hypotension prediction	Improve organ protection and generate stress profiles that guide early feeding and mobilisation strategies (Singam 2023; Zain et al. 2024)
Early postoperative	Models predicting pain crises, ileus, SSI, or delirium from monitor and lab data	Prompt escalation of regional analgesia, prokinetics, and adjustments in enteral vs parenteral nutrition (McGillion et al. 2021; McLean et al. 2023)
Post-discharge	Prediction of readmission and functional decline from app and wearable data	Tailor telemedicine schedules, home-based nutrition support, and rehabilitation intensity (Wu et al. 2023; Sierra et al. 2025)

AI Artificial Intelligence, *ERAS* Enhanced Recovery After Surgery, *EHR* Electronic Health Records, *SSI* Surgical Site Infection

15.6.3 Digital Twins and Simulation

Digital twins, computational models of a particular patient's physiology, have been studied in cardiologic and ICU practice and might eventually be employed in ERAS (Pavez Loriè et al. 2021). A surgical digital twin could include parameters related to organ performance, metabolism, gut flora, and pharmacogenomics to evaluate the impact of various anaesthesia and nutrition approaches.

In principle, digital twins could be used preoperatively to:

- Design various scenarios for the ERAS pathway, such as alternate carbohydrate loading protocols, nutritional formulas, or pain management strategies.
- Assess risks of adverse events and hospital stay duration in each scenario.
- Facilitate joint decision-making by physicians and patients.

While currently aspirational, they reflect the natural progression of AI-enabled, data-driven ERAS.

15.7 Multi-omics and Systems Biology in Integrated Anaesthesia–Nutrition ERAS

15.7.1 Genomics and Polygenic Risk

Apart from the use of pharmacogenomics, PRS have been developed for various disorders, including coronary artery disease, venous thromboembolism, and type 2 diabetes. Theoretically, it would be possible to include PRS in ERAS risk scoring models to pinpoint those patients requiring more aggressive prophylaxis against the development of blood clots, proper glycaemic control during surgery, and cardiac monitoring (Zeng et al. 2024).

15.7.2 Metabolomics and Inflammatory Signatures

Metabolomics is a measurement of metabolic status that includes the use of substrates, amino acid metabolism, and lipids. Studies of perioperative metabolomics have found patterns related to catabolic stress, insulin resistance, and organ dysfunction (Li & Shuang 2024). Combined with inflammation markers such as interleukin 6 and tumour necrosis factor alpha, such patterns can be used to detect patients prone to an excessive inflammatory or immunosuppressive response to surgery.

Tailoring nutrition in ERAS based on metabolomic and inflammatory profiles could involve:

- Modification of protein-energy goals in individuals with very high catabolism.
- Use of IMN or amino acid-specific formulations in cases of severe immune disorders.
- Alteration of fat composition in the event of particular metabolic disturbances.

15.7.3 Microbiome-Targeted Therapies

As mentioned previously, the microbiome regulates metabolism and the immune system and is affected by surgery and perioperative nutrition. The use of metagenomics and culturomics is providing knowledge on microbial species that might have beneficial uses (Armetta et al. 2025; Gopalakrishnan et al. 2025). Microbiome-focused interventions for ERAS might include:

- Pre-operative probiotic and prebiotic therapies based on initial microbiome composition and metabolic profiles.
- Post-operative nutrition protocols that promote beneficial bacteria growth and short-chain fatty acid production.
- Biomarkers in stool samples for assessing recovery of microbiome and determining treatment duration.

15.8 Implementing Personalised, Technology-Enabled ERAS

15.8.1 Multidisciplinary Governance and Leadership

The successful implementation of personalised ERAS requires effective governance with involvement of the surgical team, anaesthetists, nutritionists, nurses, physiotherapists, statisticians, and ethicists. The role of leadership entails:

- Selection and supervision of digital and AI-based technologies.
- Policy formulation for data management, privacy issues, and algorithms' transparency.
- Guaranteeing that personalisation will supplement and not contradict the principles of ERAS.

ERAS committees should have dedicated leadership roles in anaesthesia and nutrition.

15.8.2 Data Infrastructure and Interoperability

The deployment of an individualised approach to ERAS would require establishing an infrastructure capable of ingesting, integrating, and analysing data from EHR systems, medical devices, applications, and omics technologies. Some components needed include:

- Enterprise data warehouse or lake containing standardised perioperative data models.
- Interoperability of anaesthesia information management systems, nutritional intake recording, and monitoring equipment.
- Analysis and visualisation applications showing actionable insights as opposed to just raw data.

Hospitals that see value in perioperative data will be more willing to create such an infrastructure.

15.8.3 Change Management, Clinician Engagement, and Training

Engagement of clinicians is critical. Personalisation and digitisation may appear to increase cognitive load or reduce autonomy. Change management strategies that work well are:

- Designing technology together with clinicians at the frontlines.
- The phased introduction process, along with rapid feedback loops.
- Digital literacy skills training for understanding, analysing, and critically evaluating AI-generated information (Sivachalam et al. 2024; Singam 2023).

Table 15.4 describes the main barriers and their enablers with regard to the introduction of personalised technology-enhanced ERAS initiatives. The table considers various barriers, including those related to data interoperability, expense, and

Table 15.4 Barriers and enablers of personalised, technology-enabled ERAS

Domain	Common barriers	Potential enablers
Data infrastructure	Fragmented EHRs; siloed devices and apps	Enterprise integration platforms; health information exchanges; ERAS dashboards (Knight et al. 2021)
Evidence base	Few RCTs of AI/ digital tools within ERAS	Pragmatic and registry-based trials embedded in ERAS programs (Zain et al. 2024; Sauro et al. 2024)
Workforce	Limited digital and data literacy; change fatigue	Training programs; ERAS "digital champions"; protected time for innovation (Sivachalam et al. 2024)
Equity	Unequal access to devices; algorithmic bias	Subsidised technology; multilingual content; bias audits of models (Zain et al. 2024; McGillion et al. 2021)
Regulation	Uncertain liability and regulatory pathways	Regulatory sandboxes; professional society guidance; transparent reporting standards (Singam 2023; Ljungqvist 2019a, Ljungqvist 2019b)

RCTs Randomised Controlled Trials, *AI* Artificial Intelligence, *ERAS* Enhanced Recovery After Surgery, *EHRs* Electronic Health Records

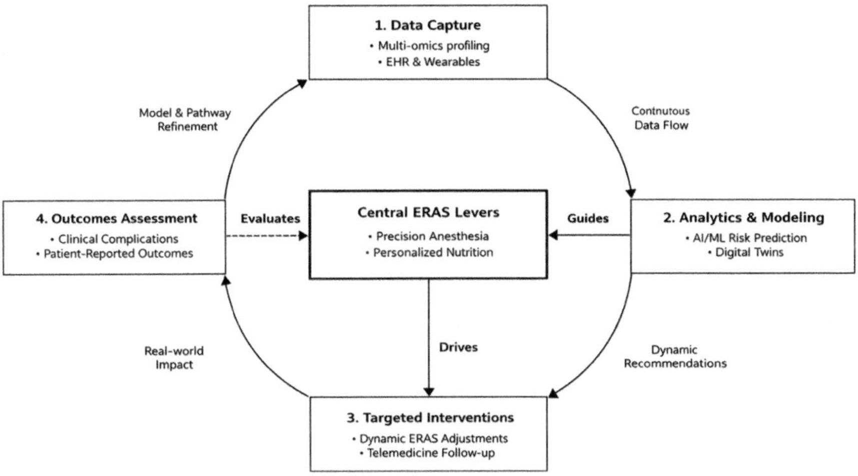

Fig. 15.2 Learning health-system model for ERAS. (Figure created by the author using draw.io (diagrams.net))

physician reluctance. These barriers come with a range of proposed remedies, including uniform data structures, interprofessional training, and ethical guidance.

The feedback mechanism entails integrating patient outcomes and multi-omics information into the learning health system framework (refer to Fig. 15.2 for an elaborate depiction of the learning health system model).

15.9 Ethical, Legal, and Equity Considerations

15.9.1 Algorithmic Fairness and Transparency

AI technologies employed to make decisions related to risk assessment or assistance in ERAS can unknowingly contribute to or worsen existing health inequalities based on biased training datasets. Marginalised patients can be misdiagnosed and/or under-medicated (Zain et al. 2024). An ethical approach to ERAS includes:

- Diverse and representative training datasets.
- Periodic assessment of model effectiveness on different demographics.
- Clarity in explaining model weaknesses to healthcare professionals and patients.

15.9.2 Data Privacy, Consent, and Secondary Use

A personalised ERAS may require comprehensive data gathering, which includes genomics, metabolomics, microbial data, and constant monitoring, posing issues regarding data security. An effective informed consent process must provide information on:

- What data is collected and why?
- How does technology impact the delivery of care?
- Will data be used to further any research? (Pavez Loriè et al. 2021)

Ownership of the data, who will have access to it, and how long it will be retained.

15.9.3 Avoiding Digital Divides

The digital health interventions could favour the younger generation, higher socioeconomic status, and individuals who are proficient with technology (McGillion et al. 2021; Shinwari et al. 2025). The personalised ERAS protocols, on the other hand, should:

- Providing low-tech options (e.g., telephonic monitoring and print material)
- Providing culturally and linguistically appropriate material
- Consideration of institutional assistance for gadgets/communication

15.10 Future Directions and Research Priorities

Several key questions must be answered to fully realise personalised, technology-enabled ERAS:

Clinical effectiveness of precision tools: Trials need to be carried out to determine whether the implementation of pharmacogenomics for analgesic use, AI for managing haemodynamic, gut microbiome for nutrition, and the use of digital technology bring about any improvement in the patients' conditions (Zain et al. 2024; Weimann et al. 2017).

Optimal combination and sequencing of interventions: The study needs to determine if there is any synergy or redundancy when these technologies are combined and how they can be used together (Sierra et al. 2025; McGillion et al. 2021).

Cost-effectiveness and scalability: For the implementation of precision medicine in ERAS, health economic evaluations will be essential to inform decision-making regarding investments in healthcare and reimbursement policies (Sauro et al. 2024).

Equity and inclusiveness: There is a need for research that examines whether the application of precision medicine in ERAS reduces or exacerbates social inequalities in outcomes among populations of varying sociodemographic backgrounds (Zain et al. 2024; McGillion et al. 2021).

Implementation strategies and governance models: Research using a mixed-methods approach would be instrumental in establishing guidelines regarding the inclusion of precision tools in ERAS implementation while ensuring that clinicians are not burdened and the fundamental aspects of ERAS are not compromised (Altman et al. 2019; Ljungqvist 2019a, Ljungqvist 2019b).

Professional associations such as the ERAS® Society and ESPEN have the expertise to organise research conducted at multiple centres, develop definitions, and establish outcomes for AI- and omics-driven ERAS (Ljungqvist 2019a, Ljungqvist 2019b; Weimann et al. 2017).

15.11 Conclusion

Enhanced Recovery After Surgery has yielded significant gains through standardisation of evidence-based care in the perioperative period. Over the coming decade, it is probable that there will be a shift from static and rigid pathways to dynamic and adaptive ones, where the individual patient's ERAS pathway can be optimised according to comprehensive information available about his or her unique bio-psycho-environmental profile.

Through the use of precise anaesthesia, perioperative nutrition, digital health tracking, and AI-driven decision-making tools, it might be possible to decrease the occurrence of complications, expedite recovery, and enhance patient outcomes while optimising the utilisation of limited resources. The implementation of this concept would necessitate proper infrastructure, inter-disciplinary cooperation, ethical considerations, and thorough testing; however, the benefits outweigh the costs. Personalised ERAS can be viewed as an extension of the core tenets of the study of integrated anaesthesia and nutrition.

References

Althans AR, Holder-Murray J, Tessler RA. The future of enhanced recovery after surgery-precision vs protocol. JAMA Netw Open. 2024;7(6):e2418968. https://doi.org/10.1001/jamanetworkopen.2024.18968.

Altman AD, Helpman L, McGee J, Samouëlian V, Auclair MH, Brar H, Nelson GS, Society of Gynecologic Oncology of Canada's Communities of Practice in ERAS and Venous Thromboembolism. Enhanced recovery after surgery: implementing a new standard of surgical care. Can Med Assoc J. 2019;191(17):E469–75. https://doi.org/10.1503/cmaj.180635.

Armetta J, Li SS, Vaaben TH, Vazquez-Uribe R, Sommer MOA. Metagenome-guided culturomics for the targeted enrichment of gut microbes. Nat Commun. 2025;16(1):663. https://doi.org/10.1038/s41467-024-55668-y.

Bellini V, Valente M, Bertorelli G, Pifferi B, Craca M, Mordonini M, Lombardo G, Bottani E, Del Rio P, Bignami E. Machine learning in perioperative medicine: a systematic review. J Anesth Analg Crit Care. 2022;2(1):2. https://doi.org/10.1186/s44158-022-00033-y.

Engelman DT, Ben Ali W, Williams JB, Perrault LP, Reddy VS, Arora RC, Roselli EE, Khoynezhad A, Gerdisch M, Levy JH, Lobdell K, Fletcher N, Kirsch M, Nelson G, Engelman RM, Gregory AJ, Boyle EM. Guidelines for perioperative care in cardiac surgery: enhanced recovery after surgery society recommendations. JAMA Surg. 2019;154(8):755–66. https://doi.org/10.1001/jamasurg.2019.1153.

Gopalakrishnan V, Kumar C, Robertsen I, Morehouse C, Sparklin B, Khader S, Henry I, Johnson LK, Hertel JK, Christensen H, Sandbu R, Greasley PJ, Sellman BR, Åsberg A, Andersson S, Löfmark RJ, Hjelmesæth J, Karlsson C, Cohen TS. A multi-omics microbiome signature is associated with the benefits of gastric bypass surgery and is differentiated from diet induced weight loss through 2 years of follow-up. Mucosal Immunol. 2025;18(4):825–35. https://doi.org/10.1016/j.mucimm.2025.04.002.

Grant MC, Engelman DT. Enhanced recovery after surgery: overarching themes of the ERAS® society guidelines & consensus statements for adult specialty surgery. Perioper Med. 2025;14(1):120. https://doi.org/10.1186/s13741-025-00590-0.

Ho C, Daud ZAM, Mohd Yusof BN, Abdul Majid H. Perioperative immunonutrition intervention on postoperative outcomes among gynecological cancer patients under enhanced recovery after surgery setting: a study protocol of explanatory mixed method study. PLoS One. 2024;19(12):e0315568. https://doi.org/10.1371/journal.pone.0315568.

Keskey R, Papazian E, Lam A, Toni T, Hyoju S, Thewissen R, Zaborin A, Zaborina O, Alverdy JC. Defining microbiome readiness for surgery: dietary pre-habilitation and stool biomarkers as predictive tools to improve outcome. Ann Surg. 2022;276(5):e361–9. https://doi.org/10.1097/SLA.0000000000004578.

Knight SR, Ng N, Tsanas A, Mclean K, Pagliari C, Harrison EM. Mobile devices and wearable technology for measuring patient outcomes after surgery: a systematic review. NPJ Digit Med. 2021;4(1):157. https://doi.org/10.1038/s41746-021-00525-1.

Li J-S, Shuang W-B. Perioperative nutrition optimization: a review of the current literature. Front Nurs. 2024;11(2):127–37. https://doi.org/10.2478/fon-2024-0014.

Ljungqvist O. Enhanced recovery after surgery and the ERAS® society. J Perioper Med. 2019a;9(1):1–7.

Ljungqvist O. Enhanced recovery after surgery and the ERAS® society. J Pancreatol. 2019b;2(3):75–82. https://doi.org/10.1097/JP9.0000000000000025.

Ljungqvist O, Scott M, Fearon KC. Enhanced recovery after surgery: a review. JAMA Surg. 2017;152(3):292–8. https://doi.org/10.1001/jamasurg.2016.4952.

Malviya AK, Khanna P. Precision medicine in anesthesia: pharmacogenomics and personalized care. National Board of Examinations. J Med Sci. 2024;2(Special Issue):S22–31. https://doi.org/10.61770/NBEJMS.2024.v02.i11.S04.

Masi D, Watanabe M, Clément K. Gut microbiome and obesity care: bridging dietary, surgical, and pharmacological interventions. Cell Rep Med. 2026;7(2):102573. https://doi.org/10.1016/j.xcrm.2025.102573.

McGillion MH, Parlow J, Borges FK, Marcucci M, Jacka M, Adili A, Lalu MM, Ouellette C, Bird M, Ofori S, Roshanov PS, Patel A, Yang H, O'Leary S, Tandon V, Hamilton GM, Mrkobrada M, Conen D, Harvey V, Lounsbury J, et al. Post-discharge after surgery Virtual Care with Remote Automated Monitoring-1 (PVC-RAM-1) technology versus standard care: randomised controlled trial. BMJ. 2021;374:n2209. https://doi.org/10.1136/bmj.n2209.

McLean KA, Sgrò A, Brown LR, Buijs LF, Daines L, Potter MA, Bouamrane MM, Harrison EM. Evaluation of remote digital postoperative wound monitoring in routine surgical practice. NPJ Digit Med. 2023;6(1):85. https://doi.org/10.1038/s41746-023-00824-9.

Pavez Loriè E, Baatout S, Choukér A, Buchheim JI, Baselet B, Dello Russo C, Wotring V, Monici M, Morbidelli L, Gagliardi D, Stingl JC, Surdo L, Yip VLM. The future of personalized medicine in space: from observations to countermeasures. Front Bioeng Biotechnol. 2021;9:739747. https://doi.org/10.3389/fbioe.2021.739747.

Sauro KM, Smith C, Ibadin S, Thomas A, Ganshorn H, Bakunda L, Bajgain B, Bisch SP, Nelson G. Enhanced recovery after surgery guidelines and hospital length of stay, readmission, complications, and mortality: a meta-analysis of randomized clinical trials. JAMA Netw Open. 2024;7(6):e2417310. https://doi.org/10.1001/jamanetworkopen.2024.17310.

Shinwari H, Kamath AG, Gill SS, Sugand K. Role and impact of telemedicine in spine surgery: a systematic review. EFORT Open Rev. 2025;10(12):894–902. https://doi.org/10.1530/EOR-2025-0020.

Sierra MC, To, H, Song WJ. Use and application of mHealth technologies in perioperative surgical care: narrative review. JMIR Mhealth Uhealth. 2025;13:e52206. https://doi.org/10.2196/52206.

Singam A. Revolutionizing patient care: a comprehensive review of artificial intelligence applications in anesthesia. Cureus. 2023;15(12):e49887. https://doi.org/10.7759/cureus.49887.

Sivachalam SN, Jeyakumar J, Elangobaalan S, Parthasarathy S. A systematic review of digital health technology in preanaesthesia assessment. Int J Med Inform. 2024;186:105415. https://doi.org/10.1016/j.ijmedinf.2024.105415.

Weimann A, Bezmarevic M, Braga M, Correia MITD, Funk-Debleds P, Gianotti L, Gillis C, Hübner M, Inciong JFB, Jahit MS, Klek S, Kori T, Laviano A, Ljungqvist O, Lobo DN, Loinaz Segurola C, Montroni I, Reddy B, Saur NM, Schweinlin A, Shi H-P, Takeuchi H, Waitzberg DL, Wallengren O, Wischmeyer PE, Ysebaert D, Bischoff SC. ESPEN guideline on clinical nutrition in surgery—Update 2025. Clin Nutr. 2025;53:222–61. https://doi.org/10.1016/j.clnu.2025.08.029.

Weimann A, Braga M, Carli F, Higashiguchi T, Hübner M, Klek S, Laviano A, Ljungqvist O, Lobo DN, Martindale R, Waitzberg DL, Bischoff SC, Singer P. ESPEN guideline: clinical nutrition in surgery. Clin Nutr. 2017;36(3):623–50. https://doi.org/10.1016/j.clnu.2017.02.013.

Williams AM, Bhatti UF, Alam HB, Nikolian VC. The role of telemedicine in postoperative care. mHealth. 2018;4:11. https://doi.org/10.21037/mhealth.2018.04.03.

Wu Y, Wang X, Gao F, Liao J, Zeng J, Fan L. Mobile nutrition and health management platform for perioperative recovery: an interdisciplinary research achievement using WeChat Applet. Front Med. 2023;10:1201866. https://doi.org/10.3389/fmed.2023.1201866.

Zain Z, Almadhoun MKIK, Alsadoun L, Bokhari SFH. Leveraging artificial intelligence and machine learning to optimize enhanced recovery after surgery (ERAS) protocols. Cureus. 2024;16(3):e56668. https://doi.org/10.7759/cureus.56668.

Zeng S, Qing Q, Xu W, Yu S, Zheng M, Tan H, Peng J, Huang J. Personalized anesthesia and precision medicine: a comprehensive review of genetic factors, artificial intelligence, and patient-specific factors. Front Med. 2024;11:1365524. https://doi.org/10.3389/fmed.2024.1365524.

Case Studies and Clinical Outcomes in Integrated Anesthesia and Nutrition Approaches to Enhanced Recovery After Surgery

16

Ravi Yadav and Debasrita Banerjee

Abstract

Enhanced Recovery After Surgery (ERAS) pathways are now increasingly adopted in many surgical fields, where they consistently prove their effectiveness by offering improved outcomes for patients in terms of lower complication rates, length of hospitalization, and expenses without compromising safety. Amongst the numerous aspects of ERAS, anesthesia/analgosedation and perioperative nutrition can be considered two of the most effective and dependent on each other factors, but which are still very frequently analyzed individually. This narrative chapter is based on data provided by clinical trials, cohort analysis, multicenter implementation studies, and prehabilitation studies showing the benefits of an integrated approach towards anesthesia and nutrition.

Clinical series and programs are examined in colorectal, upper GI, and HPB, gynecologic oncology, orthopedic arthroplasty, bariatric, and cardiothoracic surgery settings, with an emphasis on how multimodal, opioid-conserving anesthetic techniques and nutrition management work together to reduce surgical stress, maintain functional status, and enable early mobilization and feeding. Three specific case studies are presented that demonstrate how to apply this knowledge in clinical practice. Concluding the chapter is a discussion of key learnings, knowledge gaps, and practical approaches to integrating anesthetic-nutritional ERAS pathways.

R. Yadav
Department of Anesthesia & Operation Theater Technology, Medhavi Skills University, School of Health Sciences & Technology, Singtam, Sikkim, India

D. Banerjee (✉)
Department of Nutrition and Dietetics, Medhavi Skills University, Singtam, Sikkim, India

P. K. Bhattacharyya et al. (eds.), *Integrated Anesthesia and Nutrition Approaches to Enhanced Recovery after Surgery*,
https://doi.org/10.1007/978-981-92-3294-9_16

Keywords

Multimodal analgesia · Regional anesthesia · Perioperative nutrition · Carbohydrate loading · Oral nutrition supplements · Prehabilitation · Colorectal surgery · Arthroplasty

16.1 Introduction

Surgery triggers an intense neuro-endocrine and inflammatory stress response involving hypothalamic-pituitary-adrenal axis activation, sympathetic activation, insulin resistance, hyperglycemia, proteolysis, and fluid redistribution (Weimann et al. 2017; Ljungqvist and Carli 2024). Malnourished, sarcopenic-obese, or frail patients experience intensified stress responses that are linked to post-operative complications, hospital stays, and poor functional outcomes (Wischmeyer et al. 2018; Weimann 2019). Conventional approaches to perioperative care, such as extended fasting, generous fluid administration, heavy opioid dosing, and delayed mobilization and feeding, worsen the detrimental impact on metabolism (Gillis and Wischmeyer 2019; Gillis et al. 2015).

The ERAS protocols provide a multi-modal, scientifically proven approach to reduce the effect of surgery on the body and help achieve rapid recovery through standardization of care during the pre-operative, intraoperative, and post-operative stages (Ljungqvist et al. 2017; Gustafsson et al. 2025). Important components of ERAS include patient education, reduced fasting time and carbohydrate loading before surgery, opioid-sparing multi-modal anesthesia and analgesia, goal-directed fluid management, early mobilization, and early oral or enteral feeding (Gustafsson et al. 2025; Weimann et al. 2021; Wischmeyer et al. 2018). Of all these, anesthesia/analgesia and nutrition have a profound interrelationship because anesthetic methods affect gut perfusion, digestive functions, and oral food acceptance, whereas nutritional status affects drug absorption, wound healing, and immunity (Myles et al. 2019; Funk Debleds et al. 2024).

The chapter presents an intensive, clinically oriented review of enhanced recovery outcomes associated with the intentional combination of anesthetics and nutritional approaches in ERAS protocols. Instead of covering every aspect of an ERAS protocol comprehensively, this chapter emphasizes how the particular use of regional anesthesia, multimodal pain control, and goal-directed fluid management combines with preoperative nutrition assessment, carbohydrate loading, postoperative feeding, and oral nutrition supplements (ONSs). All information presented in this chapter is taken from quality guidelines and reviews such as European Society for Clinical Nutrition and Metabolism (ESPEN) guidelines and the American Society for Enhanced Recovery–Perioperative Quality Initiative consensus statements, along with specialized ERAS guidelines (Wischmeyer et al. 2018; Weimann et al. 2017, 2021; Weimann 2019).

16.2 Pathophysiologic Rationale for Integrating Anesthesia and Nutrition

16.2.1 Surgical Stress Response and Metabolic Derangements

The stress response following surgery involves alterations in endocrine, metabolic, and inflammatory mechanisms that help ensure sufficient energy supply for wound repair; however, in cases where these responses occur in excess, they cause catabolism and organ dysfunction (Weimann et al. 2017; Weimann 2019). An increase in catecholamines, cortisol, and glucagon results in an increased breakdown of proteins in muscles, which leads to insulin resistance, hyperglycemia, reduced immune response, and vulnerability to infections (Ljungqvist and Carli 2024; Funk Debleds et al. 2024). On the other hand, an increased rate of muscle proteolysis helps to facilitate the production of acute-phase proteins (Weimann et al. 2021; Gillis et al. 2015).

The impact of perioperative fasting, high-dose opioid usage, postoperative ileus, and delayed nutrition initiation exacerbates these metabolic disturbances (Gillis and Wischmeyer 2019; Funk Debleds et al. 2024). Observational studies in patients undergoing colorectal surgery, cardiac surgery, and upper gastrointestinal surgery have found insufficient postoperative nutritional intake even among patients enrolled in ERAS protocols and are related to poor patient outcomes, highlighting the importance of nutrition interventions that should be part of a larger recovery process (Gillis et al. 2015; Beaulieu et al. 2025; Hubert et al. 2021).

16.2.2 Mechanistic Synergy Between Anesthesia and Nutrition

Nutrition-related processes are affected by anesthetics and analgesics that affect central and peripheral pathways. The use of regional anesthesia or neuraxial blockade procedures, such as thoracic epidural, spinal, and peripheral nerve blocks, leads to a decreased need for systemic opioids, resulting in reduced postoperative ileus, nausea, and vomiting, which are significant obstacles to early oral feeding (Myles et al. 2019; Wong et al. 2024). Rapid recovery is promoted by the use of short-acting intravenous anesthesia, along with multimodal non-opioid pain management and effective Post Operative Nausea & Vomiting (PONV) prevention measures (Cavallaro and Bordeianou 2019; Huang et al. 2024).

Nutrition-wise, carbohydrate loading before surgery helps prevent insulin resistance, preserves glycogen, and enhances well-being, whereas early feeding and high-protein oral nutritional supplements after surgery can aid in preventing muscle catabolism and enhancing immune function (Tong and Tan 2022; Sebestyén et al. 2025; Gillis et al. 2015). Nutritional strategies can be effectively utilized in patients who are comfortable, have stable hemodynamics, are not suffering from severe nausea, and can sit upright, all of which are strongly influenced by anesthesia practices (Wischmeyer et al. 2018; Funk Debleds et al. 2024).

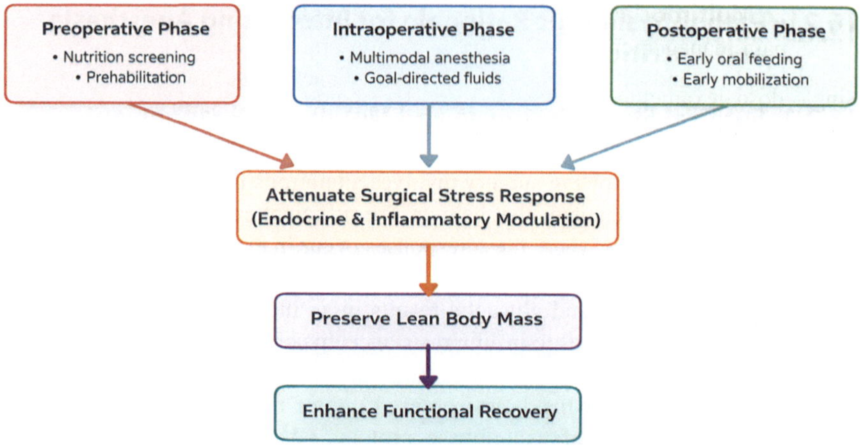

Fig. 16.1 Synergy between anesthesia and nutrition in ERAS. (Created by author using MS Word 2021)

It follows that effective perioperative management involves the careful integration of anesthesia and nutritional strategies. This would entail, for instance, the timed administration of carbohydrates in accordance with fasting protocols, the coordination of antiemetic administration with expected oral consumption, and the use of appropriate pain control measures from regional blocks and multimodal analgesia to enable early movement and nutrition, among others (Cavallaro and Bordeianou 2019; Martin et al. 2019). This interplay of perioperative phases in order to mitigate surgical stress is shown in Fig. 16.1 below.

16.3 Core Components of Integrated ERAS Pathways

16.3.1 Anesthetic Strategies in ERAS

There are certain themes that consistently emerge when examining anesthetic techniques used in various ERAS programs.

16.3.1.1 Regional and Neuraxial Anesthesia

There have been many studies demonstrating how thoracic epidural analgesia for open colorectal surgery and upper abdominal surgery can result in better pain management, reduction in the usage of opioids, as well as lower Length of Stay (LOS) and cardiopulmonary complications (Myles et al. 2019; Ljungqvist et al. 2017). For total hip replacement and knee arthroplasty, there has been evidence to suggest that neuraxial anesthesia and light sedation and peripheral nerve blocks (adductor canal block) result in lower incidences of PONV and respiratory depression, as well as early mobilization when compared to general anesthesia (Wainwright et al. 2020; Riga et al. 2023; Albrecht et al. 2026).

16.3.1.2 Multimodal, Opioid-Sparing Analgesia

ERAS pain management pathways focus on non-opioid scheduled analgesia (e.g., acetaminophen and NSAIDs), local infiltration anesthesia, gabapentinoids, and regional anesthesia modalities, using opioids only for rescue purposes (Wong et al. 2024). Multimodal analgesic bundles have been found to decrease opioid use, opioid-associated complications, and occasionally length of stay and readmissions (Wainwright et al. 2020).

16.3.1.3 Short-Acting Anesthetic Agents and Depth Monitoring

The administration of propofol TIVA (total intravenous anesthesia) or the use of low-solubility agents and depth-of-anesthesia monitoring with appropriate titration results in fast recovery with early involvement in breathing exercises and ingestion (Cavallaro and Bordeianou 2019; Myles et al. 2019).

16.3.1.4 Goal-Directed Fluid Therapy (GDFT)

Guided by dynamic indicators for hemodynamic management during surgery and early post-operative periods, GDFT prevents both under- and overhydration, thus reducing gut edema, ileus, and cardiopulmonary complications (Ljungqvist et al. 2017; Mercedes et al. 2019). Most ERAS protocols for colorectal and upper gastrointestinal procedures include GDFT as an integral element, which has proven effective in decreasing LOS and complications after surgery (Cavallaro and Bordeianou 2019; Mangone et al. 2024).

16.3.2 Nutritional Strategies in ERAS

International guidelines and consensus statements provide an organized approach to perioperative nutrition, which has increasingly been integrated into ERAS pathways:

16.3.2.1 Systematic Nutrition Screening and Risk Stratification

The ESPEN guidelines and the ASER-POQI (American Society for Enhanced Recovery–Perioperative Quality Initiative) consensus advise the use of validated screening methods, such as the Subjective Global Assessment, MUST (Malnutrition Universal Screening Tool), to screen for malnutrition risks in all patients undergoing surgical procedures (Weimann et al. 2017; Wischmeyer et al. 2018). Patients who present with high risks should be subjected to individualized nutritional assessments with the option of providing nutritional support through enteral or parenteral routes for at least 7–14 days before surgery (Weimann et al. 2021; Weimann 2019).

16.3.2.2 Minimization of Fasting and Preoperative Carbohydrate Loading

However, modern fasting instructions require clear carbohydrates for 2 hours and solid foods up to 6 hours prior to anesthetic induction instead of "nothing by mouth after midnight" protocol (Weimann et al. 2017; Gillis and Wischmeyer 2019). A meta-analysis of randomized trials proved that preoperative consumption of carbohydrate-containing liquids up to 2 hours before operations alleviates thirst, anxiety, postoperative insulin resistance, and reduces LOS when used as part of ERAS protocols (Tong and Tan 2022; Sebestyén et al. 2025; Haselton et al. 2025).

16.3.2.3 Early Postoperative Oral or Enteral Feeding

The ERAS colorectal guidelines also advise starting the intake of clear fluids a few hours after the operation, while moving towards the intake of solid foods in the evening or on the first postoperative day without any contraindication (Gustafsson et al. 2025; Cavallaro and Bordeianou 2019). The early oral feeding in colorectal and gynecological oncological patients proved to be both safe and effective, being linked with less infection and lower LOS, and allowing for better nutritional energy intake with a combination of analgesic techniques and antiemetic measures (Gillis et al. 2015; Ho et al. 2022; Funk Debleds et al. 2024).

16.3.2.4 High-Protein Oral Nutrition Supplements and Post-discharge Support

ONS (Oral Nutritional Supplements) with high protein content are essential in perioperative nutritional support, especially for those who experience low appetite and food restrictions. For colorectal ERAS patients, evidence from structured ONS interventions, such as 60 mL provided five times a day, has revealed better protein intake goals and shorter LOS (Gillis et al. 2015; Yeung et al. 2017). Observational findings suggest that patients often have deficiencies in both energy and protein consumption after discharge, thus requiring ongoing ONS and dietitian management (Hubert et al. 2021; Beaulieu et al. 2025; Funk Debleds et al. 2024).

16.3.2.5 Selective Use of Immunonutrition

Formulas enriched with nutrients that target a specific disease process (such as those containing arginine, omega-3 fatty acids, and nucleotides) have primarily been evaluated in upper gastrointestinal surgery and colorectal cancer surgery. While several studies and systematic reviews have demonstrated a decrease in infections and LOS, results vary, and safety issues persist among certain critically ill groups (Friedman et al. 2021; Weimann et al. 2017). Currently, there is evidence to support the use of immunonutrition formulas in selected malnourished individuals undergoing major abdominal cancer surgery under the ERAS protocol (Friedman et al. 2021; Weimann 2019). Summary of Key ERAS Elements is described in Table 16.1.

Table 16.1 Core anesthetic and nutritional components of an integrated ERAS pathway

Domain	Key components	Resources
Anesthesia/analgesia	Neuraxial/regional blocks, multimodal non-opioid analgesia, short-acting anesthetic agents, aggressive PONV prophylaxis, goal-directed fluid therapy	Myles et al. (2019); Wainwright et al. (2020); Wong et al. (2024)
Preoperative nutrition	Systematic nutrition screening, risk stratification, ONS or enteral nutrition for high-risk patients, micronutrient optimization	Weimann et al. (2017); Wischmeyer et al. (2018); Weimann et al. (2021)
Fasting and carbohydrate loading	Solids until 6 h, clear carbohydrate drinks until 2 h before induction	Tong and Tan (2022); Weimann et al. (2017)
Early postoperative feeding	Early oral fluids and solids as tolerated, avoidance of routine nasogastric tubes, early enteral feeding when oral route inadequate	Gustafsson et al. (2025); Cavallaro and Bordeianou (2019); Funk Debleds et al. (2024)
Post-discharge nutrition	Continued ONS, dietitian follow-up, support for adequate protein and energy intake	Hubert et al. (2021); Beaulieu et al. (2025)

16.4 Specialty-Specific Evidence and Case Studies

16.4.1 Colorectal Surgery: A Mature ERAS Model

Colorectal surgery has been the most intensively investigated area within the ERAS literature, where many randomized controlled trials and meta-analyses have shown decreases in LOS by 1–3 days and decreased complication rates when compared with traditional approaches (Table 16.2) (Al-Omari and Othman 2025; Mangone et al. 2024; Ljungqvist et al. 2017). Cavallaro and associates designed a comprehensive ERAS protocol for elective colorectal surgery cases with the following steps before surgery: ingestion of oral carbohydrates, administration of preemptive multimodal pain therapy, use of fast-acting general anesthesia, either epidural or TAP (Transversus Abdominis Plane) block anesthesia, goal-directed fluid therapy, catheter removal soon after operation, and early nutrition (Cavallaro and Bordeianou 2019). The pre- and post-intervention analysis found significant improvements in LOS and postoperative complications without an increase in readmission rates. The order of the combination therapies is illustrated in Fig. 16.2.

Gillis et al. carried out a prospective observational trial involving colorectal surgery patients who were managed using an ERAS program that focused on nutrition adequacy (Gillis et al. 2015). In this trial, solid foods were introduced on POD (Postoperative Day) 0, while protein-enriched ONS was administered five times per day at a dose of 60 mL. Additionally, patients had access to multimodal pain management and early mobilization. Gillis et al. noted that preoperative nutrition risk was highly prevalent among the participants, but the ERAS

Table 16.2 Selected clinical studies of integrated anesthesia–nutrition ERAS pathways in colorectal surgery

Study	Design and population	Integrated elements	Key outcomes
Cavallaro and Bordeianou (2019)	Single-center pre–post study, elective colorectal surgery	Preop carbohydrate drinks, multimodal analgesia, short-acting anesthesia, GDFT, early feeding	Reduced LOS and complications without increased readmissions
Gillis et al. (2015)	Prospective observational cohort, colorectal ERAS	Early solid food (POD 0), structured high-protein ONS, multimodal analgesia, early mobilization	Higher nutrition adequacy associated with shorter LOS and fewer complications
Martin et al. (2019)	Multicenter pre–post ERAS implementation	Systematic nutrition screening, ONS pre- and post-op, standardized analgesia, early mobilization	Improved nutrition care processes and reduced LOS
Mangone et al. (2024)	National registry analysis	Implementation of ERAS colorectal pathways	Reduced LOS at system level with maintained safety

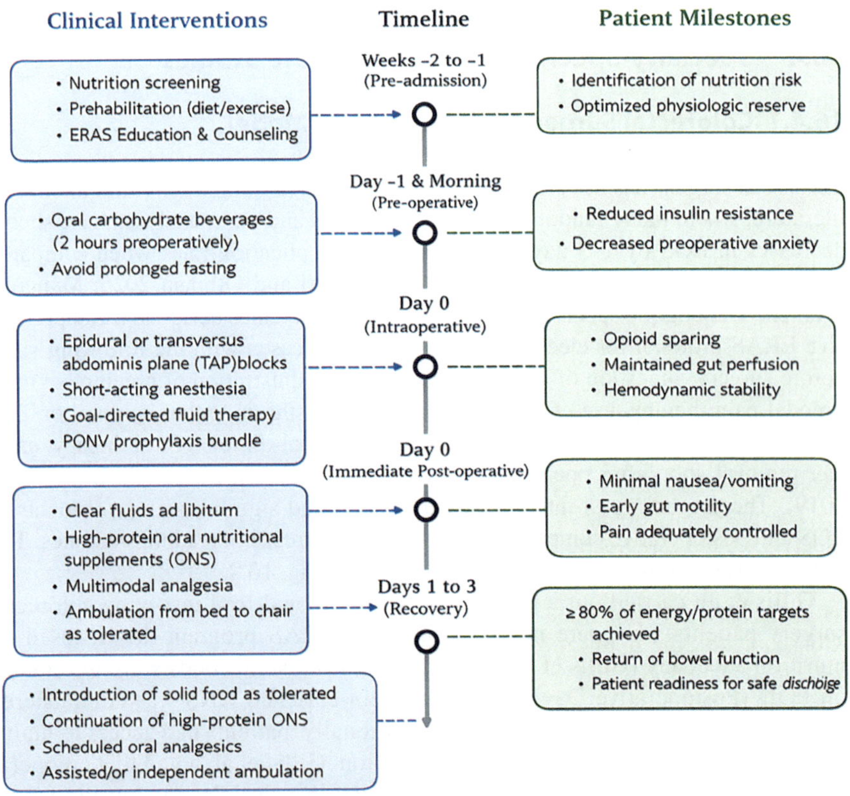

Fig. 16.2 Timeline of integrated anesthesia-nutrition interventions for elective colorectal surgery. (Created by author using MS Word 2021)

strategy allowed a significant number of participants to attain at least 60–80% of energy and protein needs in the early postoperative phase (Gillis et al. 2015; Yeung et al. 2017).

The impact of implementing ERAS on perioperative nutrition practices in elective colorectal surgery was investigated by Martin et al. via a JPEN multicenter study (Martin et al. 2019). Following the implementation of ERAS, there have been significant increases in the practice of conducting nutrition screening tests, preoperative ONS (Oral Nutritional Supplements), and postoperative ONS in addition to analgesia and mobilization protocols. All these resulted in better achievement of protein and caloric goals and shorter LOS. It is worth noting that improvements in nutrition are rarely isolated from ERAS implementation (Fig. 16.2) (Martin et al. 2019).

16.4.2 Upper Gastrointestinal and Hepatopancreatobiliary Surgery

Surgical procedures like upper gastrointestinal surgery and hepato-pancreato-biliary surgery pose a significant risk of developing catabolic state, delayed gastric emptying, and postoperative complications; therefore, the use of anesthesia and nutrition together is vital (Weimann et al. 2017; Weimann 2019). The ERAS approach for this area of surgery includes thoracic epidural or paravertebral analgesia, early ambulation, and early feeding through jejunal routes when oral feeding cannot be initiated (Weimann et al. 2021; Friedman et al. 2021).

Observational studies on pancreaticoduodenectomy and complex HPB operations suggest that ERAS protocols involving epidural anesthesia, GDFT (Goal-Directed Fluid Therapy), early mobilization, and early enteral feeding result in shorter lengths of stay (LOS) and lower incidence of complications than those observed in historical controls, but high-quality randomized evidence is still scarce (Weimann 2019; Weimann et al. 2021). ESPEN (European Society for Clinical Nutrition and Metabolism) surgical nutritional guidelines recommend the initiation of enteral nutrition within 24 hours in severely malnourished or at-risk patients if the expected oral intake is below 50%, thus highlighting the relevance of nutrition in the context of anesthetics and surgical management (Weimann et al. 2017; Weimann et al. 2021).

There is plenty of research on the topic of immunonutrition in upper gastrointestinal oncologic surgery. According to meta-analysis, perioperative immunonutrition may help decrease infection rates and LOS in malnourished patients with cancer. Nonetheless, heterogeneity and safety issues should not be disregarded. Consequently, the application of immunonutrition in upper GI (gastrointestinal) oncologic surgery should be prudent. Moreover, the effectiveness of immunonutrition will be maximized only within the ERAS program, including proper analgesia, hemodynamic management, and early rehabilitation (Friedman et al. 2021).

16.4.3 Gynecologic Oncology

Gynecologic oncology has emerged as an especially productive field for the application of ERAS protocols, emphasizing early mobility, the withdrawal of catheters and drains, and early feeding following major pelvic operations (Friedman et al. 2021; MD Anderson Cancer Center 2022). Gynecologic oncology ERAS protocols usually consist of carbohydrate loading before surgery, multimodal pain relief involving spinal or TAP block anesthesia, and early dietary intake on post-operative day zero to one (MD Anderson Cancer Center 2022).

In a study analyzing data from a clinical trial on gynecological cancer patients, Ho et al. demonstrated that adequate intake of calories and proteins during the post-operative period correlated with improved recovery rate, fewer complications, and reduced LOS (Ho et al. 2022). This effect was achieved due to effective management of pain and PONV, indicating the interrelation between the two factors. Patient education information provided by leading hospitals highlights the importance of protein intake, physical activity, and the need for oral nutrition supplementation if there is no appetite, which represents the practical application of the ERAS principles (MD Anderson Cancer Center 2022).

16.4.4 Total Hip and Knee Arthroplasty

ERAS guidelines have been widely implemented in total joint replacement surgeries, with shortening the hospital stay and early discharge being specific goals (Wainwright et al. 2020; Riga et al. 2023; AAOS 2026). According to the guidelines of the ERAS society, patients should receive full educational training, neuraxial anesthesia with minimal sedation, peripheral nerve block, multimodal pain management, restrictive fluid management, and immediate ambulation within hours of surgery (Wainwright et al. 2020).

Nutritional aspects of ERAS protocols used in arthroplasty involve fasting reduction, preoperative carbohydrate drinks, early oral food intake, and ONS in patients considered to be at high risk of complications or suffering from malnutrition (Riga et al. 2023; Weimann et al. 2017). According to Albrecht et al. (2026), an ERAS protocol was developed for primary hip and knee arthroplasty that included neuraxial anesthesia, adductor canal and tibial nerve blockade, dexamethasone and NSAID administration intraoperatively, early mobilization, and early feeding. In their study, the authors noted that there were no problems implementing the neuraxial anesthesia technique, reduced use of opioids, and safe early ambulation and discharge, which shows that nutritional and anesthesia techniques can complement each other in early rehabilitation (AAOS 2026).

The Haselton et al. study on randomized trials of carbohydrate loading before surgery as part of an ERAS pathway for elective total hip replacement has shown that there were positive effects on metabolic markers and recovery following surgery when compared to fasting. These results correlate with other studies done in general surgery and would favor including carbohydrate drinks in orthopedic ERAS pathways (Haselton et al. 2025).

16.4.5 Bariatric and Metabolic Surgery

Patients who undergo bariatric surgery have other metabolic disorders like insulin resistance, nutritional deficiencies, and sleep apnea, which make them excellent candidates for the ERAS multidisciplinary care approach (Friedman et al. 2021; Funk Debleds et al. 2024). The ERAS bariatric protocol focuses on multimodal analgesia, minimal use of opioids, early mobility, and early administration of protein-containing liquids or ONS and subsequent gradual transition to texture-modified diets (Friedman et al. 2021; Dietitians in Bariatric and Upper GI Surgery 2020).

While there is a lack of evidence-based randomized controlled trials directly testing anesthetic and nutritional management in bariatric surgery, observational series indicate that ERAS application may improve outcomes, including LOS and complication rates, compared to historical controls, especially when integrated with nutrition counseling and early oral intake alongside regional anesthetic techniques and PONV management interventions (Weimann et al. 2017).

16.4.6 Cardiac and Thoracic Surgery

ERACS (Enhanced Recovery After Cardiac Surgery) and ERAS for Thoracic Surgery are two areas where integrated anesthesia-nutrition strategies show promise, although their evidence base is currently developing (Weimann 2019; Beaulieu et al. 2025). The principles of ERACS encourage the early removal of breathing tubes, use of multiple analgesics, hemodynamics monitoring, early mobility, early oral or enteral feeding, and nutritional screening (Weimann 2019; Wischmeyer et al. 2018).

In one prospective study conducted among cardiac surgery patients treated using an ERAS protocol, it was observed that the amount of food consumed orally after surgery was often inadequate, underscoring the importance of formulating ONS orders along with the involvement of a dietitian in integrated care (Beaulieu et al. 2025). In thoracic ERAS protocols, the emphasis is placed on regional anesthesia, such as epidural or paravertebral block, lung-protective ventilation, rapid weaning from chest drains, and early feeding (Table 16.3) (Weimann 2019; Ljungqvist et al. 2017).

Table 16.3 Integrated anesthesia–nutrition themes across surgical specialties

Specialty	Key anesthetic elements	Key nutritional elements	Representative outcomes
Colorectal	Epidural/TAP blocks, multimodal analgesia, GDFT	Preop carbohydrate drinks, early solids, high-protein ONS	Reduced LOS and complications (Cavallaro and Bordeianou 2019; Gillis et al. 2015; Martin et al. 2019)
Upper GI/ HPB	Thoracic epidural, GDFT	Early enteral feeding, immunonutrition in selected patients	Reduced LOS and infections in observational series (Weimann 2019)
Gynecologic oncology	Neuraxial/TAP blocks, multimodal analgesia	Preop carbohydrate drinks, early oral intake, ONS	Faster functional recovery when intake goals met (Ho et al. 2022)
Arthroplasty	Neuraxial anesthesia, nerve blocks, multimodal analgesia	Minimized fasting, carbo drinks, early oral intake	Safe early discharge, lower complications (Wainwright et al. 2020; Albrecht et al. 2026)

16.5 Prehabilitation and Postoperative Rehabilitation

16.5.1 Multimodal Prehabilitation

Prehabilitation programs that include both aerobic and resistance training, nutritional optimization, and psychological strategies have emerged in recent years and are now considered an expansion of the ERAS protocol (Gillis et al. 2022; Lau et al. 2020; Widanage et al. 2025). In patients with colorectal cancer, meta-analyses show evidence that multimodal prehabilitation may enhance pre- and post-surgical functioning and potentially minimize adverse outcomes depending on intensity and customization of exercises (see Fig. 16.3) (Lau et al. 2020; Widanage et al. 2025).

Such programs usually involve personalized exercise, high-protein ONS, or nutritional advice to address higher protein requirements, and education concerning ERAS principles, pain management, and early nutrition (Table 16.4) (Gillis et al. 2022; Kallikourdis et al. 2023). The involvement of anesthetists, surgeons, dietitians, and physiotherapists in prehabilitation programs helps enhance both cardiorespiratory capacity and nutritional status prior to the procedure, thus enhancing tolerance of anesthesia and surgery (Weimann 2019; Ljungqvist and Carli 2024).

16.5.2 Patient Perspectives and Engagement

According to qualitative research conducted by Gillis et al., patients consider prehabilitation to be an empowering aspect of the ERAS approach, where patients have a

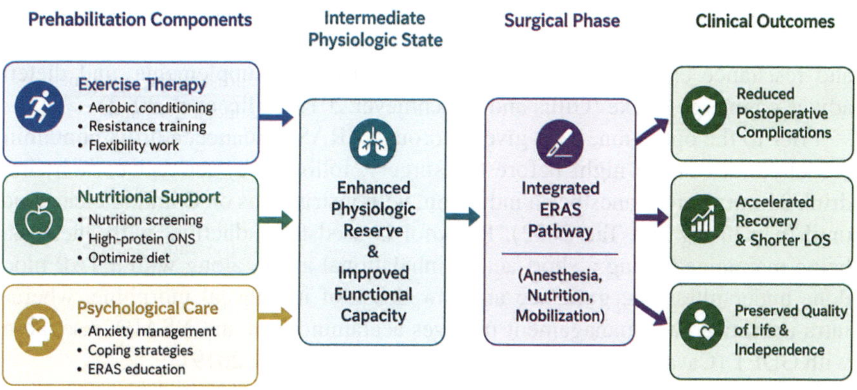

Fig. 16.3 Multimodal prehabilitation components and perioperative outcomes. (Created by author using MS PowerPoint 2021)

Table 16.4 Typical components of a multimodal prehabilitation program

Component	Description	Resources
Exercise training	Supervised and home-based aerobic and resistance training 3–5 times per week	Lau et al. (2020); Widanage et al. (2025)
Nutritional optimization	High-protein ONS, individualized dietitian counseling, and correction of micronutrient deficiencies	Gillis and Wischmeyer (2019); Weimann (2019)
Psychological support	Coping strategies, anxiety management, and expectation setting	Gillis et al. (2021)
Education on ERAS	Information on early feeding, mobilization, pain control, and self-management	Gillis et al. (2022); Kallikourdis et al. (2023)

chance to prepare themselves physically and nutritionally before surgery, as well as get information on how to use their efforts along with medical assistance (Gillis et al. 2021). It is important for patients to receive adequate information regarding early mobilization and nutrition, get family members involved in their preparation for surgery, and find ways to deal with anorexia and exhaustion (Funk Debleds et al. 2024; Gillis et al. 2021).

16.6 Representative Clinical Vignettes

16.6.1 Case 1: Laparoscopic Sigmoid Colectomy in a Malnourished Older Adult

The patient is a 72-year-old male with a history of left-sided colorectal cancer, involuntary weight loss of 8% over the past 3 months, and low grip strength. The patient was identified as being at high risk for malnutrition through the Malnutrition Screening Tool and also satisfies the guidelines provided by ESPEN for preoperative nutritional intervention (Weimann et al. 2017). This patient is to undergo a two-week period of prehabilitation involving a combination of walking and resistance exercises, high-protein oral nutritional supplements, and dietetic advice on energy intake (Gillis and Wischmeyer 2019; Gillis et al. 2022).

Prior to the operation, he is given thorough ERAS guidance, a drink containing carbohydrates in the night before the surgery, followed by another carbohydrate drink 2 hours before anesthesia induction, with instructions on drinking clear fluids until then (Tong and Tan 2022). Propofol is used for induction, with anesthesia being maintained using a short-acting inhalational agent, along with a TAP block done under ultrasonic guidance and low doses of intrathecal morphine, whereas intra-operative pain management involves acetaminophen and NSAIDs use, along with GDFT (Cavallaro and Bordeianou 2019; Myles et al. 2019).

Pain scores at rest and on coughing are low, PONV is prevented by preoperative administration of dexamethasone and ondansetron, and postoperative intake of clear fluids and high-protein ONS starts on the day of surgery, followed by soft foods on POD 1 (Cavallaro and Bordeianou 2019; Gillis et al. 2015). Mobilization to sitting position occurs in less than 6 hours after extubation, and ambulation with assistance occurs on POD 1 (Gillis et al. 2015; Martin et al. 2019). The patient reaches almost 80% of his energy and protein requirements within 3 days of the post-operative period, with dietetic consultation every day (Gillis et al. 2015; Martin et al. 2019).

This scenario demonstrates the integration of the ESPEN and ERAS guidelines, with the use of prehabilitation, glucose loading, multimodal pain management, and organized ONS to enhance the results in a vulnerable patient due to malnutrition (Weimann et al. 2017; Gillis et al. 2015; Gillis et al. 2022).

16.6.2 Case 2: Primary Total Knee Arthroplasty in an Obese, High-Risk Patient

A 65-year-old female with obesity, type 2 diabetes, and severe osteoarthritis of the knee joint requires a procedure of unilateral total knee arthroplasty. The patient participates in ERAS education, which includes information about the use of regional anesthesia and blocks, early mobilization, nutrition, and analgesia (Wainwright et al. 2020; AAOS 2026). Screening of nutrition demonstrates poor protein consumption and low levels of vitamin D, thus, initiating supplementation of the patient with high-protein ONS and micronutrients before surgery for 3 weeks (Weimann et al. 2017; Weimann 2019).

On the day of surgery, she takes carbohydrate drinks in accordance with fasting instructions and undergoes spinal anesthesia under mild sedation, adductor canal nerve block, and multi-modal systemic pain control that consists of acetaminophen, non-steroidal anti-inflammatory drugs (NSAIDs), and low-dose opioids (Haselton et al. 2025; Albrecht et al. 2026). Dexamethasone intraoperatively serves as both an antiemetic and an anti-inflammatory drug, while GDFT is performed to avoid fluid overloading. Postoperatively, she starts receiving food orally, including high-protein ONS, in the recovery room and proceeds with a regular diet by the first postoperative day (POD 1) (Riga et al. 2023; Albrecht et al. 2026).

She rises from bed and walks under the supervision of physiotherapy in the operating room. She is discharged at POD 1 with a defined pain management protocol and a continued nutrition program, which involves ONS for 2 weeks and advice about high-protein diet foods. This scenario brings out the benefits of neuraxial anesthesia, peripheral nerve block, and multimodal analgesia that facilitate immediate mobility and early oral ingestion, with optimal nutritional status preoperatively and postoperatively, enhancing wound healing and glucose control (Wainwright et al. 2020; Haselton et al. 2025).

16.6.3 Case 3: Pancreaticoduodenectomy in a Severely Malnourished Patient

This is a 60-year-old man who has adenocarcinoma of the head of the pancreas. This patient underwent neoadjuvant chemotherapy followed by significant weight loss. He will undergo a pancreatectomy. His nutritional status showed poor protein-calorie nutrition with sarcopenia. Thus, he was given 10 days of preoperative enteral feeding through nasogastric tube along with a high-protein diet, and also underwent exercises and physiotherapy (Weimann et al. 2017; Weimann 2019).

The thoracic epidural block is done prior to induction, and anesthesia management is by short-acting anesthetics and GDFT to maintain splanchnic blood flow (Myles et al. 2019; Weimann 2019). In the postoperative period, adequate epidural analgesia will allow for effective respiration and early walking and starting jejunal feedings using a high-protein and energy diet within 24 hours after surgery (Weimann et al. 2021; Friedman et al. 2021).

Within the first week after surgery, he advances to intake of small amounts of clear liquids followed by a soft oral diet with enteral feeding to meet a protein intake goal of 1.5 g/kg/day. The patient's LOS is less than average and without any significant complications, thus showing how anesthesia and nutrition work together in an approach that uses ESPEN/ERAS principles for upper GI oncological patients (Weimann et al. 2017; Weimann et al. 2021; Weimann 2019).

16.7 Cross-Cutting Lessons and Implementation Considerations

16.7.1 Importance of Adherence to Bundled Protocols

Regardless of specialty, the effect size seen with the ERAS protocol is strongly associated with protocol compliance. The literature shows that high levels of compliance with various bundled protocols, including anesthesia, analgesia, and nutritional components, lead to significant decreases in LOS, complications, and even mortality after colorectal surgery for cancer (Cavallaro and Bordeianou 2019;

Mangone et al. 2024; Ripollés et al. 2019). In contrast, the nutritional components of early feeding and reaching protein goals have been identified as some of the least complied with components of the ERAS bundle (Martin et al. 2019; Hubert et al. 2021).

16.7.2 Tailoring to Nutrition Risk, Frailty, and Sarcopenia

The integration of the nutritional and anesthesia management in cases where there is already preexisting malnutrition, sarcopenic obesity, or frailty is particularly beneficial for such patients, though each of them will need individual care with regard to the prolonged period of prehabilitation, higher doses of nutritional interventions, and titrated anesthesia (Weimann et al. 2017; Weimann et al. 2024). The latest recommendations provided in the ESPEN guidelines highlight the necessity to assess the patient's nutrition, frailty, and sarcopenia prior to the development of individual nutrition and rehabilitation programs (Weimann et al. 2024).

16.7.3 Systems-Level Implementation Strategies

The integration of anesthesia and nutrition into the ERAS pathway requires a systems-based approach, rather than individual initiatives by clinicians. Important techniques include forming interdisciplinary ERAS management teams; incorporating anesthesia and nutritional orders within electronic order sets; offering preoperative courses that provide patients with information regarding the importance of anesthesia, pain management, and nutrition; and conducting constant audits and feedback (Wischmeyer et al. 2018; Mangone et al. 2024; Martin et al. 2019). Resource adjustment is important, especially in LMICs (low- and middle-income countries), where essential ERAS practices, such as reduced fasting, multimodal analgesia, early nutrition, and mobility, can still be observed, even without the latest equipment, like hemodynamic monitors (Al-Omari and Othman 2025; Wong et al. 2024).

16.7.4 Research Priorities

Critical unanswered questions include how long and what kind of nutrition support should be used in patients with different levels of nutrition risk and surgical procedures' complexity, which combination of regional anesthesia and analgesia, along with anti-emetics is most efficient to help with early feeding and ambulation; and how such integrated anesthesia-nutrition enhanced recovery pathways affect quality of life, functionality, and cancer outcomes in the long term (after 30 days or even 90 days) (Ljungqvist and Carli 2024; Weimann 2019; Funk Debleds et al. 2024). Pragmatic studies are needed to investigate the effectiveness and scalability of integrated pathways (Mangone et al. 2024; Widanage et al. 2025).

16.8 Conclusion

It is evident from the data collected through ERAS pathways for colorectal surgery, upper GI surgery, gynecological surgery, orthopedic surgery, bariatric surgery, and cardiac/thoracic surgery that anesthetic and nutritional approaches are key factors in ensuring improved recovery. Multimodal, opioid-sparing anesthesia/analgesia makes it possible to move on to early activity and feeding, whereas nutritional intervention ensures maintenance of muscle mass, immunocompetence, and prevention of catabolism.

When anesthesia and nutrition therapies are carefully designed together and applied in concert in ERAS protocols, as opposed to being adopted on a case-by-case basis, patients are likely to stay in hospitals for less time, have fewer adverse outcomes, and recover more quickly, without any additional readmissions. Further optimization, customization, and expansion of such strategies, combined with comprehensive auditing, active participation, and rigorous investigation, will be key to fully exploiting the benefits of ERAS programs.

Ethics Statement The current chapter represents a narrative review of literature and case studies derived from real-life situations. There was no need for an ethical committee to approve any experiments involving human subjects because there were no new studies conducted.

References

AAOS. ERAS applies evidence-based, multimodal care to reduce complications and length of stay in total joint arthroplasty. AAOS Now; 2026. AAOS article.

Albrecht E, Oliveira M, Addor V, Wegrzyn J. Implementation of an ERAS® programme for total hip and knee arthroplasty in a high-volume university hospital. J Clin Med. 2026;15(2):836. https://doi.org/10.3390/jcm15020836.

Al-Omari AY, Othman RA. Effect of enhanced recovery after surgery protocols on postoperative length of stay and complication rates in elective colorectal surgery: a systematic review and meta-analysis of randomized controlled trials. Int Surg J. 2025;12(10):1745–52. https://doi.org/10.18203/2349-2902.isj20253026.

Beaulieu B, Lamarche Y, Rousseau-Saine N, Ferland G. Adequacy of oral intakes after cardiac surgery within an ERAS pathway: a prospective observational study. Nutr Clin Pract. 2025;40(3):605–15. https://doi.org/10.1002/ncp.11258.

Cavallaro P, Bordeianou L. Implementation of an ERAS pathway in colorectal Surgery. Clin Colon Rectal Surg. 2019;32(2):102–8. https://doi.org/10.1055/s-0038-1676474.

Dietitians in Bariatric and Upper GI Surgery. Nutrition support following enhanced recovery after surgery protocol. J Nutr. 2020;76(2):123–30. Retrieved from http://jnl.calorie-smile.jp

Friedman J, et al. Enhanced recovery after surgery (ERAS) and immunonutrition: an evidence-based approach. Pract Gastroenterol. 2021;45(1):20–32. Retrieved from https://practicalgastro.com

Funk Debleds P, Chambrier C, Slim K. Postoperative nutrition in the setting of enhanced recovery programmes. Eur J Surg Oncol. 2024;50(5):106866. https://doi.org/10.1016/j.ejso.2023.03.006.

Gillis C, Nguyen TH, Liberman AS, Carli F. Nutrition adequacy in enhanced recovery after surgery: a single academic center experience. Nutr Clin Pract. 2015;30(3):414–9. https://doi.org/10.1177/0884533614562840.

Gillis C, Wischmeyer PE. Preoperative nutrition and the elective surgical patient: why, how and what? Anaesthesia. 2019;74(Suppl. 1):27–35. https://doi.org/10.1111/anae.14506.

Gillis C, et al. Patients' perspectives of prehabilitation as an extension of enhanced recovery after surgery: a qualitative study. Can J Surg. 2021;64(6):E578–86. https://doi.org/10.1503/cjs.005220.

Gillis C, et al. Prehabilitation, enhanced recovery after surgery, or both? Br J Anaesth. 2022;128(5):e287–9. https://doi.org/10.1016/j.bja.2021.10.025.

Gustafsson UO, Scott MJ, Hübner M, et al. Guidelines for perioperative care in elective colorectal surgery: Enhanced Recovery After Surgery (ERAS®) Society recommendations (updated). Surgery. 2025;184:109397. https://doi.org/10.1016/j.surg.2025.109397.

Haselton SD, Chadayammuri VP, Emerson RH. Preoperative carbohydrate loading as part of an enhanced recovery after surgery (ERAS) protocol confers early postoperative benefits following elective total hip arthroplasty. Clin Nutr ESPEN. 2025;68:602–7. https://doi.org/10.1016/j.clnesp.2025.05.049.

Ho CY, et al. Postoperative dietary intake achievement: a secondary analysis of a randomized controlled trial. Nutrients. 2022;14(1):222. https://doi.org/10.3390/nu14010222.

Huang L, et al. Postoperative multimodal analgesia strategy for enhanced recovery after colorectal cancer surgery in older patients. Pain Ther. 2024;13:745. PMCID: PMC11254899

Hubert M, et al. Energy and protein intake after return home in colorectal surgery patients with an enhanced recovery program: a prospective observational study. Nutr Clin Pract. 2021;36(3):655–64. https://doi.org/10.1002/ncp.10617.

Kallikourdis A, et al. Perioperative nutrition for gastrointestinal surgery: on the crossroad between ERAS and prehabilitation. Nutr Clin Pract. 2023;38(1):15–28. https://doi.org/10.1002/ncp.10970.

Lau CSM, et al. Prehabilitation programs improve exercise capacity in patients undergoing gastrointestinal cancer surgery: a systematic review and meta-analysis. Surg Oncol. 2020;34:98–109. https://doi.org/10.1016/j.suronc.2020.05.003.

Ljungqvist O, Carli F. Contemporary perioperative nutritional care. Annu Rev Nutr. 2024;44:1–24. https://doi.org/10.1146/annurev-nutr-062222-021228.

Ljungqvist O, Scott M, Fearon KC. Enhanced recovery after surgery: a review. JAMA Surg. 2017;152(3):292–8. https://doi.org/10.1001/jamasurg.2016.4952.

Mangone L, et al. Outcomes before and after implementation of the ERAS protocol in colorectal surgery. Curr Oncol. 2024;31:2907. PMCID: PMC11202664

Martin L, Gillis C, Atkins M, et al. Implementation of an enhanced recovery after surgery program can change nutrition care practice: a multicenter experience in elective colorectal surgery. JPEN J Parenter Enteral Nutr. 2019;43(2):206–19. https://doi.org/10.1002/jpen.1417.

MD Anderson Cancer Center. ERAS: nutrition for gynecologic oncology patients; 2022. Retrieved from https://www.mdanderson.org

Mercedes CO, et al. Implementation of an enhanced recovery after surgery program reduces length of stay in colorectal cancer surgery. Surg Oncol. 2019;30:79–85. https://doi.org/10.1016/j.suronc.2018.11.004.

Myles PS, et al. Regional anesthetic and analgesic techniques and their role in enhanced recovery after colorectal surgery. Reg Anesth Pain Med. 2019;47:282. PMCID: PMC6395101[^12]

Riga M, et al. Enhanced recovery after surgery (ERAS) protocols for total joint arthroplasty: current evidence and future directions. SICOT-J. 2023;9:5. https://doi.org/10.1051/sicotj/2023005.

Ripollés-Melchor J, Ramírez-Rodríguez JM, Casans-Francés R, Aldecoa C, Abad-Motos A, Logroño-Egea M, García-Erce JA, Camps-Cervantes Á, Ferrando-Ortolá C, Suarez de la Rica A, Cuellar-Martínez A, Marmaña-Mezquita S, Abad-Gurumeta A, Calvo-Vecino JM, POWER Study Investigators Group for the Spanish Perioperative Audit and Research Network (REDGERM). Association between use of enhanced recovery after surgery protocol and postoperative complications in colorectal surgery: the postoperative outcomes within enhanced recovery after surgery protocol (POWER) study. JAMA Surg. 2019;154(8):725–36. https://doi.org/10.1001/jamasurg.2019.0995.

Sebestyén AR, et al. Preoperative carbohydrate loading reduces length of stay in major non-cardiac surgery: a systematic review and meta-analysis. Sci Rep. 2025;15:12345. https://doi.org/10.1038/s41598-025-00767-z.

Tong E, Tan X. Effects of preoperative carbohydrate loading on recovery after elective surgery: a systematic review and Bayesian network meta-analysis of randomized controlled trials. Front Nutr. 2022;9:951676. https://doi.org/10.3389/fnut.2022.951676.

Wainwright TW, Immins T, Middleton RG, et al. Consensus statement for perioperative care in total hip replacement and total knee replacement surgery: Enhanced Recovery After Surgery (ERAS®) Society recommendations. Acta Orthop. 2020;91(1):3–19. https://doi.org/10.1080/17453674.2019.1683790.

Weimann A. Is there a rationale for perioperative nutrition therapy in the times of ERAS? Innov Surg Sci. 2019;4(4):152–7. https://doi.org/10.1515/iss-2019-0012.

Weimann A, Braga M, Carli F, et al. ESPEN guideline: clinical nutrition in surgery. Clin Nutr. 2017;36(3):623–50. https://doi.org/10.1016/j.clnu.2017.02.013.

Weimann A, Braga M, Carli F, et al. ESPEN practical guideline: clinical nutrition in surgery. Clin Nutr. 2021;40(7):4745–61. https://doi.org/10.1016/j.clnu.2021.03.031.

Weimann A, et al. ESPEN guideline on clinical nutrition in surgery (update). Clin Nutr. 2024;43(2):345–90. https://doi.org/10.1016/j.clnu.2022.10.012.

Widanage N, et al. The effects of multimodal prehabilitation on postoperative outcomes in colorectal surgery: a systematic review and meta-analysis. Cureus. 2025;17(10):e95032. https://doi.org/10.7759/cureus.95032.

Wischmeyer PE, Carli F, Evans DC, et al. American Society for Enhanced Recovery and Perioperative Quality Initiative joint consensus statement on nutrition screening and therapy within a surgical enhanced recovery pathway. Anesth Analg. 2018;126(6):1883–95. https://doi.org/10.1213/ANE.0000000000002743.

Wong CRJ, et al. Multimodal analgesia as part of enhanced recovery after surgery in colorectal surgery. Malays J Anaesthesiol. 2024;3(2):100–8. https://doi.org/10.35119/myja.v3i2.70.

Yeung SE, et al. Protein intakes are associated with reduced length of stay: an analysis within an ERAS framework. Am J Clin Nutr. 2017;106(1):44–51. https://doi.org/10.3945/ajcn.116.136259.

GPSR Compliance

The European Union's (EU) General Product Safety Regulation (GPSR) is a set of rules that requires consumer products to be safe and our obligations to ensure this.

If you have any concerns about our products, you can contact us on ProductSafety@springernature.com

In case Publisher is established outside the EU, the EU authorized representative is:

Springer Nature Customer Service Center GmbH
Europaplatz 3
69115 Heidelberg, Germany

Batch number: 10732076

Printed by Printforce, the Netherlands